PN Maternal Newborn Nursing
REVIEW MODULE EDITION 12.0

W9-BTS-698

Contributors

Alissa Althoff, Ed.D, MSN, RN

Michelle E. Cawley, MSN, RN

Mendy Gearhart, DNP, MSN, CCCE

Norma Jean Henry, MSN/Ed., RN

Honey C. Holman, MSN, RN

Janean Johnson, DNP, RN, CNE

Beth Cusatis Phillips, PhD,
RN, CNE, CHSE

Pamela Roland, MSN, MBA, RN

LaKeisha Wheless MSN, RN

Consultants

Stephanie L. Belim, PhD, RN, CNE

Jessica L. Johnson, DNP, MSN, RN

Kelly Migler, DNP, RN, CNE

INTELLECTUAL PROPERTY NOTICE

Director of content review: Kristen Lawler

Director of development: Derek Prater

Project management: Meri Ann Mason

Coordination of content review: Alissa Althoff, Honey C. Holman

Copy editing: Kelly Von Lunen, Tricia Lunt, Bethany Robertson, Kya Rodgers, Rebecca Her, Sam Shiel, Alethea Surland, Graphic World

Layout: Bethany Robertson, Maureen Bradshaw, Haylee Hedge, scottie. o

Illustrations: Randi Hardy, Graphic World

Online media: Brant Stacy, Ron Hanson, Britney Frerking, Trevor Lund

Interior book design: Spring Lenox

IMPORTANT NOTICE TO THE READER

User's Guide

Welcome to the Assessment Technologies Institute®️ PN Maternal Newborn Nursing Review Module Edition 12.0. The mission of ATI's Content Mastery Series®️ Review Modules is to provide user-friendly compendiums of nursing knowledge that will:

- Help you locate important information quickly.
- Assist in your learning efforts.
- Provide exercises for applying your nursing knowledge.
- Facilitate your entry into the nursing profession as a newly licensed nurse.

ORGANIZATION

This Review Module is organized into units covering antepartum, intrapartum, postpartum, and newborn nursing care. Chapters within these units conform to one of three organizing principles for presenting the content.

- Nursing concepts
- Procedures
- Complications of pregnancy

Nursing concepts chapters begin with an overview describing the central concept and its relevance to nursing. Subordinate themes are covered in outline form to demonstrate relationships and present the information in a clear, succinct manner.

Procedures chapters include an overview describing the procedure(s) covered in the chapter. These chapters provide nursing knowledge relevant to each procedure, including indications, nursing considerations, and complications.

Complications of pregnancy chapters include an overview describing the complication; assessment, including risk factors and expected findings; and patient-centered care, including nursing care, medications, and client education.

ACTIVE LEARNING SCENARIOS AND APPLICATION EXERCISES

Each chapter includes opportunities for you to test your knowledge and to practice applying that knowledge. Active Learning Scenario exercises pose a nursing scenario and then direct you to use an ATI Active Learning Template (included both in the chapter and in the Appendix) to record the important knowledge a nurse should apply to the scenario. An example is then provided to which you can compare your completed Active Learning Template. Application exercises throughout the chapters include NCLEX-style questions, such as multiple-choice and multiple-select items, providing you with opportunities to practice answering the kinds of questions you might expect to see on ATI assessments or the NCLEX. Answers and rationales are provided to further your learning.

NCLEX®️ CONNECTIONS

To prepare for the NCLEX-PN, it is important to understand how the content in this Review Module is connected to the NCLEX-PN test plan. You can find information on the detailed test plan at the National Council of State Boards of Nursing's website, www.ncsbn.org. When reviewing content in this Review Module, regularly ask yourself, "How does this content fit into the test plan, and what types of questions related to this content should I expect?"

To help you in this process, we've included NCLEX Connections at the beginning of each unit and with each question in the Application Exercises Answer Keys. The NCLEX Connections at the beginning of each unit point out areas of the detailed test plan that relate to the content within that unit. The NCLEX Connections attached to the Application Exercises Answer Keys demonstrate how each exercise fits within the detailed content outline.

These NCLEX Connections will help you understand how the detailed content outline is organized, starting with major client needs categories and subcategories and followed by related content areas and tasks. The major client needs categories are:

- Safe and Effective Care Environment
  - Management of Care
  - Safety and Infection Control
- Health Promotion and Maintenance
- Psychosocial Integrity
- Physiological Integrity
  - Basic Care and Comfort
  - Pharmacological and Parenteral Therapies
  - Reduction of Risk Potential
  - Physiological Adaptation

An NCLEX Connection might, for example, alert you that content within a unit is related to:

- Health Promotion and Maintenance
  - Ante-/Intra-/Postpartum and Newborn Care
    - Assess client psychosocial response to pregnancy.

QSEN COMPETENCIES

As you use the Review Modules, you will note the integration of the Quality and Safety Education for nurses (QSEN) competencies throughout the chapters. These competencies are integral components of the curriculum of many nursing programs in the United States and prepare you to provide safe, high-quality care as a newly licensed nurse. Icons appear to draw your attention to the six QSEN competencies.

Safety: The minimization of risk factors that could cause injury or harm while promoting quality care and maintaining a secure environment for clients, self, and others.

Patient-Centered Care: The provision of caring and compassionate, culturally sensitive care that addresses clients' physiological, psychological, sociological, spiritual, and cultural needs, preferences, and values.

Evidence-Based Practice: The use of current knowledge from research and other credible sources, on which to base clinical judgment and client care.

Informatics: The use of information technology as a communication and information-gathering tool that supports clinical decision-making and scientifically based nursing practice.

Quality Improvement: Care related and organizational processes that involve the development and implementation of a plan to improve health care services and better meet clients' needs.

Teamwork and Collaboration: The delivery of client care in partnership with multidisciplinary members of the health care team to achieve continuity of care and positive client outcomes.

ICONS

Icons are used throughout the Review Module to draw your attention to particular areas. Keep an eye out for these icons.

(N) This icon is used for NCLEX Connections.

(G) This icon indicates gerontological considerations, or knowledge specific to the care of older adult clients.

Qs This icon is used for content related to safety and is a QSEN competency. When you see this icon, take note of safety concerns or steps that nurses can take to ensure client safety and a safe environment.

QPCC This icon is a QSEN competency that indicates the importance of a holistic approach to providing care.

QEBP This icon, a QSEN competency, points out the integration of research into clinical practice.

QI This icon is a QSEN competency and highlights the use of information technology to support nursing practice.

QQI This icon is used to focus on the QSEN competency of integrating planning processes to meet clients' needs.

QTC This icon highlights the QSEN competency of care delivery using an interprofessional approach.

SDoH This icon highlights content related to social determinants of health.

M◇ This icon appears at the top-right of pages and indicates availability of an online media supplement, such as a graphic, animation, or video. If you have an electronic copy of the Review Module, this icon will appear alongside clickable links to media supplements. If you have a hard copy version of the Review Module, visit www.atitesting.com for details on how to access these features.

FEEDBACK

ATI welcomes feedback regarding this Review Module. Please provide comments to comments@atitesting.com.

As needed updates to the Review Modules are identified, changes to the text are made for subsequent printings of the book and for subsequent releases of the electronic version. For the printed books, print runs are based on when existing stock is depleted. For the electronic versions, a number of factors influence the update schedule. As such, ATI encourages faculty and students to refer to the Review Module addendums for information on what updates have been made. These addendums, which are available in the Help/FAQs on the student site and the Resources/eBooks & Active Learning on the faculty site, are updated regularly and always include the most current information on updates to the Review Modules.

Table of Contents

NCLEX® Connections   73

UNIT 2   *Intrapartum Nursing Care*

SECTION: *Labor and Delivery*   75

Newborn Nursing Care

UNIT 4

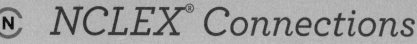

When reviewing the following chapters, keep in mind the relevant topics and tasks of the NCLEX outline.

Health Promotion and Maintenance

ANTE-/INTRA-/POSTPARTUM AND NEWBORN CARE
Assist in performing client non-stress test.

Reinforce client teaching on infant care skills.

DATA COLLECTION TECHNIQUES: Collect data for health history.

HEALTH PROMOTION/DISEASE PREVENTION: Identify clients in need of immunizations.

HIGH-RISK BEHAVIORS: Reinforce client teaching related to client high risk behavior.

LIFESTYLE CHOICES
Recognize client need/desire for contraception.

Reinforce teaching with client on healthy lifestyle choices.

Basic Care and Comfort

NONPHARMACOLOGICAL COMFORT INTERVENTIONS
Provide nonpharmacological measures for pain relief.

Pharmacological Therapies

ADVERSE EFFECTS/CONTRAINDICATIONS/ SIDE EFFECTS/ INTERACTIONS
Reinforce client teaching on possible effects of medications.

Monitor client for actual and potential adverse effects of medications.

EXPECTED ACTIONS/OUTCOMES
Identify client expected response to medication.

Evaluate client response to medication.

PHARMACOLOGICAL PAIN MANAGEMENT: Identify client need for pain medication.

Reduction of Risk Potential

DIAGNOSTIC TESTS: Reinforce client teaching about diagnostic tests.

LABORATORY VALUES
Monitor diagnostic or laboratory test results.

Compare client laboratory values to normal laboratory values.

POTENTIAL FOR ALTERATIONS IN BODY SYSTEMS
Identify signs or symptoms of potential prenatal complications.

Perform focused data collection based on client condition.

THERAPEUTIC PROCEDURES: Reinforce client teaching on treatments and procedures.

Physiological Adaptation

ALTERATIONS IN BODY SYSTEMS: Provide care for a client experiencing complications of pregnancy/labor and/or delivery.

CHAPTER 1 *Contraception*

Contraception refers to strategies or devices used to reduce the risk of fertilization/implantation or to prevent pregnancy. The human ovum can be fertilized 24 hr after ovulation. Motile sperm's ability to fertilize the ovum lasts an average of 48 to 72 hr.

A nurse should identify clients' need, desire, and preference for contraception. A thorough discussion of benefits, risks, and alternatives of each method should be discussed. ⓆPCC

Sexual partners often make a joint decision regarding a desired preference (vasectomy or tubal ligation). Postpartum discharge instructions should include the discussion of future contraceptive plans.

Prior the initiation of some contraceptives, the provider may recommend a comprehensive physical examination (Pap smear, blood tests [Hgb, Hct], and STI screening). A client history should be documented and include medical and obstetric history.

Expected outcomes for family planning methods consist of preventing pregnancy until a desired time. Nurses should support clients in making the decision that is best for their individual situations.

Some of the methods of contraception include natural family planning; fertility awareness, barrier, hormonal, and intrauterine methods; and surgical procedures.

NATURAL FAMILY PLANNING (FERTILITY AWARENESS-BASED METHODS)

Abstinence

Abstaining from having sexual intercourse eliminates the possibility of sperm entering the vagina.

CLIENT EDUCATION: Refrain from sexual intercourse. Discuss permissible sexual activities with partners.

ADVANTAGES
- Most effective method of birth control
- No chemicals involved or introduction of foreign objects into the body
- Abstinence during fertile periods (rhythm method) can be used, but it requires an understanding of the menstrual cycle and fertility awareness.
- Can eliminate the risk of sexually transmitted infections (STIs) if there is no genitalia contact

DISADVANTAGES:
- Requires self-control
- High failure rate due to lack of adherence

RISKS: If complete abstinence is maintained, there are no risks.

Coitus interruptus (withdrawal)

Withdrawal of penis from vagina prior to ejaculation

CLIENT EDUCATION: Be aware that pre-ejaculatory fluid can leak from the penis prior to ejaculation. It can contain sperm, which can fertilize an ovum.

ADVANTAGES: Possible choice for monogamous couples who do not have any other contraceptives available

DISADVANTAGES
- One of the least effective methods of contraception
- No protection against STIs

RISKS: Possible pregnancy

Calendar rhythm method

Involves determining fertile days by tracking the menstrual cycle to estimate the time of ovulation, which occurs about 14 days before the onset of the next menstrual cycle. This method can be used to facilitate conception or be used as a natural contraceptive. If trying to conceive, the client would have intercourse during the fertile period. If trying to prevent pregnancy, the client would abstain from intercourse during the fertile period.

CLIENT EDUCATION

- Maintain a diary. Accurately record the number of days in each menstrual cycle, counting from the first day of menses for a period of at least six menstrual cycles.
- The start of the fertile period is figured by subtracting 18 days from the number of days in the shortest menstrual cycle.
- The end of the fertile period is established by subtracting 11 days from the number of days of the longest cycle.

> For example:
> Shortest cycle, 26 – 18 = 8th day
> Longest cycle, 30 – 11 = 19th day
> Fertile period is days 8 through 19.
> Refrain from intercourse during these
> days to avoid conception.

ADVANTAGES

- Most useful when combined with basal body temperature or cervical mucus method
- Inexpensive

DISADVANTAGES

- Not a very reliable technique
- Does not protect against STIs
- Requires accurate record-keeping
- Requires adherence regarding abstinence during fertile periods

RISKS

- Various factors can affect and change the time of ovulation and cause unpredictable menstrual cycles.
- Possible pregnancy due to miscalculating fertile period or not abstaining from intercourse during fertile days.

Standard days method (cycle beads)

More modern form of the calendar method that uses a standard number of fertile days for each cycle. The cycle beads are color-coded and located on a stringed necklace.

CLIENT EDUCATION

- Start the first day of the menstrual cycle. Use the rubber ring to advance one bead per day.
- Red bead: the first bead and marks the first day of the menstrual cycle.
- Brown beads: nonfertile days.
- White beads: fertile days.

ADVANTAGES

- Increased adherence by using a visual aid
- Mobile app available
- Easy to understand

DISADVANTAGES

- Unreliable for menstrual cycles longer than 32 days or shorter than 26 days
- Can lose track of the days

RISKS/POSSIBLE COMPLICATIONS

- Do not use if menstrual cycles are short or long
- Possible pregnancy
- Less effective if used with hormonal contraceptives or breastfeeding

Basal body temperature (BBT)

BBT is the temperature of the body at rest. Prior to ovulation, the temperature drops slightly and rises during ovulation. Identifying the time of ovulation is a symptom-based method that can be used to facilitate or avoid conception.

CLIENT EDUCATION

- Take temperature immediately after waking up and before getting out of bed. If working at night, take temperature after awakening from the longest sleep cycle. Use a thermometer that records temperature to the tenths. Record the temperatures on a specialized graph.
- During ovulation as the progesterone rises some clients may see a slight elevation in their basal body temperature. Fertility extends through 3 consecutive days of temperature elevations.
- Use this method with the calendar method to increase effectiveness.

ADVANTAGES: Inexpensive, convenient, and no adverse effects

DISADVANTAGES

- Reliability can be influenced by many variables that can cause inaccurate interpretation of temperature changes (stress, fatigue, illness, alcohol, warmth of sleeping environment).
- Does not protect against STIs.

RISKS: Possible pregnancy

Cervical mucus ovulation detection method

Fertility awareness method (also known as Billings method) is a symptom-based method in which the client analyzes cervical mucous to determine ovulation.

- Following ovulation, the cervical mucus becomes thin and flexible under the influence of estrogen and progesterone to allow for sperm viability and motility.
- The ability for the mucus to stretch between the fingers is greatest during ovulation. This known as spinnbarkeit.
- The fertile period begins when the cervical mucus is thin, slippery, and lasts 3 to 4 after the last day of cervical mucus having this appearance.

CLIENT EDUCATION

- Use this method with the calendar method to increase effectiveness.
- Engage in good hand hygiene prior to and following assessment.
- Begin examining mucus from the last day of the menstrual cycle.
- Mucus is obtained from the vaginal introitus. It is not necessary to reach into the vagina to the cervix.
- Use fingers or tissue paper to examine the cervical mucus.
- The stretchy consistency of egg whites is a good example of how cervical mucus will appear during ovulation.
- Do not use a douche prior to assessment.

ADVANTAGES

- A client can become knowledgeable in recognizing their own mucus characteristics at ovulation, and self-evaluation can be very accurate.
- Self-evaluation of cervical mucus can be diagnostically helpful in determining the start of ovulation while breastfeeding and planning a desired pregnancy.

DISADVANTAGES

- Some clients are uncomfortable with touching their genitals and mucus, and therefore find this method objectionable.
- Self-analysis of cervical mucus can be difficult.
- Does not protect against STIs.

RISKS/POSSIBLE COMPLICATIONS

- Data collection of cervical mucus characteristics can be inaccurate if mucus is mixed with semen, blood, contraceptive foams, or discharge from infections.
- Sexual arousal or intercourse (thins secretions), or use of deodorants, douches, medication, or lubricants can alter cervical mucus appearance and affect accuracy.
- Possible pregnancy.

2-day method

A symptom-based method that involves checking for vaginal secretions daily, with no analysis of secretions. After 2 days without the presence of secretions, the fertile period has passed.

CLIENT EDUCATION: If vaginal secretions are present 2 days in a row, avoid unprotected intercourse to prevent pregnancy.

ADVANTAGES: Simple and easy to use

DISADVANTAGES: Requires daily assessment for vaginal secretions

RISK: Possible pregnancy

LACTATION AMENORRHEA METHOD (LAM)

Suppression of ovulation and menstruation while breastfeeding

CLIENT EDUCATION

- Criteria for use and increase the effectiveness of method:
  - Infant less than 6 months
  - Must exclusive breastfeed at least every 4 hr and every 6 hours during bedtime
  - No supplemental feeding
  - Absence of menses

ADVANTAGES

Natural method–no chemicals used

DISADVANTAGES

Effective for at least 6 months (after 6 months my need to consider another contraceptive method)

RISKS/POSSIBLE COMPLICATIONS

Possible pregnancy (if not consistent with exclusive breastfeeding)

BARRIER METHODS

Penile condom

A thin sheath used to cover the penis during sexual intercourse as a contraceptive or as protection against infection. Male condoms can be made of latex rubber, polyurethane, or natural membrane.

CLIENT EDUCATION

- Place a condom on the erect penis, leaving an empty space at the tip for a sperm reservoir.
- Following ejaculation, withdraw the penis from the vagina while holding the rim of the condom to prevent any semen spillage to the vulva or vaginal area.
- Can use in conjunction with spermicidal gel or cream to increase effectiveness.
- Check expiration date prior to use.
- Latex and polyurethane condoms protect against STI, but natural skin (lamb tissue) condoms do not because they have small pores. Polyurethane condoms can slip or lose shape more easily than latex, and therefore might not be as effective.
- Only water-soluble lubricants should be used with latex condoms, to avoid condom breakage.

ADVANTAGES

- Protects against most STIs
- Involves partner in contraceptive method
- No adverse effects
- Readily accessible

DISADVANTAGES

- High rate of nonadherence
- Can reduce spontaneity of intercourse
- Decreased sensation
- The penis must be erect to apply a condom.
- Withdrawing the penis while still erect can interfere with sexual intercourse.
- Does not protect against STIs that are transmitted from lesions on the skin or mucus membranes (HPV, HSV, syphilis).
- Condoms have a one-time usage, which creates a replacement cost.

RISKS/POSSIBLE COMPLICATIONS/CONTRAINDICATIONS

- Condoms can rupture or leak, potentially resulting in pregnancy.
- Condoms made of latex should not be worn by those who are sensitive or allergic to latex.

Vaginal condom

Vaginal sheath made of nitrile, a nonlatex synthetic rubber with flexible rings on both ends that is pre-lubricated with a spermicide.

CLIENT EDUCATION

- The closed end of the condom pouch is inserted into the vagina by the client prior to intercourse and anchored around the cervix. The open ring of the condom covers the labia. The condom is removed and thrown away after each act of intercourse.
- Do not use in conjunction with a male condom.

ADVANTAGES

- Offers protection against pregnancy and STIs
- Offers some protection against STI transmitted by skin-to-skin contact (HPV, HSV, syphilis)

DISADVANTAGES

- Complicated to use
- Bulky
- Noisy during intercourse
- More expensive than male condoms

Spermicide

Chemical barrier that is available in a variety of forms and destroys sperm before they can enter the cervix. It causes the vaginal flora to be more acidic, which is not favorable for sperm survival.

CLIENT EDUCATION

- Plan to insert spermicide 15 min before intercourse. Spermicide is only effective for 1 hr after insertion, but should not be removed until 6 hr after intercourse.
- Fold films prior to use and insert in the vagina, where it will dissolve.

ADVANTAGES

- No prescription needed
- Increases the effectiveness of other methods of contraception when used together
- Various preparations (suppositories, foams, creams, gel, films)

DISADVANTAGES

- Messy
- Must reapply after each act of intercourse
- Does not protect against STIs

RISKS/CONTRAINDICATIONS

- Contraindicated in clients who have cervical infections.
- Spermicides that contain nonoxynol-9 (N-9) can cause lesions and increase the risk of HIV if used more than twice daily. Clients at high risk for STI should not use products containing N-9.

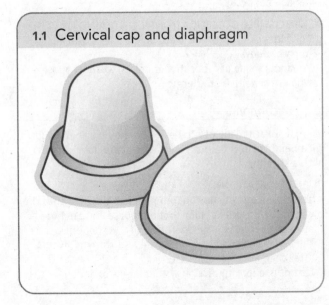

1.1 Cervical cap and diaphragm

Diaphragm

A dome-shaped cup with a flexible rim made of silicone that fits snugly over the cervix. The effectiveness is increased with the use of a spermicidal cream or gel placed into the dome and around the rim. Diaphragms are available in different sizes.

CLIENT EDUCATION

- Be properly fitted with a diaphragm by a provider.
- Replace every 2 years and refit for a 20% weight fluctuation, after abdominal or pelvic surgery, and after every pregnancy.
- The diaphragm requires proper insertion and removal. Prior to coitus, the diaphragm is inserted vaginally over the cervix with spermicidal jelly or cream that is applied to the cervical side of the dome and around the rim. The diaphragm can be inserted up to 6 hr before intercourse and must stay in place 6 hr after intercourse but for no more than 24 hr.
- Spermicide must be reapplied with each act of coitus.
- Empty the bladder prior to insertion of the diaphragm, to decrease pressure on the urethra.
- The diaphragm should be washed with mild soap and warm water after each use.

ADVANTAGES

- Gives a client more control over contraception
- Easy to insert

DISADVANTAGES

- Inconvenient, interfere with spontaneity, and require reapplication with spermicidal gel, cream, or foam with each act of coitus to be effective
- Requires a prescription and a visit to a provider
- Must be inserted correctly to be effective
- Does not protect against STIs

RISKS/POSSIBLE COMPLICATIONS/CONTRAINDICATIONS

- Not recommended for clients who have a history of toxic shock syndrome (TSS), cystocele, uterine prolapse, or frequent, recurrent urinary tract infections.
- Increased risk of acquiring TSS, which is caused by a bacterial infection. Clinical findings include high fever, a faint feeling, drop in blood pressure, watery diarrhea, headache, macular rash, and muscle aches.
- Proper hand hygiene aids in prevention of TSS, as well as removing the diaphragm promptly 6 to 8 hr following coitus.
- Risk of allergic reaction and UTIs.

Cervical cap

Silicone rubber cap that fits tightly around the base of the cervix. This serves as a physical barrier against sperm entering the cervix. Use with a spermicide increases its effectiveness. Cervical caps come in three sizes.

CLIENT EDUCATION

- Insert up to 6 hr before intercourse and leave in place at least 6 hr after intercourse but for no more than 48 hr at a time.
- Replace every 2 years and refit after any gynecological surgery, birth, or any major weight fluctuation.

ADVANTAGES

- Extended period of use
- No additional application of spermicide needed

DISADVANTAGES

- Possible risk of acquiring TSS
- Risk of allergic reaction
- Does not protect against STIs

RISKS/POSSIBLE COMPLICATIONS/CONTRAINDICATIONS:
Not for clients who have abnormal Pap test results or those who have a history of TSS.

Contraceptive sponge

Small, round, concave-shaped, polyurethane sponge containing spermicide. It fits over the cervix and acts as a physical/chemical barrier against sperm from entering the vagina.

CLIENT EDUCATION

- One size fits all.
- Moisten with water prior to insertion in the vagina.
- Should be left in place for 6 hr after the last act of intercourse and provides protection for up to 24 hr.

ADVANTAGES

- Can have repeated acts of intercourse
- Easy to insert

DISADVANTAGES: Does not protect against STIs

RISKS/COMPLICATIONS: Risk of TSS if left in the vagina greater than 24 hr.

HORMONAL METHODS

Combined oral contraceptives (COCs)

Hormonal contraception containing estrogen and progestin, which acts by suppressing ovulation, thickening the cervical mucus to block semen, altering the uterine decidua to prevent implantation.

CLIENT EDUCATION

- Medication requires a prescription and follow-up appointments with the provider.
- Routine Pap smears and breast examination might be needed.
- Medication requires consistent and proper use to be effective.
- Regular menstrual cycles should occur during the last 7 days.
- Observe for and report manifestations of complications (chest pain, shortness of breath, leg pain [thromboembolism], headache, vision changes [stroke], hypertension).
- In the event of missing a dose, if one pill is missed, take one as soon as possible; if two or three pills are missed, follow the manufacturer's instructions. Instruct the client on the use of alternative forms of contraception or abstinence to prevent pregnancy until regular dosing is resumed.
- If nausea occurs, take at bedtime.

ADVANTAGES

- Highly effective if taken correctly and consistently, preferably at the same time each day.
- Hormonal contraception containing low-dose estrogen (less than 35 mcg) has other therapeutic effects, including decreased menstrual blood loss, decreased iron deficiency anemia, regulation of menorrhagia and irregular cycles, and reduced incidence of dysmenorrhea and premenstrual findings.
- Offers protection against endometrial, ovarian, and colon cancer, reduces the incidence of benign breast disease, improves acne, and protects against the development of functional ovarian cysts.

DISADVANTAGES

- Does not protect against STIs.
- Can increase the risk of thromboembolism, stroke, heart attack, hypertension, gallbladder disease, and liver tumor.
- Exacerbates conditions affected by fluid retention (migraine, epilepsy, asthma, kidney or heart disease).
- Adverse effects include headache, nausea, breast tenderness, and breakthrough bleeding.
  - Estrogen can cause nausea, breast tenderness, and fluid retention.
  - Progestin can cause increased appetite, fatigue, depression, breast tenderness, oily skin and scalp, and hirsutism.

RISKS/POSSIBLE COMPLICATIONS/CONTRAINDICATIONS

- Clients who have a history of thromboembolic disorders, stroke, heart attack, coronary artery disease, gallbladder disease, cirrhosis or liver tumor, headache with focal neurologic findings, uncontrolled hypertension, diabetes mellitus with vascular involvement, breast or estrogen-related cancers, pregnancy, lactating, less than 6 weeks postpartum, or smoking (if over 35 years of age) are advised not to take oral contraceptive medications.
- Oral contraceptive effectiveness decreases when taking medications that affect liver enzymes (anticonvulsants, antifungals, some antibiotics).

Progestin-only pills (minipill)

Oral progestins that provide the same action as combined oral contraceptives, which decreases the chance of fertilization and implantation

CLIENT EDUCATION

- Take the pill at the same time daily to ensure effectiveness secondary to a low dose of progestin.
- Do not miss a pill.
- Might need another form of birth control during the first month of use to prevent pregnancy.

ADVANTAGES

- Fewer adverse effects when compared with a combined oral contraceptive
- Considered safe to take while breastfeeding

DISADVANTAGES
- Less effective in suppressing ovulation than combined oral contraceptives.
- No protection against STIs.
- Adverse effects include breakthrough, irregular, vaginal bleeding (frequently reported/most common); headache; nausea; and breast tenderness.

RISKS/POSSIBLE COMPLICATIONS/CONTRAINDICATIONS
- Oral contraceptive effectiveness decreases when taking medications that affect liver enzymes (anticonvulsants, some antibiotics).
- Contraindications include severe cirrhosis, liver tumors, and current or past breast cancer.

Emergency oral contraceptive

Morning-after pill that prevents fertilization from taking place by inhibiting ovulation and the transport of sperm

CLIENT EDUCATION
- The pill is taken within 72 hr after unprotected coitus.
- A provider will recommend an over-the-counter antiemetic to be taken 1 hr prior to each dose to counteract the adverse effects of nausea that can occur with high doses of estrogen and progestin.
- Be evaluated for pregnancy if menstruation does not begin within 21 days.
- Consider counseling about contraception and modification of sexual behaviors that are risky.
- A copper IUD can be used up to 5 days following unprotected intercourse as an emergency contraceptive, but a prescription is required.

ADVANTAGES
- This method is not taken on a regular basis.
- Anyone, regardless of age, is allowed to purchase emergency oral contraceptive at a pharmacy.
- Directions are easy to understand.

DISADVANTAGES
- Nausea, heavier than normal menstrual bleeding, lower abdominal pain, fatigue, and headache
- Does not provide long-term contraception
- Does not terminate an established pregnancy
- Does not protect against STIs

RISKS/POSSIBLE COMPLICATIONS/CONTRAINDICATIONS:
Method is contraindicated if a client is pregnant or has undiagnosed abnormal vaginal bleeding.

Transdermal contraceptive patch

Contains estrogen and progesterone or progestin, which is delivered at continuous levels through the skin into subcutaneous tissue. Inhibits ovulation by thickening cervical mucus.

CLIENT EDUCATION
- Apply the patch to dry skin overlying subcutaneous tissue of the buttock, abdomen, upper arm, or torso, excluding breast area.
- Requires patch replacement once a week.
- Apply the patch the same day of the week for 3 weeks with no application on the fourth week.

ADVANTAGES
- Maintains consistent blood levels of hormone
- Avoids liver metabolism of medication because it is not absorbed in the gastrointestinal tract
- Decreases risk of forgetting a daily pill
- Can be used while in water, such as when swimming

DISADVANTAGES
- Does not protect against STIs.
- Same adverse effects as oral contraceptives.
- Skin reaction can occur from patch application.
- Can cause breast discomfort.

RISKS/POSSIBLE COMPLICATIONS/CONTRAINDICATIONS
- Same as those of oral contraceptives
- Avoid applying of patch to skin rashes or lesions
- Less effective in clients who are obese

Injectable progestins

Medroxyprogesterone is an intramuscular or subcutaneous injection given to a female client every 11 to 13 weeks. It inhibits ovulation and thickens cervical mucus.

CLIENT EDUCATION
- Start of injections should be during the first 5 days of the menstrual cycle and every 11 to 13 weeks thereafter. Injections in postpartum nonbreastfeeding clients should begin within 5 days following delivery. For breastfeeding clients, injections should start in the sixth week postpartum.
- Keep follow-up appointments.
- Maintain an adequate intake of calcium, vitamin D, and engage in weight-bearing exercise to decrease the risk of osteoporosis.
- Do not massage after IM injections because it decreases the absorption and effectiveness of the medication.

ADVANTAGES
- Very effective and requires only four injections per year
- Does not impair lactation
- Decreased risk of uterine cancer if used long-term

DISADVANTAGES
- Adverse effects include decreased bone mineral density, weight gain, increased depression, amenorrhea, headache, and irregular vaginal spotting or bleeding.
- Does not protect against STIs.
- Return to fertility can be delayed as long as up to 18 months after discontinuation.
- Should only be used as a long-term method of birth control (more than 2 years) if other birth control methods are inadequate.

RISKS/POSSIBLE COMPLICATIONS/CONTRAINDICATIONS
- Avoid massaging injection site following administration to avoid accelerating medication absorption, which will shorten the duration of its effectiveness.
- Contraindications include breast cancer, evidence of current cardiovascular disease, abnormal liver function, liver tumors, and unexplained vaginal bleeding.
- This method can impair glucose tolerance for clients who have diabetes mellitus and increase diabetes risk for clients who do not have diabetes mellitus.

Contraceptive vaginal ring

A flexible silicone ring that contains etonogestrel and ethinyl estradiol, which are delivered at continuous levels vaginally.

CLIENT EDUCATION
- Insert the ring vaginally.
- Perform ring replacement after 3 weeks, and placement of new vaginal ring within 7 days. Insertion should occur on the same day of the week monthly.
- If removed for greater than 4 hr, replace with new ring and use a barrier method of contraception for 7 days.

ADVANTAGES
- Does not have to be fitted
- Decreases the risk of forgetting to take the pill
- Vaginal route of delivery increases bioavailability of hormones, enabling lower dose and reducing adverse effect

DISADVANTAGES
- Method does not protect against STIs.
- Method has the same adverse effects as oral contraceptives.
- Some clients report discomfort during intercourse. The ring can be removed for up to 3 hr without compromising its effectiveness.
- Prescription is required.

RISKS/POSSIBLE COMPLICATIONS/CONTRAINDICATIONS
- Blood clots, hypertension, stroke, heart attack
- Vaginal irritation/discomfort, increased vaginal secretions

Implantable progestin

Small, thin rods consisting of progestin that are implanted by the provider under the skin of the inner upper aspect of the arm. Prevents pregnancy by suppressing the ovulatory cycle and thickening cervical mucus.

CLIENT EDUCATION
- Avoid trauma to the area of implantation.
- A client should report to the provider late or abnormal spotting or bleeding, abdominal pain or pain with intercourse, abnormal or foul-smelling vaginal discharge, fever, chills, a change in string length, or if IUD cannot be located.
- Wear condoms for protection against STIs.

ADVANTAGES
- Effective continuous contraception for 3 years
- Can be inserted immediately after spontaneous or elective abortion, childbirth, while breastfeeding
- Reversible

DISADVANTAGES
- Does not protect against STIs.
- Adverse effects include irregular and unpredictable menstruation (most common), mood changes, headache, acne, depression, decreased bone density, and weight gain.
- Scarring at insertion site can warrant the need for removal.

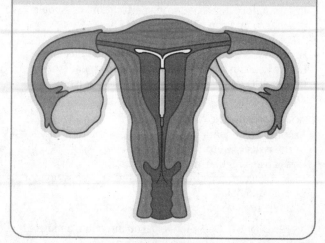

1.2 Intrauterine device

RISKS/POSSIBLE COMPLICATIONS/CONTRAINDICATIONS
- Contraindications include unexplained vaginal bleeding.
- Infection can occur at site.

Intrauterine device (IUD)

A chemically active T-shaped device that is inserted through the cervix and placed in the uterus by the provider (1.1). Releases a chemical substance that damages sperm in transit to the uterine tubes and prevents fertilization. The most effective contraceptive methods at preventing pregnancy are the long-acting reversible contraceptive (LARC) methods: implant and IUDs. IUDs can be used by nulliparous and multiparous female clients.

CLIENT EDUCATION
- The device must be monitored monthly by clients after menstruation to ensure the presence of the small string that hangs from the device into the upper part of the vagina to rule out migration or expulsion of the device.
- Sign a consent form prior to insertion.
- Pregnancy test, Pap smear, and cervical cultures should be negative prior to insertion.
- If pregnancy is suspected after IUD insertion, a sonogram can be needed to rule out ectopic pregnancy.

ADVANTAGES
- An IUD can maintain effectiveness for 3 to 10 years (hormonal IUD 3 to 5 years; copper IUD 10 years).
- Insertion can be immediately after elective or spontaneous abortion, childbirth, and while breastfeeding.
- Contraception can be reversed with immediate return to fertility.
- Does not interfere with spontaneity.
- Hormonal IUDs decrease menstrual pain and heavy bleeding.
- Copper IUD contains no hormones, so it's safe for clients cautioned against hormonal birth control methods.

DISADVANTAGES

- This method can increase the risk of pelvic inflammatory disease, uterine perforation, or ectopic pregnancy and can be expelled.
- This method does not protect from STIs.
- Hormonal IUD includes spotting, irregular bleeding, headache, nausea, depression, and breast tenderness.
- Copper IUD includes increase in menstrual pain and bleeding.

RISKS/CONTRAINDICATIONS

- Best used by clients in a monogamous relationship due to the risks of STIs
- Can cause irregular menstrual bleeding
- Risk of bacterial vaginosis, PID, uterine perforation, or uterine expulsion
- Must be removed in the event of pregnancy

CONTRAINDICATIONS: Active pelvic infection, abnormal uterine bleeding, severe uterine distortion

TRANSCERVICAL STERILIZATION

Insertion of small flexible agents through the vagina and cervix into the fallopian tubes. This results in the development of scar tissue in the tubes, preventing conception. The FDA recently reports that manufacturer has discontinued production of device. ○EBP

Therefore this method is not currently used. Examination must be done after 3 months to ensure fallopian tubes are blocked.

Client education

ADVANTAGES

- Quick procedure that requires no general anesthesia.
- Nonhormonal means of birth control and is 99.8% effective in preventing pregnancy.
- Rapid return to normal activities of daily living.

DISADVANTAGES

- Not reversible.
- Delay in effectiveness for 3 months. An alternative means of birth control should be used until confirmation of blocked fallopian tubes occurs.
- Does not protect against STIs.

RISKS/POSSIBLE COMPLICATIONS/CONTRAINDICATIONS

- Expulsion and perforation can occur.
- Unwanted pregnancy can occur if a client has unprotected sexual intercourse during the first 3 months following the procedure.
- Increased risk of ectopic pregnancy if pregnancy occurs.

SURGICAL METHODS

Tubal ligation (bilateral tubal ligation–BTL)

A surgical procedure consisting of severance and/ or burning or blocking the fallopian tubes to prevent fertilization. If using federal funding for procedure, the client must be at least 21 years of age, provide informed consent, and wait about 30 days after providing consent to have procedure. **(1.3)**

PROCEDURE: The cutting, burning, or blocking of the fallopian tubes to prevent the ovum from being fertilized by the sperm.

ADVANTAGES

- Permanent, immediate contraception.
- This method can be done within 24 to 48 hr after childbirth.
- Sexual function is unaffected.

DISADVANTAGES

- A surgical procedure carrying risks related to anesthesia, complications, infection, hemorrhage, trauma
- Considered irreversible in the event that a client desires conception
- Does not protect against STIs

RISKS: Risk of ectopic pregnancy if pregnancy occurs

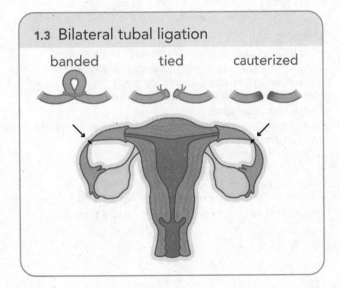

1.3 Bilateral tubal ligation

banded tied cauterized

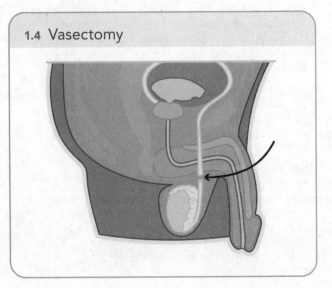

1.4 Vasectomy

Vasectomy

A surgical procedure consisting of ligation and severance of the vas deferens, which prevents sperm from traveling (1.4)

PROCEDURE: The cutting of the vas deferens in the male as a form of permanent sterilization.

CLIENT EDUCATION
- Following the procedure, scrotal support, and moderate activity for a couple of days is recommended to reduce discomfort.
- Sterility is delayed until the proximal portion of the vas deferens is cleared of all remaining sperm (approximately 20 ejaculations).
- Alternate forms of birth control must be used until the vas deferens is cleared of sperm.
- Follow up with the provider for sperm count testing. Sperm count must be zero on two consecutive tests to confirm sterility.
- Reversal can be done by complicated and expensive procedure.
- Prior to procedure, sperm can be banked for future use.

ADVANTAGES
- Method is permanent.
- Procedure is short, safe, and simple.
- Sexual function is not impaired.

DISADVANTAGES
- Surgery is required.
- Reversal is possible but not always successful.
- This method does not protect against STIs.
- Accumulation of sperm can cause granulomas.

COMPLICATIONS: Rare, but can include bleeding, infection, anesthesia reaction, hematomas at site, kidney stones, chronic pain (might need reversal)

Application Exercises

1. A nurse is discussing the use of a penile condom with a client. Which of the following information should the nurse include in the teaching as a disadvantage of using a penile condom? (Select all that apply.)
   A. Reduces spontaneity of intercourse
   B. Offers low rate of nonadherence
   C. Usage one time
   D. Protects against HSV
   E. Decreases sensation

2. A nurse in a provider's office is answering a call from a client who had unprotected sexual relations and is requesting additional information about emergency contraception. What information should the nurse provide the client?

3. A nurse is reinforcing teaching with a client about the disadvantages of various contraceptives. Match each disadvantage to corresponding contraceptive.

   A. Cervical cap
   B. Transdermal patch
   C. Implantable progesterone
   D. Intrauterine device
   E. Bilateral tubal ligation

   1. Considered irreversible
   2. Increase the risk of pelvic inflammatory disease
   3. Decreases bone density
   4. Skin reaction can occur from patch application
   5. Possible risk of acquiring TSS

Active Learning Scenario

A nurse is reinforcing teaching with a client who is considering a vasectomy. Which of the following should be included in the teaching? Use the ATI Active Learning Template: Therapeutic Procedure to complete this item.

DESCRIPTION OF PROCEDURE: Define the procedure.

INDICATIONS: Describe one advantage and one disadvantage of this form of contraception.

CLIENT EDUCATION: Describe two teaching points for this client.

Active Learning Scenario Key

Using the ATI Active Learning Template: Therapeutic Procedure

DESCRIPTION OF PROCEDURE: Surgical procedure involving ligation and severance of the vas deferens

INDICATIONS

Advantages
- Method is permanent.
- Procedure is short, safe, and simple.
- Sexual function is not impaired.

Disadvantages: A surgical procedure; considered irreversible.

CLIENT EDUCATION
- Scrotal support and moderate activity are recommended for several days after the procedure to improve comfort.
- An alternate form of contraception should be used for approximately 20 ejaculations to ensure that the vas deferens is cleared of remaining sperm.
- A follow-up sperm count should be done.

Ⓝ *NCLEX® Connection: Health Promotion and Maintenance, Lifestyle Choices*

Application Exercises Key

1. A, C, E. **CORRECT:** The nurse should discuss with the client the disadvantages of using a penile condom which includes reduced spontaneity of intercourse, one time usage, decreased sensation during intercourse.
   B. The use of condoms offers a high rate of nonadherence and does not protect against HSV, HSV, and syphilis that can be transmitted from lesions on the skin or mucus membranes.
   D. The use of condoms offers a high rate of nonadherence and does not protect against HSV, HSV, and syphilis that can be transmitted from lesions on the skin or mucus membranes.

Ⓝ *NCLEX® Connection: Health Promotion and Maintenance, Lifestyle Choices*

2. Emergency contraceptives should be taken with 72 hr after unprotected coitus. The provider recommends taking an over-the-counter antiemetic 1 hr prior to each dose to decrease that nausea that occurs with high doses of progestin and estrogen. Additionally, a follow up with the provider to test for pregnancy if menstruation does not begin within 21 days.

Ⓝ *NCLEX® Connection: Health Promotion and Maintenance, Lifestyle Choices*

3. A, 5; B, 4; C, 3; D, 3; E, 1

   A disadvantage of an intrauterine device is that it is considered irreversible. A disadvantage of an intrauterine device it can increase the risk of pelvic inflammatory disease. A disadvantage of an implantable progesterone is that it can decrease bone density. A disadvantage of a transdermal patch is it can cause a skin reaction from the patch application. A disadvantage of a cervical cap is it can possibly increase the risk of acquiring TSS.

Ⓝ *NCLEX® Connection: Health Promotion and Maintenance, Lifestyle Choices*

When reviewing the following chapters, keep in mind the relevant topics and tasks of the NCLEX outline.

Health Promotion and Maintenance

ANTE-/INTRA-/POSTPARTUM AND NEWBORN CARE
Assist in performing client non-stress test.

Reinforce client teaching on infant care skills.

DATA COLLECTION TECHNIQUES: Collect data for health history.

HEALTH PROMOTION/DISEASE PREVENTION: Identify clients in need of immunizations.

HIGH-RISK BEHAVIORS: Reinforce client teaching related to client high risk behavior.

LIFESTYLE CHOICES
Recognize client need/desire for contraception.

Reinforce teaching with client on healthy lifestyle choices.

Basic Care and Comfort

NONPHARMACOLOGICAL COMFORT INTERVENTIONS: Provide nonpharmacological measures for pain relief.

Pharmacological Therapies

ADVERSE EFFECTS/CONTRAINDICATIONS/SIDE EFFECTS/ INTERACTIONS
Reinforce client teaching on possible effects of medications.

Monitor client for actual and potential adverse effects of medications.

EXPECTED ACTIONS/OUTCOMES
Identify client expected response to medication.

Evaluate client response to medication.

PHARMACOLOGICAL PAIN MANAGEMENT: Identify client need for pain medication.

Reduction of Risk Potential

DIAGNOSTIC TESTS: Reinforce client teaching about diagnostic tests.

LABORATORY VALUES
Monitor diagnostic or laboratory test results.

Compare client laboratory values to normal laboratory values.

POTENTIAL FOR ALTERATIONS IN BODY SYSTEMS
Identify signs or symptoms of potential prenatal complications.

Perform focused data collection based on client condition.

THERAPEUTIC PROCEDURES: Reinforce client teaching on treatments and procedures.

Physiological Adaptation

ALTERATIONS IN BODY SYSTEMS: Provide care for a client experiencing complications of pregnancy/labor or delivery.

UNIT 1   ANTEPARTUM NURSING CARE
SECTION: CHANGES DURING PREGNANCY

CHAPTER 2   *Expected Physiological Changes During Pregnancy*

Recognizing changes during pregnancy is helpful for both clients and nurses. The nurse and provider collect data during the client's initial prenatal visit.

Signs of pregnancy are classified into three groups: presumptive, probable, and positive.

The nurse calculates the delivery date, determines the number of pregnancies, and evaluates the physiological status of a client who is pregnant.

SIGNS OF PREGNANCY QEBP

PRESUMPTIVE SIGNS

Presumptive signs are changes the client experiences that make them think that they might be pregnant. These changes might be subjective manifestations or objective findings. Signs also might be a result of physiological factors other than pregnancy (peristalsis, infections, stress).

- **Amenorrhea**
- **Fatigue**
- **Nausea and vomiting**
- **Urinary frequency**
- **Breast changes:** darkened areolae, enlarged Montgomery's glands
- **Quickening:** slight fluttering movements of the fetus felt by the client, usually between 16 to 20 weeks of gestation
- **Uterine enlargement**

PROBABLE SIGNS

Probable signs are changes that make the examiner suspect a client is pregnant (primarily related to physical changes of the uterus). Signs can be caused by physiological factors other than pregnancy (pelvic congestion, tumors).

- **Abdominal enlargement** related to changes in uterine size, shape, and position
- **Hegar's sign:** softening and compressibility of lower uterus
- **Chadwick's sign:** deepened violet-bluish color of cervix and vaginal mucosa
- **Goodell's sign:** softening of cervical tip

- **Ballottement:** rebound of unengaged fetus
- **Braxton Hicks contractions:** false contractions that are painless, irregular, and usually relieved by walking
- **Positive pregnancy test**

POSITIVE SIGNS

Positive signs are those that can be explained only by pregnancy.

- **Fetal heart sounds**
- **Visualization of fetus by ultrasound**
- **Fetal movement** palpated by an experienced examiner

VERIFYING PREGNANCY

Blood and urine tests provide an accurate assessment for the presence of human chorionic gonadotropin (hCG). hCG production can start as early as the day of implantation and can be detected as early as 7 to 8 days before expected menses.

- Production of hCG begins with implantation, peaks at about 60 to 70 days of gestation, declines until around 100 to 130 days of pregnancy, and then plasma levels remain at this lower level for the remainder of the pregnancy.
- Higher levels of hCG can indicate multifetal pregnancy, ectopic pregnancy, hydatidiform mole (gestational trophoblastic disease), or a genetic abnormality such as Down syndrome.
- Lower blood levels of hCG might suggest a miscarriage or ectopic pregnancy.
- Some medications (anticonvulsants, diuretics, tranquilizers) can cause false-positive or false-negative pregnancy results.
- Home pregnancy test: Urine samples should be first-voided morning specimens and follow the directions for accuracy.

CALCULATING DELIVERY DATE AND DETERMINING NUMBER OF PREGNANCIES FOR PREGNANT CLIENT

Naegele's rule: Take the first day of the client's last menstrual cycle, subtract 3 months, and then add 7 days and 1 year, adjusting for the year as necessary.

Measurement of fundal height in centimeters from the symphysis pubis to the top of the uterine fundus (between 18 and 30 weeks of gestation approximates the gestational age, plus or minus 2 gestational weeks.

Gravidity: number of pregnancies.
- **Nulligravida:** a client who has never been pregnant
- **Primigravida:** a client in their first pregnancy
- **Multigravida:** a client who has had two or more pregnancies

Parity: number of pregnancies in which the fetus or fetuses reach at least 20 weeks of pregnancy, not the number of fetuses. Parity is not affected whether the fetus is born stillborn or alive. Nullipara: no pregnancy beyond the stage of viability

- **Primipara:** has completed one pregnancy with a fetus or fetuses who have reached at least 20 weeks of gestation
- **Multipara:** has completed two or more pregnancies to 20 weeks of gestation or more

Viability: the point in time when an infant has the capacity to survive outside the uterus. There is not a specific weeks of gestation; however, infants born between 22 to 25 weeks are considered on the threshold of viability.

GTPAL acronym
- Gravidity
- Term births (37 weeks or more)
- Preterm births (from viability up to 37 weeks)
- Abortions/miscarriages (prior to viability)
- Living children

PHYSIOLOGICAL STATUS OF PREGNANT CLIENT

BODY SYSTEMS

Reproductive

Ovulation and menses cease during pregnancy. Uterus increases in size and changes shape and position.

Cardiovascular

Cardiac output increases (30% to 50%) and blood volume increases (40% to 50% at term) to meet the greater metabolic needs. Heart rate increases during pregnancy beginning around week 5 and reaches a peak (15 to 20/min above prepregnancy rate) around 32 weeks of pregnancy.

Respiratory

Maternal oxygen needs increase. During the last trimester, the size of the chest might enlarge, allowing for lung expansion, as the uterus pushes upward. Respiratory rate increases and total lung capacity decreases.

Musculoskeletal

Body alterations and weight increase necessitate an adjustment in posture. Pelvic joints relax.

Gastrointestinal

Nausea and vomiting might occur due to hormonal changes and/or an increase of pressure within the abdominal cavity as the pregnant client's stomach and intestines are displaced within the abdomen. Constipation might occur due to increased transit time of food through the gastrointestinal tract and, thus, increased water absorption.

Renal

Filtration rate increases secondary to the influence of pregnancy hormones and an increase in blood volume and metabolic demands. The amount of urine produced remains the same. Urinary frequency is common during pregnancy.

Endocrine

The placenta becomes an endocrine organ that produces large amounts of hCG, progesterone, estrogen, human placental lactogen, and prostaglandins. Hormones are very active during pregnancy and function to maintain pregnancy and prepare the body for delivery.

BODY IMAGE CHANGES

- Due to physical and psychological changes that occur, the pregnant client requires support from their provider and family members.
- In the first trimester of pregnancy, physiological changes are not obvious. Many clients look forward to the changes so that the pregnancy will be more noticeable.
- During the second trimester, there are rapid physical changes due to the enlargement of the abdomen and breasts. These changes can affect a client's mobility. Skin changes also occur (stretch marks, hyperpigmentation). They might find themselves losing their balance and feeling back or leg discomfort and fatigue. These factors might lead to a negative body image. The client might make statements of resentment toward the pregnancy and express anxiousness for the pregnancy to be over soon.

EXPECTED VITAL SIGNS Q EBP

Blood pressure

- Blood pressure measurements are within the prepregnancy range during the first trimester.
- **Systolic:** slight or no increase from prepregnancy levels
- **Diastolic:** slight decreases around 24 to 32 weeks; will gradually return to prepregnancy level by the end of the pregnancy.
- The position of the pregnant client also might affect blood pressure. In the supine position, blood pressure might appear to be lower due to the weight and pressure of the gravid uterus on the vena cava, which decreases venous blood flow to the heart. Maternal hypotension and fetal hypoxia might occur, which is referred to as supine hypotensive syndrome or supine vena cava syndrome. Manifestations include dizziness, lightheadedness, pallor, and clammy skin. Encourage the client to engage in maternal positioning on the left-lateral side, semi-Fowler's position, or, if supine, with a wedge placed under one hip to alleviate pressure to the vena cava.

Pulse

Pulse increases 10 to 15/min around 32 weeks of gestation and remains elevated throughout the remainder of the pregnancy.

Respirations

Respirations are unchanged or slightly increased. Respiratory changes in pregnancy are attributed to the elevation of the diaphragm by as much as 4 cm, as well as changes to the chest wall to facilitate increased maternal oxygen demands. Some shortness of breath might be noted.

EXPECTED FINDINGS QEBP

- Fetal heart tones are heard at a normal baseline rate of 110 to 160/min with reassuring FHR accelerations noted, which indicates an intact fetal CNS.
- The client's heart changes in size and shape with resulting cardiac hypertrophy to accommodate increased blood volume and increased cardiac output. Heart sounds also change to accommodate the increase in blood volume with a more distinguishable splitting of S1 and S2, with S3 more easily heard following 20 weeks of gestation. Murmurs also might be auscultated. Heart size and shape should return to normal shortly after delivery.
- Uterine size changes from a uterine weight of 50 to 1,000 g (0.1 to 2.2 lb). By 36 weeks of gestation, the top of the uterus and the fundus will reach the xiphoid process. This might cause the pregnant client to experience shortness of breath as the uterus pushes against the diaphragm.
- Cervical changes are obvious as a purplish-blue color extends into the vagina and labia, and the cervix becomes markedly soft.
- Breast changes occur due to hormones of pregnancy, with the breasts increasing in size and the areolae darkening.

SKIN CHANGES
- Chloasma: an increase of pigmentation on the face
- Linea nigra: dark line of pigmentation from the umbilicus extending to the pubic area
- Striae gravidarum: stretch marks most notably found on the abdomen and thighs

NURSING INTERVENTIONS

- Acknowledge the client's concerns about pregnancy and encourage sharing of these feelings while providing an atmosphere free of judgment.
- Discuss with the client the expected physiological changes and a possible timeline for a return to the prepregnant state.
- Assist the client in setting goals for the postpartum period in regard to self-care and newborn care.
- Assist with referring the client to counseling if body image concerns appear to have a negative impact on the pregnancy. Qᴛᴄ
- Reinforce education about the expected physiological and psychosocial changes. Common discomforts of pregnancy and ways to resolve those discomforts are reviewed during prenatal visits.
- The client is encouraged to keep all follow-up appointments and to contact the provider immediately if there is any bleeding, leakage of fluid, or contractions at any time during the pregnancy. Qs

Application Exercises

1. A nurse is discussing signs of pregnancy with a newly licensed nurse. Which findings should the nurse include related to presumptive, probable, and positive signs of pregnancy?

   A. Hegar's sign

   B. Fetal movement

   C. Positive pregnancy test

   D. Amenorrhea

2. A nurse is caring for a client who is pregnant and states that their last menstrual period was September 9th. What is the client's estimated date of delivery?

3. Sort the following items into physiological changes of endocrine, renal, and musculoskeletal.

   A. Urinary frequency

   B. Filtration rate increases

   C. Large amounts of hCG

   D. Pelvic joints relax

4. Discuss body image changes which occur during pregnancy to include psychological and physiological changes.

Active Learning Scenario

A nurse is caring for a client who is in the fourth week of gestation. The client asks about skin and breast changes that can occur during pregnancy. What information should the nurse include when reinforcing teaching? Use the ATI Active Learning Template: Basic Concept to complete this item.

RELATED CONTENT: Describe at least three changes that occur to the skin and breasts during pregnancy.

UNDERLYING PRINCIPLES: Describe the basis for these changes.

Active Learning Scenario Key

Using the ATI Active Learning Template: Basic Concept

RELATED CONTENT
- **Skin changes:** hyperpigmentation; linea nigra; chloasma (mask of pregnancy) on the face; striae gravidarum (stretch marks), most pronounced on abdomen and thighs
- **Breast changes:** darkening of the areola, enlarged Montgomery's glands, increase in size and heaviness, increased sensitivity

UNDERLYING PRINCIPLES: Increase in estrogen and progesterone occurring during pregnancy

Ⓝ *NCLEX® Connection: Physiological Adaption, Alterations in Body Systems*

Application Exercises Key

1. **PRESUMPTIVE:** D; **PROBABLE:** A, C; **POSITIVE:** B

   The nurse should include in the discussion that Amenorrhea is a presumptive sign of pregnancy. While Hegar's sign and a positive pregnancy test are probable signs of pregnancy. Fetal movement is a positive sign of pregnancy.

   Ⓝ *NCLEX® Connection: Health Promotion and Maintenance, Data Collection Techniques*

2. Naegele's rule: Take the first day of the client's last menstrual cycle, subtract 3 months, and then add 7 days and 1 year, adjusting for the year as necessary. Therefore, September 9th minus 3 months plus 7 days and 1 year equals an estimated date of delivery of June 16th.

   Ⓝ *NCLEX® Connection: Health Promotion and Maintenance, Data Collection Techniques*

3. **MUSCULOSKELETAL:** D; **ENDOCRINE:** C; **RENAL:** A, B

   Many physiological changes occur during pregnancy. The filtration rate increases and urinary frequency are common renal changes. Pelvic joint relaxation is a musculoskeletal change that can occur. Also, large amounts of hCG are excreted by the endocrine system.

   Ⓝ *NCLEX® Connection: Health Promotion and Maintenance, Data Collection Techniques*

4. The client can experience both psychological and physiological body image changes during pregnancy. During the first trimester, it is not obvious that physiological changes are occurring. However, during the second trimester, psychological changes can include anxiousness, and even resentment toward the pregnancy if it was unplanned. Physiological changes include skin changes such as hyperpigmentation and stretch marks. Enlargement of the breasts and abdomen occurs. A client's mobility can be affected, loss of balance and feelings of discomfort in legs and back, and fatigue. All of these factors can lead to a negative body image.

   Ⓝ *NCLEX® Connection: Health Promotion and Maintenance, Data Collection Techniques*

CHAPTER 3 *Prenatal Care*

Prenatal care involves data collection and reinforcement of education for pregnant clients. When providing prenatal care, nurses must take into account cultural considerations.

The reinforcement of prenatal education encompasses information provided to a client who is pregnant. Major areas of focus include assisting the client in self-care of the discomforts of pregnancy, promoting a safe outcome to pregnancy, and fostering positive feelings by the pregnant client and their family regarding the childbearing experience.

Prenatal care dramatically reduces infant and maternal morbidity and mortality rates by early detection and treatment of potential problems. A majority of birth defects occur between 2 and 8 weeks of gestation. Q̲EBP

DATA COLLECTION

Nurses play an integral role in determining a client's current knowledge, previous pregnancies, and birthing experiences.

CLIENT HISTORY

Nursing data collection in prenatal care includes obtaining information regarding:

- **Reproductive and obstetrical history** (contraception use, gynecological diagnoses, history of STIs, previous pregnancies, obstetrical difficulties).
- **Medical history**, including physical preexisting conditions, surgical procedures, any handicapping conditions, and the client's immune status (rubella and hepatitis B).
- **Nutritional history**, a complete dietary data collection can alert the practitioner to deficient practices and food allergies. Good nutrition is important and has a direct effect on the growth and development of the fetus.
- **Family history**, such as genetic disorders or conditions that could affect the mother or fetus.
- Any recent or current illnesses or infections.
- **Current medications**, including substance use and alcohol consumption. The nurse should display a nonjudgmental, matter-of-fact demeanor when interviewing a client regarding substance use and observe for clinical findings such as lack of grooming.

- **Psychosocial history** (a client's emotional response to pregnancy, adolescent pregnancy, spouse, support system, history of depression, domestic violence issues).
- Any hazardous environmental exposures; current work conditions. Q̲s
- Current exercise and lifestyle.
- **Abuse history or risk**; check all clients for all forms, including physical, sexual, or psychological abuse, because the risk increases during pregnancy.

BIRTH PLAN

The nurse should provide information regarding birthing methods, such as Lamaze, and pain control options (epidural, natural childbirth). Q̲PCC

PRENATAL DATA COLLECTION

Prenatal care begins with an initial visit (within the first 12 weeks) and continues throughout pregnancy. In an uneventful pregnancy, prenatal visits are scheduled monthly for weeks 16 through 28, every 2 weeks from 29 through 36 weeks, and every week from 36 weeks until birth.

Initial prenatal visit

- Determine the estimated date of birth based on the last menstrual period.
- Obtain medical and nursing history to include social supports and review of systems (to determine risk factors).
- Collect physical data to include a client's baseline weight, vital signs, and pelvic examination.
- Obtain initial laboratory tests, including hemoglobin, hematocrit, WBC, blood type and Rh, rubella titer, urinalysis, renal function test, Pap test, cervical cultures, HIV antibody, hepatitis B surface antigen, toxoplasmosis, and RPR or VDRL.

Ongoing prenatal visits

- Monitor weight, blood pressure, and urine for glucose, protein, and leukocytes.
- Monitor for the presence of edema.
- Monitor fetal development.
  - FHR can be detected at early appointments by ultrasound. The heartbeat can be heard by Doppler late in the first trimester. Listen at the midline, right above the symphysis pubis, by holding the Doppler firmly on the abdomen.
  - Measure fundal height starting in the second trimester. From weeks 18 to 30, the fundal height in centimeters is approximately the same as the number of weeks gestation.
  - Fetal health data collection: Begin monitoring for fetal movement between 16 and 20 weeks of gestation.
- Reinforce education for self-care to include management of common discomforts and concerns of pregnancy (nausea and vomiting, fatigue, backache, varicosities, heartburn, activity, sexuality).

Nursing care

- Assist with Leopold maneuvers to palpate presentation and position of the fetus.
- Assist the provider with the gynecological examination. This examination is performed to determine the status of a client's reproductive organs and birth canal. Pelvic measurements determine whether the pelvis will allow for the passage of the fetus at delivery. Qᴛᴄ
  - The nurse has the client empty their bladder and take deep breaths during the examination to decrease discomfort.
- Administer Rh₀(D) immune globulin IM around 28 weeks of gestation for clients who are Rh-negative.

Routine laboratory tests

Blood type, Rh factor, and presence of irregular antibodies: Determines the risk for maternal-fetal blood incompatibility (erythroblastosis fetalis) or neonatal hyperbilirubinemia. Indirect Coombs' test identifies clients sensitized to Rh-positive blood. For clients who are Rh-negative and not sensitized, the indirect Coombs' test is repeated between 24 and 28 weeks of gestation.

CBC with differential, Hgb, and Hct: Detects infection and anemia.

Hgb electrophoresis: Identifies hemoglobinopathies (sickle cell anemia and thalassemia).

Rubella titer: Determines immunity to rubella.

Hepatitis B screen: Identifies carriers of hepatitis B.

Group B Streptococcus (GBS): Vaginal and rectal cultures are performed at 36 0/7 and up to 37 6/7 weeks of gestation.

Urinalysis with microscopic examination of pH, specific gravity, color, sediment, protein, glucose, albumin, RBCs, WBCs, casts, acetone, and human chorionic gonadotropin: Identifies pregnancy, diabetes mellitus, gestational hypertension, renal disease, and infection.

One-hour glucose tolerance (oral ingestion with venous sample taken 1 hr later [fasting not necessary]): Identifies hyperglycemia; done at initial visit for at-risk clients and at 24 to 28 weeks of gestation for all pregnant clients (greater than 140 mg/dL requires follow up).

Three-hour glucose tolerance (fasting overnight prior to oral ingestion or IV administration of concentrated glucose with a venous sample taken 1, 2, and 3 hr later): Used in clients who have elevated 1-hr glucose test as a screening tool for diabetes mellitus. A diagnosis of gestational diabetes requires two elevated blood-glucose readings.

Glycosylated hemoglobin (HbA1c): Indicated for clients who have diabetes mellitus prior to pregnancy.

- HbA1c is the best indicator of an average blood glucose level for the past 120 days.
- Assists in evaluating treatment effectiveness and adherence to the diet plan, medication regimen, and exercise schedule.
- 6.5% to 8% indicates diabetes.
- Greater than 8% indicates poor control of diabetes.
- EXPECTED REFERENCE RANGE: 5.7% or less indicates that the client does not have diabetes mellitus.

Papanicolaou (Pap) test: Used as a screening tool for cervical cancer. HPV co-testing can also be done.

Vaginal/cervical culture: Detects streptococcus beta-hemolytic, bacterial vaginosis, or sexually transmitted infections (gonorrhea and chlamydia).

PPD (tuberculosis screening), chest x-ray after 20 weeks of gestation with a positive PPD test: Identifies exposure to tuberculosis.

Venereal disease research laboratory (VDRL) or Rapid plasma reagent (RPR): Syphilis screening mandated by law.

HIV: Detects HIV infection (the Centers for Disease Control and Prevention and the American College of Obstetricians and Gynecologists recommend testing all clients who are pregnant unless the client refuses testing).

Toxoplasmosis, other infections, rubella, cytomegalovirus, and herpes virus (TORCH) screening when indicated: Screening for a group of infections capable of crossing the placenta and adversely affecting fetal development.

Maternal serum alpha-fetoprotein (MSAFP): Screening occurs between 15 to 22 weeks of gestation. Used to rule out Down syndrome (low level) and neural tube defects (high level). The provider might decide to use a more reliable indicator and opt for the Quad screen instead of the MSAFP at 16 to 18 weeks of gestation. This includes AFP, inhibin-A, a combination analysis of human chorionic gonadotropin and estriol.

CLIENT EDUCATION

Prenatal reinforcement of teaching includes health promotion, preparation for pregnancy and birth, common discomforts of pregnancy, and warning/danger signs to report.

HEALTH PROMOTION

Preconception and prenatal education reinforcement emphasizes healthy behaviors that promote the health of the pregnant client and their fetus. Qᴘᴄᴄ

- Avoid all over-the-counter medications, supplements, and prescription medications unless the provider who is supervising their care has knowledge of this practice.
- Alcohol (birth defects) and tobacco (low birth weight) are contraindicated during pregnancy.
- Substance use of any kind is to be avoided during pregnancy and lactation. Strategies to reduce or eliminate substance use are reviewed.
- Exercise during pregnancy yields positive benefits and should consist of 30 min of moderate exercise (walking or swimming) daily if not medically or obstetrically contraindicated.
- Avoid the use of hot tubs or saunas.
- Consume at least 8 to 10 glasses (2.5 L) of water each day.

The nurse reinforces anticipatory teaching to a client about the following.
- Need for flu vaccine
- Tdap (whooping cough) vaccines given at 27 to 35 weeks for client. Any family members caring for newborn should also receive it.
- COVID vaccine should be given according to CDC recommendations
- Smoking cessation
- Treatment of current infections
- Genetic testing and counseling
- Exposure to hazardous materials

PREPARATION FOR PREGNANCY AND BIRTH

- Nurses reinforce to the pregnant client and their family about the following.
  - Physical and emotional changes during pregnancy and interventions that can be implemented to provide relief.
  - Indications of complications to report to the provider.
  - Birthing options available to enhance the birthing process.
- Maternal adaptation to pregnancy and the attainment of the maternal role—whereby the idea of pregnancy is accepted and assimilated into the client's way of life—includes hormonal and psychological aspects.
  - Emotional lability is experienced by many clients with unpredictable mood changes and increased irritability, tearfulness, and anger alternating with feelings of joy and cheerfulness. This might result from hormonal changes.
  - A feeling of ambivalence about the pregnancy, which is a normal response, might occur early in the pregnancy and resolve before the third trimester. It consists of conflicting feelings (joy, pleasure, sorrow, hostility) about the pregnancy. These feelings can occur simultaneously, whether the pregnancy was planned or not.
- The nurse anticipates reviewing prenatal education topics with a client based on their current knowledge and previous pregnancy and birth experiences. The client's readiness to learn is enhanced when the nurse provides reinforcement during the appropriate trimester based on learning needs. Using a variety of methods (pamphlets, videos) to provide information and having the client verbalize and demonstrate learned topics will ensure that learning has taken place. Qpcc

FIRST TRIMESTER
- Physical and psychosocial changes
- Common discomforts of pregnancy and measures to provide relief
- Lifestyle: exercise, stress, nutrition, sexual health, dental care, over-the-counter and prescription medications, tobacco, alcohol, substance use, and STIs (encourage safe sexual practices)
- Possible complications and indications to report (preterm labor)
- Fetal growth and development
- Prenatal exercise
- Expected laboratory testing

SECOND TRIMESTER
- Benefits of breastfeeding
- Common discomforts and relief measures
- Lifestyle: sex and pregnancy, rest and relaxation, posture, body mechanics, clothing, seat belt safety and travel Qs
- Fetal movement
- Complications (preterm labor, gestational hypertension, gestational diabetes mellitus, premature rupture of membranes)
- Preparation for childbirth and childbirth education classes
- Review of birthing methods
- Development of a birth plan (verbal or written agreement about what the client wishes during labor and delivery)

THIRD TRIMESTER
- Childbirth preparation QEBP
  - Childbirth classes or birth plan
  - Coping methods
  - Breathing and relaxation techniques
  - Use of effleurage and counter pressure
  - Application of heat/cold, touch and massage, and water therapy
  - Use of transcutaneous electrical nerve stimulation (TENS)
  - Acupressure and acupuncture
  - Music and aromatherapy
  - Discussion regarding pain management during labor and birth (natural childbirth, epidural)
  - Use of a doula to provide support to the client and family during labor and birth
  - Indications of preterm labor and labor
  - Labor process
  - Infant care
  - Postpartum care
- Fetal movement/kick counts to ascertain fetal well-being: A client should be instructed to count and record fetal movements or kicks daily. There are several different methods to complete kick counts.
  - One method: Clients should count fetal activity two or three times a day for 2 hr after meals or bedtime. Fetal movements of less than 3 per hr or movements that cease entirely for 12 hr indicate a need for further evaluation.
- Diagnostic testing for fetal well-being (nonstress test, biophysical profile, ultrasound, and contraction stress test)

COMMON DISCOMFORTS OF PREGNANCY

Nausea and vomiting might occur during the first trimester. The client should eat crackers or dry toast before rising in the morning to relieve discomfort. Instruct the client to avoid having an empty stomach and ingesting spicy, greasy, or gas-forming foods. Encourage the client to drink fluids between meals.

Breast tenderness might occur during the first trimester. The client should wear a bra that provides adequate support.

Urinary frequency might occur during the first and third trimesters. The client should empty the bladder frequently, decrease fluid intake before bedtime, and use perineal pads. The client is taught how to perform Kegel exercises (alternate tightening and relaxation of pubococcygeal muscles) to reduce stress incontinence (leakage of urine with coughing and sneezing).

Urinary tract infections (UTIs) are common during pregnancy because of renal changes and the vaginal flora becoming more alkaline.

- UTI risks can be decreased by encouraging the client to wipe the perineal area from front to back after voiding, avoiding bubble baths, wearing cotton underpants, avoiding tight-fitting pants, and consuming plenty of water (8 glasses per day). Q EBP
- The client should urinate before and after intercourse to flush bacteria from the urethra that are present or introduced during intercourse.
- Advise the client to urinate as soon as the urge occurs because retaining urine provides an environment for bacterial growth.
- Advise the client to notify the provider if their urine is foul-smelling, contains blood, or appears cloudy.

Fatigue might occur during the first and third trimesters. The client is encouraged to engage in frequent rest periods.

Heartburn might occur during the second and third trimesters due to the stomach being displaced by the enlarging uterus and a slowing of gastrointestinal tract motility and digestion brought about by increased progesterone levels. The client should eat small, frequent meals, not allow the stomach to get too empty or too full, and check with the provider prior to using any over-the-counter antacids. The client should not immediately lie down after eating, as this can exacerbate reflux.

Constipation might occur during the second and third trimesters. The client is encouraged to drink plenty of fluids, eat a diet high in fiber, and exercise regularly.

Hemorrhoids might occur during the second and third trimesters. A warm sitz bath, witch hazel pads, and application of topical ointments will help relieve discomfort.

Backaches are common during the second and third trimesters. The client is encouraged to exercise regularly, perform pelvic tilt exercises (alternately arching and straightening the back), use proper body mechanics by using the legs to lift rather than the back, and use the side-lying position.

Shortness of breath and dyspnea might occur because of the enlarged uterus, which limits inspiration. The client should maintain good posture, sleep with extra pillows, and contact the provider if manifestations worsen.

Leg cramps during the third trimester might occur due to the compression of lower-extremity nerves and blood vessels by the enlarging uterus. This can result in poor peripheral circulation, as well as an imbalance in the calcium/phosphorus ratio. The client should extend the affected leg, keeping the knee straight, and dorsiflex the foot (toes toward head). Application of heat over the affected muscle or a foot massage while the leg is extended can help relieve cramping. The client should notify the provider if frequent cramping occurs.

Varicose veins and lower-extremity edema can occur during the second and third trimesters. The client should rest with the legs and hips elevated, avoid constricting clothing, wear support hose, avoid sitting or standing in one position for extended periods of time, and not sit with the legs crossed at the knees. The client should sleep in the left-lateral position and exercise moderately with frequent walking to stimulate venous return.

Gingivitis, nasal stuffiness, and epistaxis (nosebleed) can occur as a result of elevated estrogen levels causing increased vascularity and proliferation of connective tissue. The client should gently brush their teeth, observe good dental hygiene, use a humidifier, and use normal saline nose drops or spray.

Braxton Hicks contractions, which occur from the first trimester onward, might increase in intensity and frequency during the third trimester. Inform the client that a change of position and walking should cause contractions to subside. If contractions increase in intensity and frequency (true contractions) with regularity, the client should notify the provider.

Supine hypotension occurs when a client lies on their back and the weight of the gravid uterus compresses the vena cava. This reduces blood supply to the fetus. The client might experience feelings of lightheadedness and faintness. Reinforce to the client to lie in a side-lying or semi-sitting position with the knees slightly flexed.

DANGER SIGNS DURING PREGNANCY

The following indicate potential dangerous situations that should be reported to the provider immediately.

FIRST TRIMESTER
- Burning on urination (infection)
- Severe vomiting (hyperemesis gravidarum)
- Diarrhea (infection)
- Fever or chills (infection)
- Abdominal cramping and/or vaginal bleeding (miscarriage, ectopic pregnancy)

SECOND AND THIRD TRIMESTER

- Gush of fluid from the vagina (rupture of amniotic fluid) prior to 37 weeks of gestation
- Vaginal bleeding (placental problems such as abruption or previa)
- Abdominal pain (premature labor, abruptio placentae, or ectopic pregnancy)
- Changes in fetal activity (decreased fetal movement might indicate fetal distress)
- Persistent vomiting (hyperemesis gravidarum)
- Severe headaches (gestational hypertension)
- Elevated temperature (infection)
- Dysuria (urinary tract infection)
- Blurred vision (gestational hypertension)
- Edema of face and hands (gestational hypertension)
- Epigastric pain (gestational hypertension)
- Concurrent occurrence of flushed dry skin, fruity breath, rapid breathing, increased thirst and urination, and headache (hyperglycemia)
- Concurrent occurrence of clammy pale skin, weakness, tremors, irritability, and lightheadedness (hypoglycemia)

Active Learning Scenario

A nurse is caring for a client at 14 weeks of gestation and is reviewing self-care concepts regarding the prevention of urinary tract infections (UTIs). What should the nurse reinforce with the client? Use the ATI Active Learning Template: Basic Concept to complete this item.

UNDERLYING PRINCIPLES: Describe two.

NURSING INTERVENTIONS: Describe two actions that decrease the risk of UTIs as they relate to each of the following types of interventions: When? Why? and How?

Application Exercises

1. A nurse is preparing to draw laboratory tests from a client who is 8 weeks of gestation and at the initial prenatal visit. Which of the following tests should the nurse anticipate obtaining? (Select all that apply.)
   - A. CBC with differential
   - B. Rubella titer
   - C. Blood type, Rh factor
   - D. Maternal serum alpha-fetoprotein (MSAFP)
   - E. One-hour glucose tolerance

2. A nurse is reinforcing teaching with a client who is at 6 weeks of gestation about common discomforts of pregnancy. Which of the following findings should the nurse include? (Select all that apply.)
   - A. Breast tenderness
   - B. Urinary frequency
   - C. Epistaxis
   - D. Dysuria
   - E. Epigastric pain

3. A nurse is reinforcing teaching with a group of clients who are pregnant about measures to relieve backache during pregnancy. Which of the following measures should the nurse include?

4. A nurse is reinforcing teaching with a client who is pregnant and reviewing manifestations of complications the client should promptly report to the provider. Which of the following complications should the nurse include?
   - A. Vaginal bleeding
   - B. Swelling of the ankles
   - C. Heartburn after eating
   - D. Lightheadedness when lying on back

Active Learning Scenario Key

Using the ATI Active Learning Template: Basic Concept

UNDERLYING PRINCIPLES: UTIs are common because of renal changes during pregnancy and the vaginal flora becoming more alkaline.

NURSING INTERVENTIONS

Decrease risk of UTIs by:

- How, When: Encouraging client to wipe the perineal area from front to back after voiding.
- How: Avoiding bubble baths.
- How: Wearing cotton underpants, avoiding tight-fitting pants.
- How: Consuming at least 8 glasses of water per day.
- How, Why: Instructing the client to urinate before and after intercourse to flush bacteria from the urethra that are present or introduced during intercourse.
- How, Why: Advising the client to urinate as soon as the urge occurs because retaining urine provides an environment for bacterial growth.
- When, Why: Advising the client to notify the provider if their urine is foul-smelling, contains blood, or is cloudy, so evaluation and early treatment can be initiated.

Ⓝ *NCLEX® Connection: Reduction of Risk Potential, Potential for Alterations in Body Systems*

Application Exercises Key

1. A, B, C. **CORRECT:** The nurse should anticipate collecting a blood sample to test for rubella titer, CBC with differential, and blood type, RH factor. All of these laboratory tests should be collected during the initial prenatal visit. The one-hour glucose tolerance test is obtained between 24 and 28 weeks of gestation and maternal serum alpha-fetoprotein (MSAFP) is collected between 15 to 22 weeks of gestation.

Ⓝ *NCLEX® Connection: Reduction of Risk Potential, Laboratory Values*

2. A, B, C. **CORRECT:** The nurse should discuss common discomforts during the first trimester of pregnancy which include breast tenderness, urinary frequency, and epistaxis. Dysuria is a complication that might occur during pregnancy. Instruct the client to report this finding to the provider. Epigastric pain is a clinical finding of pregnancy-induced hypertension. Instruct the client to report this finding to the provider.

Ⓝ *NCLEX® Connection: Physiological Adaptation, Alterations in Body Systems*

3. The nurse should instruct the client to use the following measures to relieve backache during pregnancy. The pelvic rock or tilt exercise stretches the muscles of the lower back and helps relieve lower-back pain. The use of proper body mechanics prevents back injury that can occur with incorrect use of muscles when lifting.

Ⓝ *NCLEX® Connection: Basic Care and Comfort, Nonpharmacological Comfort Interventions*

4. A. **CORRECT:** The nurse should instruct the client to notify the provider immediately if vaginal bleeding occurs. Vaginal bleeding could indicate a potential complication of the placenta such as a placenta previa or an abruptio placenta. Swelling of the ankles, heartburn after eating, and lightheadedness when lying supine are common occurrence during pregnancy.

Ⓝ *NCLEX® Connection: Reduction of Risk Potential, Potential for Alterations in Body Systems*

CHAPTER 4 # Nutrition During Pregnancy

Adequate nutritional intake during pregnancy is essential to promoting fetal and maternal health.

Recommended weight gain during pregnancy, based on a single pregnancy, is usually 11.5 to 16 kg (25 to 35 lb). The general rule is that clients should gain 0.9 to 1.8 kg (2 to 4 lb) during the first trimester and after that approximately 0.5 kg (1 lb) per week for the last two trimesters. This varies for underweight, average, and overweight clients.

Excessive weight gain can lead to abnormal fetal growth and labor complications. Inability to gain weight could result in low birth weight of the newborn.

It is important for the nurse to identify the pregnant client's nutritional choices, possible risk factors, and diet history. The nurse also should review specific nutritional guidelines for at-risk clients. Assistance is given to clients to develop a postpartum nutritional plan.

NURSING DATA COLLECTION AND INTERVENTIONS

DATA COLLECTION

Obtain subjective and objective dietary information.
- Journal of the client's food habits, eating pattern, and cravings
- Nutrition-related questionnaires
- Health history, including contraceptive history, previous pregnancies, chronic diseases
- The client's weight on first prenatal visit and follow-up visits
- Laboratory findings (Hgb, iron levels)

Determine the client's caloric intake. QPCC
Have the client record everything eaten during a 24-hr period. The nurse, dietitian, or client can identify the caloric value of each item. This record can provide better objective data about the client's nutrition status. (4.1)

CLIENT EDUCATION

Reinforce about adhering to and maintaining the following during pregnancy.
- **Increase calories:** An increase of 340 calories/day is recommended during the second trimester. An increase of 452 calories/day is recommended during the third trimester. If the client is breastfeeding during the postpartum period, additional caloric intake is advised. The American Academy of Pediatrics (AAP) recommends that breastfeeding clients who are well-nourished should add 450 to 500 calories/day to a balanced diet.
- **Increasing protein intake** is essential to basic growth.
- **Folic acid** is crucial for neurologic development and the prevention of fetal neural tube defects. Folate found naturally in foods is converted to folic acid. Foods high in folate include leafy vegetables, dried peas and beans, seeds, and orange juice. Breads, cereals, and other grains are fortified with folic acid. The March of Dimes recommends that clients who wish to become pregnant and clients of childbearing age take 400 mcg of folic acid and clients who become pregnant take 600 mcg of folic acid. QEBP
- **Iron supplements** are often added to the prenatal plan to facilitate an increase of the maternal RBC mass. Iron is best absorbed between meals and when given with a source of vitamin C (orange juice). Milk and caffeine interfere with the absorption of iron supplements. Food sources of iron include beef liver, red meats, fish, poultry, dried peas and beans, and fortified cereals and breads. A stool softener might need to be added to decrease constipation experienced with iron supplements.
- **Calcium**, which is important to a developing fetus, is involved in bone and teeth formation. Sources of calcium include milk, calcium-fortified soy milk, fortified orange juice, nuts, legumes, and dark green leafy vegetables. Daily recommendation is 1,000 mg/day for pregnant and nonpregnant clients 19 to 50 years of age, and 1,300 mg/day for those under 19 years of age.

4.1 Reviewing plan of care for a pregnant client

Expected outcomes
The client will consume the recommended dietary allowances/nutrients during their pregnancy.

Evaluation of the plan
Is there adequate weight gain?
Is the client compliant with the nursing plan of care?

Interventions
The nurse checks the client's dietary journal during prenatal visits.

The nurse provides educational materials regarding nutritional benefits to the mother and their newborn.

The nurse provides encouragement and answers questions that the client has regarding their dietary plans.

The nurse weighs the client and monitors for findings of inadequate weight gain.

The nurse should notify the charge nurse if a referral if needed.

- **Fluid:** 8 to 10 glasses (2.3 L) of fluid are recommended daily. Preferred fluids are water and milk.
- **Limit caffeine:** The American College of Obstetricians and Gynecologists (ACOG) and March of Dimes recommend a daily intake of no more than 300 mg of caffeine. Excessive intake of caffeine can contribute to infertility, spontaneous abortion, or intrauterine growth restriction (IUGR). Ⓠᴇʙᴘ
- It is recommended that clients abstain from alcohol consumption during pregnancy.

RISK FACTORS

Age, culture, education, and socioeconomic issues could affect adequate nutrition during pregnancy. Also, certain conditions specific to each client might inhibit adequate caloric intake.

- Adolescents might have poor nutritional habits (a diet low in vitamins and protein, not taking prescribed iron supplements).
- Clients who follow a vegetarian diet might have decreased intake of protein, calcium, iron, zinc, and vitamin B$_{12}$.
- Nausea and vomiting during pregnancy
- Anemia
- Eating disorders (anorexia nervosa, bulimia nervosa)
- Pica (craving to eat nonfood substances such as dirt or red clay); this disorder might diminish the amount of nutritional foods ingested.
- Inability to purchase/access food. Ⓠᴛᴄ

DIETARY COMPLICATIONS DURING PREGNANCY

Nausea and constipation

Nausea and constipation are common during pregnancy.

CLIENT EDUCATION
- For nausea, eat small amounts frequently (every 2 to 3 hr) to avoid large meals that distend the stomach, and avoid alcohol, caffeine, and fried, fatty, and spicy foods. Also avoid consuming excessive amounts of fluid, and DO NOT take a medication to control nausea without first checking with the provider. Ginger (ginger ale soda, ginger tea, ginger candies) and herbal tea (peppermint, raspberry) might also be helpful.
- For constipation, increase fluid consumption, perform physical activity, and include extra fiber in the diet. Fruits, vegetables, and whole grains all contain fiber.

Maternal phenylketonuria

Maternal phenylketonuria (PKU) is a maternal genetic disease in which high levels of phenylalanine pose a danger to the fetus (intellectual disability, behavioral problems).

- It is important for the client to resume the PKU diet for at least 3 months prior to pregnancy and continue the diet throughout pregnancy.
- The diet includes foods that are low in phenylalanine. Foods high in protein (fish, poultry, meat, eggs, nuts, dairy products) must be avoided due to high phenylalanine levels. Aspartame, which contains phenylalanine, should be avoided by pregnant clients who have PKU.
- The client's blood phenylalanine levels are monitored during pregnancy.

Diabetes mellitus

Both preexisting diabetes mellitus and gestational diabetes mellitus are complications that require nutritional interventions.

- Monitor the amount of carbohydrates in the diet and keep glucose levels within target range.
- Limit the amount of sweets and desserts, which typically have large amounts of carbohydrates.
- Meet with a registered dietitian.

NUTRITION DURING POSTPARTUM

- A lactating client's nutritional plan includes reinforcement of the following instructions.
  - Increase protein and calorie intake while adhering to a recommended, well-balanced diet.
  - Increase oral fluids, but avoid alcohol and caffeine.
  - Avoid food substances that do not agree with the newborn.
  - Take calcium supplements if unable to consume an adequate amount of dietary calcium.
- A nutritional plan for a client who is not breastfeeding should include resumption of a previously recommended well-balanced diet.
- Discuss with the charge nurse about referring clients who need financial assistance to Women, Infants, and Children (WIC), which are federally funded state programs for pregnant clients and their children (up to 5 years old). Ⓠᴛᴄ

Application Exercises

1. A nurse in a prenatal clinic is assisting with caring for four clients. Which of the following clients' weight gain should the nurse report to the provider?

   A. 1.8 kg (4 lb) weight gain and is in the first trimester

   B. 3.6 kg (8 lb) weight gain and is in the first trimester

   C. 6.8 kg (15 lb) weight gain and is in the second trimester

   D. 11.3 kg (25 lb) weight gain and is in the third trimester

2. A nurse is discussing with a client who is 6 weeks of gestation food sources high in dietary content for folate and iron. (Sort the below food source to folate or iron)

   A. Beef liver

   B. Leafy vegetables

   C. Orange juice

   D. Poultry

3. A nurse in a clinic is teaching a client of childbearing age about recommended folic acid supplements. Which of the following defects can occur in the fetus or neonate as a result of folic acid deficiency?

   A. Iron deficiency anemia

   B. Poor bone formation

   C. Abnormal fetal growth

   D. Neural tube defects

4. A nurse in a prenatal clinic is providing education to a client who is at 8 weeks of gestation. The client states, "I don't like milk." Which of the following foods should the nurse recommend as a good source of calcium?

   A. Dark green leafy vegetables

   B. Deep red or orange vegetables

   C. White breads and rice

   D. Meat, poultry, and fish

Active Learning Scenario

A nurse is assisting a charge nurse in a prenatal clinic is preparing an in-service education program for a group of newly licensed nurses about risk factors preventing adequate nutrition during pregnancy. What information should the nurse include in this presentation? Use the ATI Active Learning Template: Basic Concept to answer this item.

UNDERLYING PRINCIPLES

• Identify one that is age-related.

• Identify two that are related to culture/lifestyle.

• Identify one that is related to a socioeconomic factor.

• Identify two that are related to dietary complications during pregnancy.

NURSING INTERVENTIONS: Describe a federal program that is available to women and children to provide nutrition support.

Active Learning Scenario Key

Using the ATI Active Learning Template: Basic Concept

UNDERLYING PRINCIPLES

- **Age-related:** Adolescents can have poor nutritional habits during pregnancy.
- **Culture/lifestyle:** Vegetarians may have diets low in protein, calcium, zinc, and vitamin B_{12}. Excessive weight gain can lead to macrosomia and labor complications.
- **Socioeconomic factor:** Inability to purchase or access foods can limit nutrition during pregnancy.
- **Dietary complications:** Nausea and vomiting during pregnancy, anemia, eating disorders (anorexia nervosa or bulimia nervosa), inability to gain weight, presence of the appetite disorder pica.

NURSING INTERVENTIONS: Women, Infants, and Children (WIC) is a federally-funded state program that provides nutritional support to pregnant women and their children (up to 5 years old).

(N) *NCLEX® Connection: Health Promotion and Maintenance, Health Promotion/Disease Prevention*

Application Exercises Key

1. B. **CORRECT:** The nurse should report to the provider the client who gained 3.6 kg (8lb) during the first trimester to the provider because the client has exceeded the expected 3 to 4 lb weight gain of a client in the first trimester. The client who gained 1.8 kg (4 lb) during the first trimester has gained the appropriate weight of 2 to 4 lb for a client in the first trimester. The client who gained 6.8 kg (15 lb) and is in the second trimester has gained the appropriate amount of weight which is approximately 1 lb per week. The client who gained 11.3 kg (25 lb) and is in the third trimester has gained the recommended weight.

(N) *NCLEX® Connection: Health Promotion and Maintenance, Data Collection Techniques*

2. **FOLATE:** B, C; **IRON:** A, D

   The nurse should discuss food sources high in dietary folate and iron with a client who is 6 weeks of gestation. Beef liver and poultry are good sources of dietary protein. Leafy vegetables and orange juice are high is dietary folate.

(N) *NCLEX® Connection: Health Promotion and Maintenance, Health Promotion/Disease Prevention*

3. D. **CORRECT:** The nurse should discuss folic acid supplements with clients of childbearing age. Neural tube defects are caused by folic acid deficiency. Food sources of folic acid include fresh green leafy vegetables, liver, peanuts, cereals, and whole-grain breads. The following factors do not result as a deficiency of folic acid. Maternal obesity can lead to a abnormal fetal growth, poor bone formation (calcium does), and iron deficiency anemia results in the lack of iron-rich-dietary food sources such as meat, chicken, and fish.

(N) *NCLEX® Connection: Health Promotion and Maintenance, Health Promotion/Disease Prevention*

4. A. **CORRECT:** The nurse should recommend dark, green leafy vegetables such as kale, artichokes, and turnips greens as a good source of calcium for fetal bone and teeth formation. Deep red or orange vegetables are good sources of vitamins C and A. White breads and rice do not contain high levels of calcium. Meat, poultry, and fish are sources of protein but do not contain high levels of calcium.

(N) *NCLEX® Connection: Basic Care and Comfort, Nutrition and Oral Hydration*

CHAPTER 5   Assessment of Fetal Well-Being

This chapter includes data collection tools that determine the well-being of a fetus during pregnancy. Diagnostic procedures include ultrasound (abdominal, transvaginal, Doppler), biophysical profile, nonstress test, contraction stress test (nipple, oxytocin), and amniocentesis. Additional diagnostic procedures for high-risk pregnancy include percutaneous umbilical cord blood sampling, chorionic villus sampling, quad marker screening, and maternal alpha-fetoprotein blood levels.

Ultrasound (abdominal, transvaginal, and Doppler)

Ultrasound is a procedure lasting approximately 20 min that consists of high-frequency sound waves used to visualize internal organs and tissues by producing a real-time, three-dimensional image of the developing fetus and maternal structures (fetal heart rate [FHR], pelvic anatomy). An ultrasound allows for early diagnosis of complications, permits earlier interventions, and thereby decreases neonatal and maternal morbidity and mortality. There are three types of ultrasound: external abdominal, transvaginal, and Doppler.

External abdominal ultrasound

A safe, noninvasive, painless procedure whereby an ultrasound transducer is moved over the client's abdomen to obtain an image. An abdominal ultrasound is more useful after the first trimester when the gravid uterus is larger. The client should have a full bladder for the procedure. Ⓠ EBP

Transvaginal ultrasound

An invasive procedure in which a probe is inserted vaginally to allow for a more accurate evaluation. An advantage of this procedure is that it does not require a full bladder.
- It is especially useful in clients who are obese and those in the first trimester to detect an ectopic pregnancy, identify abnormalities, and to establish gestational age.
- A transvaginal ultrasound also can be used in the third trimester in conjunction with abdominal scanning to evaluate for preterm labor.

Doppler ultrasound blood flow analysis

A noninvasive external ultrasound method to study the maternal-fetal blood flow by measuring the velocity at which RBCs travel in the uterine and fetal vessels by using a handheld ultrasound device that reflects sound waves from a moving target. It is especially useful in fetal intrauterine growth restriction (IUGR) and poor placental perfusion and as an adjunct in pregnancies at risk because of hypertension, diabetes mellitus, multiple fetuses, or preterm labor.

Two-dimensional (2D): standard medical scan; black, white, or shades of gray

Three-dimensional (3D): multiple pictures at once; almost as clear as a photograph; images look more lifelike than standard ultrasound images

Four-dimensional (4D): like 3D but also shows fetal movements in a video

INDICATIONS

POTENTIAL DIAGNOSES

- Confirming pregnancy
- Confirming gestational age by biparietal diameter (side-to-side) measurement
- Identifying multifetal pregnancy
- Determining site of fetal implantation (uterine, ectopic)
- Evaluating fetal growth and development
- Checking maternal structures
- Confirming fetal viability or death
- Ruling out or verifying fetal abnormalities
- Locating the site of placental attachment
- Determining amniotic fluid volume
- Observing fetal movement (fetal heartbeat, breathing, and activity)
- Determining fetal position
- Placental grading (evaluating placental maturation)
- Adjunct for other procedures (amniocentesis, biophysical profile)

CLIENT PRESENTATION

- Vaginal bleeding evaluation
- Questionable fundal height measurement in relationship to gestational weeks
- Reports of decreased fetal movements
- Preterm labor
- Questionable rupture of membranes

CONSIDERATIONS

NURSING ACTIONS

Abdominal ultrasound

CLIENT PREPARATION
- Explain the procedure and that it presents no known risk to self or fetus.
- Advise the client to drink 1 quart of water prior to the ultrasound to fill the bladder, lift and stabilize the uterus, displace the bowel, and act as an echolucent to better reflect sound waves to obtain a better image of the fetus.
- Assist the client into a supine position with a small pillow under their head and knees.

ONGOING CARE
- Apply an ultrasonic/transducer gel to the client's abdomen before the transducer is moved over the skin to obtain a better fetal image, ensuring that the gel is at room temperature or warmer.
- Allow the client to empty their bladder at the termination of the procedure.
- Provide the client with a washcloth or tissues to wipe away gel after completion of ultrasound.

Transvaginal ultrasound

CLIENT PREPARATION: Assist the client into a lithotomy position. The vaginal probe is covered with a protective device such as a condom, lubricated with a water-soluble gel, and inserted by the client or examiner.

ONGOING CARE
- During the procedure, the position of the probe or tilt of the table can be changed to facilitate the complete view of the pelvis.
- Inform the client that they might feel pressure as the probe is moved.

CLIENT EDUCATION

Fetal and maternal structures can be pointed out as the ultrasound procedure is performed.

Biophysical profile

Biophysical profile (BPP) uses a real-time ultrasound to visualize physical and physiological characteristics of the fetus and observe for fetal biophysical responses to stimuli. It combines FHR monitoring (nonstress test) and fetal ultrasound. $\bigcirc$EBP

INDICATIONS

POTENTIAL DIAGNOSES

- Nonreactive nonstress test
- Suspected oligohydramnios or polyhydramnios
- Suspected fetal hypoxemia or hypoxia

CLIENT PRESENTATION

- Premature rupture of membranes
- Maternal infection
- Decreased fetal movement
- Intrauterine growth restriction

CONSIDERATIONS

NURSING ACTIONS: Prepare the client following the same nursing management principles as those used for an ultrasound.

INTERPRETATION OF FINDINGS

BPP checks fetal well-being by measuring five variables with a score of 2 for each normal finding and 0 for each abnormal finding for each variable.

VARIABLES

FHR
- Reactive (nonstress test) = 2
- Nonreactive = 0

Fetal breathing movements
- At least 1 episode of greater than a 30 sec duration in 30 min = 2
- Absent or less than a 30 sec duration = 0

Gross body movements
- At least 3 body or limb movements within 30 min = 2
- Less than 3 episodes = 0

Fetal tone
- At least 1 episode of extension with return to flexion = 2
- Slow extension and flexion, lack of flexion, or absent movement = 0

Qualitative amniotic fluid volume
- At least 1 pocket of fluid that measures at least 2 cm in 2 perpendicular planes = 2
- Pockets absent or less than 2 cm = 0

TOTAL SCORE FINDINGS

8 TO 10: normal, low risk of chronic fetal asphyxia

4 TO 6: abnormal, suspect chronic fetal asphyxia

LESS THAN 4: abnormal, strongly suspect chronic fetal asphyxia

Nonstress test

Nonstress test (NST) is the most widely used technique for antepartum evaluation of fetal well-being performed during the third trimester. It is a noninvasive procedure that monitors response of the FHR to fetal movement. A Doppler transducer (used to monitor FHR) and a tocotransducer (used to monitor uterine contractions) are attached externally to a client's abdomen to obtain tracing strips. The client pushes a button attached to the monitor whenever they feel a fetal movement, which is then noted on the tracing. This allows a nurse to check the FHR in relationship to the fetal movement.

Disadvantages of an NST include a high rate of false nonreactive results with the fetal movement response blunted by sleep cycles of the fetus, fetal immaturity, maternal medications, and nicotine use disorder. ⓠEBP

INDICATIONS

POTENTIAL DIAGNOSES

- Checking for an intact fetal CNS during the third trimester
- Ruling out the risk for fetal death in clients who have diabetes mellitus. Used twice a week, starting at 28 to 32 weeks of gestation

CLIENT PRESENTATION

- Decreased fetal movement
- Intrauterine growth restriction
- Postmaturity
- History of gestational hypertension or diabetes mellitus
- Systematic lupus erythematosus
- Kidney disease
- Intrahepatic cholestasis
- Oligohydramnios
- Multiple gestation

CONSIDERATIONS

NURSING ACTIONS

CLIENT PREPARATION

- Seat the client in a reclining chair, or place client in a semi-Fowler's or left-lateral position.
- Apply conduction gel to the client's abdomen.
- Apply two belts to the client's abdomen, and attach the ultrasound transducer and tocotransducer.

ONGOING CARE

- Instruct the client to press the button on the handheld event marker each time they feel the fetus move.
- If there are no fetal movements (fetus sleeping), vibroacoustic stimulation (sound source, usually laryngeal stimulator) can be activated for 3 seconds on the maternal abdomen over the fetal head to awaken the sleeping fetus.
- This test is typically completed within 20 to 30 min.

5.1 Reactive nonstress test

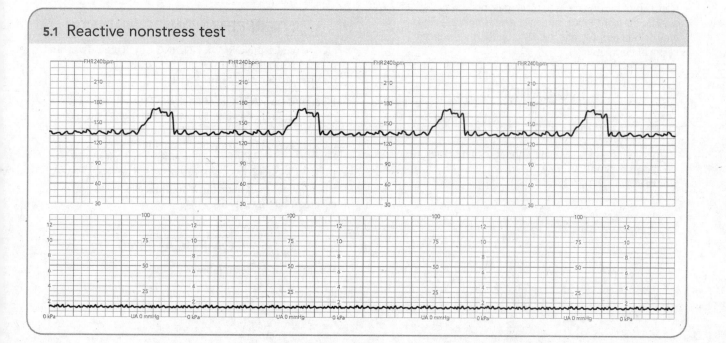

INTERPRETATION OF FINDINGS

- The NST is interpreted as reactive if the FHR accelerates at least 15/min (10/min prior to 32 weeks) above baseline for at least 15 seconds (10 seconds prior to 32 weeks) and occurs two or more times during a 20-min period.
- Nonreactive NST is a test that does not demonstrate at least two qualifying accelerations in a 20-min window. If this is so, a further evaluation, such as a contraction stress test (CST) or BPP, is indicated (5.1).

Contraction stress test

Nipple-stimulated contraction test

Consists of a client lightly brushing their palm across the nipple for 2 min, which causes the pituitary gland to release endogenous oxytocin, and then stopping the nipple stimulation when a contraction begins. The same process is repeated after a 5-min rest period.

- Analysis of the FHR response to contractions (which decrease placental blood flow) determines how the fetus will tolerate the stress of labor. A pattern of at least three contractions within a 10-min time period with duration of 40 to 60 seconds each must be obtained to use for data collection.
- Tachysystole of the uterus (uterine contraction longer than 90 seconds or five or more contractions in 10 min) should be avoided by stimulating the nipple intermittently with rest periods in between and avoiding bimanual stimulation of both nipples unless stimulation of one nipple is unsuccessful.

Oxytocin-stimulated contraction test

Also known as an oxytocin challenge test (OCT), it consists of the IV administration of oxytocin to induce uterine contractions.

- Contractions started with oxytocin can be difficult to stop and can lead to preterm labor.
- Contraindications include placenta previa, vasa previa, preterm labor, multiple gestations, previous classic incision from a cesarean birth, and reduced cervical competence.

INDICATIONS

POTENTIAL DIAGNOSES

- High-risk pregnancies (gestational diabetes mellitus, postterm pregnancy)
- Nonreactive stress test

CLIENT PRESENTATION

- Decreased fetal movement
- Intrauterine growth restriction
- Postmaturity
- Diabetes mellitus
- Hypertension
- History of previous fetal demise
- Systematic lupus erythematosus
- Kidney disease
- Intrahepatic cholestasis
- Oligohydramnios
- Multiple gestation

CONSIDERATIONS

NURSING ACTIONS

CLIENT PREPARATION
- Obtain and document a baseline of the maternal BP, FHR, fetal movement, and contractions for 10 to 20 min.
- Reinforce the procedure to the client, and assist in obtaining informed consent. Qᴘᴄᴄ

ONGOING CARE
- Monitor and provide adequate rest periods for the client to avoid tachysystole of the uterus.
- Monitor BP frequently during procedure.
- Monitor for contractions during testing period.

INTERVENTIONS
If tachysystole of the uterus or preterm labor occurs, do the following. Qᴇʙᴘ
- Monitor for contractions lasting longer than 90 seconds or occurring more frequently than every 2 min.
- Assist with administering tocolytics as prescribed.
- Maintain bed rest during the procedure.
- Observe the client for 30 min afterward to see that contractions have ceased and preterm labor does not begin.

INTERPRETATION OF FINDINGS

NEGATIVE CST (NORMAL FINDING): Indicated if within a 10-min period, with three uterine contractions, there are no late decelerations of the FHR

POSITIVE CST (ABNORMAL FINDING): Indicated with persistent and consistent late decelerations with 50% or more of the contractions. This is suggestive of uteroplacental insufficiency. Variable deceleration can indicate cord compression, and early decelerations can indicate fetal head compression. Based on these findings, the provider may determine to induce labor or perform a cesarean birth. (5.2)

COMPLICATIONS

Potential for preterm labor

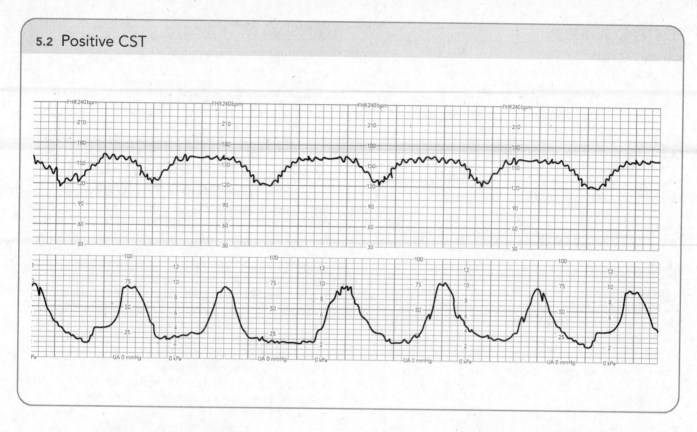

Amniocentesis

The aspiration of amniotic fluid for analysis by insertion of a needle transabdominally into a client's uterus and amniotic sac under direct ultrasound guidance locating the placenta and determining the position of the fetus. It may be performed after 14 weeks of gestation.

Alpha-fetoprotein (AFP) can be measured from the amniotic fluid between 15 and 20 weeks (16 to 18 weeks of gestation is ideal) and can be used to check for neural tube defects in the fetus or chromosomal disorders. Can be evaluated to follow up a high level of AFP in maternal blood

INDICATIONS

POTENTIAL DIAGNOSES

- Previous birth with a chromosomal anomaly
- A parent who is a carrier of a chromosomal anomaly
- A family history of neural tube defects
- Prenatal diagnosis of a genetic disorder or congenital anomaly of the fetus
- AFP level for fetal abnormalities
- Lung maturity evaluation
- Fetal hemolytic disease

CONSIDERATIONS

PREPROCEDURE

NURSING ACTIONS: Reinforce the procedure to the client, and assist in obtaining informed consent.

CLIENT EDUCATION
- If greater than 20 weeks of gestation, empty the bladder prior to the procedure to reduce its size and reduce the risk of inadvertent puncture.
- Prior to 20 weeks of gestation, a full bladder may be needed to support the uterus during the procedure. Qs

INTRAPROCEDURE

NURSING ACTIONS
- Obtain and document baseline vital signs and FHR prior to the procedure.
- Assist client into a supine position. If client is at 20 weeks of gestation or greater, place a wedge under the right hip to displace the uterus off the vena cava. Place a drape over the client, exposing only the abdomen.
- Prepare client for an ultrasound to locate the placenta.
- Cleanse client's abdomen with an antiseptic solution prior to the administration of a local anesthetic by the provider.

CLIENT EDUCATION: There will be a feeling of slight pressure as the needle is inserted. Continue breathing, because holding breath will lower the diaphragm against the uterus and shift the intrauterine contents.

POSTPROCEDURE

NURSING ACTIONS
- Allow the client to rest after the procedure.
- Administer Rho(D) immune globulin to the client if they are Rh-negative (standard practice after an amniocentesis for all clients who are Rh-negative to protect against Rh isoimmunization). Q̲EBP

CLIENT EDUCATION: Report to the provider if experiencing fever, chills, leakage of fluid or bleeding from the insertion site, decreased fetal movement, vaginal bleeding, or uterine contractions after the procedure.

INTERPRETATION OF FINDINGS

Alpha-fetoprotein

HIGH LEVELS: Associated with neural tube defects, such as anencephaly (incomplete development of fetal skull and brain), spina bifida (open spine), or omphalocele (abdominal wall defect). High AFP levels also can be present with normal multifetal pregnancies.

LOW LEVELS: Associated with chromosomal disorders (Down syndrome) or gestational trophoblastic disease (hydatidiform mole)

Fetal lung maturity

Tests for fetal lung maturity can be performed if gestation is less than 37 weeks, in the event of a rupture of membranes, for preterm labor, or for a complication indicating a cesarean birth. Amniotic fluid is tested to determine whether the fetal lungs are mature enough to adapt to extrauterine life or whether the fetus will likely have respiratory distress. Determination is made whether the fetus should be removed immediately or requires more time in utero with the administration of glucocorticoids to promote fetal lung maturity.

LECITHIN/SPHINGOMYELIN (L/S) RATIO: A 2:1 ratio indicates fetal lung maturity (2.5:1 or 3:1 for a client who has diabetes mellitus).

PHOSPHATIDYLGLYCEROL (PG): Absence of PG is associated with respiratory distress.

COMPLICATIONS

- Amniotic fluid emboli
- Maternal or fetal hemorrhage
- Fetomaternal hemorrhage with Rh isoimmunization
- Maternal or fetal infection
- Inadvertent fetal damage or anomalies involving limbs
- Fetal death
- Inadvertent maternal intestinal or bladder damage
- Miscarriage or preterm labor
- Leakage of amniotic fluid

NURSING ACTIONS
- Monitor FHR, uterine contractions, and vaginal discharge for amniotic fluid or bleeding.
- Administer medication as prescribed.
- Offer support and reassurance.

High-risk pregnancy: Percutaneous umbilical blood sampling

Percutaneous umbilical blood sampling, commonly called cordocentesis, is the most common method used for fetal blood sampling and transfusion. This procedure obtains fetal blood from the umbilical cord by passing a fine-gauge, fiber-optic scope (fetoscope) into the amniotic sac using the amniocentesis technique. The needle is advanced into the umbilical cord under ultrasound guidance, and blood is aspirated from the umbilical vein. Blood studies from the cordocentesis can consist of:
- Kleihauer-Betke test that ensures that fetal blood was obtained
- CBC count with differential
- Indirect Coombs' test for Rh antibodies
- Karyotyping (visualization of chromosomes)
- Blood gases

INDICATIONS

- Determining fetal blood type
- Anemia screening

POTENTIAL DIAGNOSES
- Fetal chromosomal disorders
- Karyotyping of malformed fetuses
- Fetal infection
- Altered acid-base balance of fetuses with IUGR

CONSIDERATIONS

NURSING ACTIONS
- Administer medication as prescribed.
- Offer support.
- Monitor the FHR as prescribed following the procedure.

CLIENT EDUCATION: Count fetal movements.

INTERPRETATION OF FINDINGS

- Evaluates for isoimmune fetal hemolytic anemia
- Determines the need for a fetal blood transfusion
- Determines specifics regarding genetic mutations

COMPLICATIONS

- Cord laceration
- Preterm labor
- Hematoma
- Fetomaternal hemorrhage

High-risk pregnancy: Chorionic villus sampling

- Chorionic villus sampling (CVS) is the evaluation of a portion of the developing placenta (chorionic villi), which is aspirated through a thin sterile catheter or syringe inserted through the abdominal wall or intravaginally through the cervix under ultrasound guidance.
- CVS is a first-trimester alternative to amniocentesis with one of its advantages being an earlier diagnosis of any abnormalities. CVS is ideally performed at 10 to 13 weeks of gestation.
- The advantage of an earlier diagnosis should be weighed against the increased risk of fetal anomalies and death.

INDICATIONS

POTENTIAL DIAGNOSES: Risk for giving birth to a neonate who has a genetic chromosomal abnormality

CONSIDERATIONS

NURSING ACTIONS
- Assist in obtaining informed consent.
- Provide ongoing reinforcement and support.

CLIENT EDUCATION: Drink 1 to 2 glasses of fluid prior to the test and avoid urination for several hours prior to testing. A full bladder is necessary for testing.

COMPLICATIONS

- Spontaneous abortion
- Risk for fetal limb loss (greatest risk prior to 9 weeks of gestation)
- Miscarriage
- Chorioamnionitis and rupture of membranes
- Rh sensitization
- Bleeding

High-risk pregnancy: Quad marker screening

A blood test that ascertains information about the likelihood of fetal birth defects. It does not diagnose the actual defect. It can be performed instead of the maternal AFP blood level yielding more reliable findings. Includes testing for:
- **Human chorionic gonadotropin (hCG):** a hormone produced by the placenta
- **Alpha-fetoprotein (AFP):** a protein produced by the fetus
- **Estriol:** a protein produced by the fetus and placenta
- **Inhibin A:** a protein produced by the ovaries and placenta

INDICATIONS

CLIENT PRESENTATION
- Preferred at 15 to 22 weeks gestation
- Risk for giving birth to a neonate who has a genetic chromosomal abnormality

INTERPRETATION OF FINDINGS

- Low levels of AFP can indicate a risk for Down syndrome.
- High levels of AFP can indicate a risk for neural tube defects.
- Levels higher than the expected reference range of hCG and inhibin A indicate a risk for Down syndrome.
- Lower levels than the expected reference range of estriol can indicate a risk for Down syndrome.

High-risk pregnancy: Maternal alpha-fetoprotein (MSAFP)

A screening tool used to detect neural tube defects. Clients who have abnormal findings should be referred for a quad marker screening, genetic counseling, ultrasound, and an amniocentesis.

INDICATIONS

POTENTIAL DIAGNOSES: All pregnant clients, preferably between 16 and 18 weeks of gestation

CONSIDERATIONS

PREPROCEDURE NURSING ACTIONS
- Discuss testing with the client.
- Draw blood sample.
- Offer support and education as needed.

INTERPRETATION OF FINDINGS

- High levels can indicate a neural tube defect or open abdominal defect.
- Low levels can indicate Down syndrome.
- This is only used as a screening tool. Abnormal results should be confirmed with further testing.

Active Learning Scenario

A nurse in a prenatal clinic is assisting with the orientation of a newly licensed nurse about how to perform a nonstress test (NST). What should the nurse include in the teaching about the procedure? Use the ATI Active Learning Template: Diagnostic Procedure to complete this item.

INDICATIONS: Identify three that relate to the status of the fetus.

INTERPRETATION OF FINDINGS: Describe a nonreactive NST.

NURSING INTERVENTIONS: Identify two that are preprocedure and one that is intraprocedure.

Application Exercises

1. A nurse is reviewing findings of a client's biophysical profile (BPP). The nurse should expect which of the following variables to be included in this test? (Select all that apply.)

   A. Fetal weight

   B. Fetal breathing movement

   C. Fetal tone

   D. Fetal position

   E. Amniotic fluid volume

2. A nurse is assisting with the care of a client who is pregnant and undergoing a nonstress test. The client asks why the nurse is using an acoustic vibration device. Which of the following responses should the nurse make?

   A. "It is used to stimulate uterine contractions."

   B. "It will decrease the incidence of uterine contractions."

   C. "It lulls the fetus to sleep."

   D. "It awakens a sleeping fetus."

3. A nurse is assisting with the care of a client who is pregnant and is to undergo a contraction stress test (CST). Which of the following findings are indications for this procedure? (Select all that apply.)

   A. Decreased fetal movement

   B. Intrauterine growth restriction (IUGR)

   C. Postmaturity

   D. Placenta previa

   E. Amniotic fluid emboli

4. A nurse is discussing with a client who is pregnant about the amniocentesis procedure. Which of the following statements should the nurse include?

   A. "You will lay on your right side during the procedure."

   B. "You should not eat anything for 24 hours prior to the procedure."

   C. "You should empty your bladder prior to the procedure."

   D. "The test is done to determine gestational age."

5. A nurse is caring for a client who is in preterm labor and is scheduled to undergo an amniocentesis. The nurse should evaluate which of the following tests to assess fetal lung maturity?

   A. Alpha-fetoprotein (AFP)

   B. Lecithin/sphingomyelin (L/S) ratio

   C. Kleihauer-Betke test

   D. Indirect Coombs' test

Application Exercises Key

1. **B, C, E. CORRECT:** A nurse reviewing findings of a client's biophysical profile should expect the following variables to be included in the test: fetal breathing movements, fetal tone, and amniotic fluid volume. Fetal weight and fetal position are not variables included in the BPP.

   Ⓝ *NCLEX® Connection: Reduction of Risk Potential, Diagnostic Tests*

2. **D. CORRECT:** The nurse should respond to the client's questioning about the reason for using an acoustic vibration device, which includes "It awakes a sleeping fetus." The acoustic vibration device is activated for 3 seconds on the client's abdomen over the fetal head to awaken a sleeping fetus. It does not stimulate the uterus. It has no effect on the uterine muscles.

   Ⓝ *NCLEX® Connection: Reduction of Risk Potential, Diagnostic Tests*

3. **A, B, C. CORRECT:** The nurse should understand that the following conditions during pregnancy are an indication for a contraction stress test (CST): decreased fetal movement, intrauterine growth restriction (IUGR) and postmaturity. A contraction stress test is contraindicated for clients who have a placenta previa. Also, there is no indication for a CST for a client who has an amniotic fluid emboli.

   Ⓝ *NCLEX® Connection: Reduction of Risk Potential, Diagnostic Tests*

4. **C. CORRECT:** A nurse is discussing with a client about an amniocentesis and should instruct the client to empty their bladder to avoid an inadvertent puncture during the procedure. Assisting the client into a supine position is an appropriate position. The client does not need to be NPO for 24 hr prior to the procedure. Amniotic fluid is tested to identify fetal genetic defects. It does not determine gestational age.

   Ⓝ *NCLEX® Connection: Health Promotion and Maintenance, Ante-/Intra-/Postpartum and Newborn Care*

5. **B. CORRECT:** The nurse is reviewing the results for an amniocentesis for a client who is in preterm labor. The nurse should evaluate Lecithin/sphingomyelin to assess for fetal lung maturity. A test of the L/S ratio is done as a part of an amniocentesis to determine fetal lung maturity. An AFP is a test to assess for fetal neural tube defects or chromosome disorders. A Kleihauer-Betke test is used to verify that fetal blood is present during a percutaneous umbilical blood sampling procedure. An indirect Coombs' test detects Rh antibodies in the mother's blood.

   Ⓝ *NCLEX® Connection: Reduction of Risk Potential, Diagnostic Tests*

Active Learning Scenario Key

Using the ATI Active Learning Template: Diagnostic Procedure

INDICATIONS
- Check for intact fetal CNS during the third trimester.
- Decreased fetal movement
- Intrauterine growth restriction
- Postmaturity

INTERPRETATION OF FINDINGS: Nonreactive NST is a test that does not demonstrate at least two qualifying accelerations in a 20-minute window. If this is so, a further data collection (contraction stress test, biophysical profile) is indicated.

NURSING INTERVENTIONS

Preprocedure
- Seat the client in a reclining chair in a semi-Fowler's or left-lateral position.
- Apply conduction gel to the client's abdomen.
- Apply the ultrasound transducer and the tocotransducer.

Intraprocedure: Instruct the client to depress the event marker button each time they feel fetal movement.

Ⓝ *NCLEX® Connection: Reduction of Risk Potential, Diagnostic Tests*

When reviewing the following chapters, keep in mind the relevant topics and tasks of the NCLEX outline.

Health Promotion and Maintenance

ANTE-/INTRA-/POSTPARTUM AND NEWBORN CARE
Assist in performing client non-stress test.

Reinforce client teaching on infant care skills.

DATA COLLECTION TECHNIQUES: Collect data for health history.

HEALTH PROMOTION/DISEASE PREVENTION: Identify clients in need of immunizations.

HIGH-RISK BEHAVIORS: Reinforce client teaching related to client high risk behavior.

LIFESTYLE CHOICES
Recognize client need/desire for contraception.

Reinforce teaching with client on healthy lifestyle choices.

Basic Care and Comfort

NONPHARMACOLOGICAL COMFORT INTERVENTIONS: Provide nonpharmacological measures for pain relief.

Pharmacological Therapies

ADVERSE EFFECTS/CONTRAINDICATIONS/SIDE EFFECTS/ INTERACTIONS
Reinforce client teaching on possible effects of medications.

Monitor client for actual and potential adverse effects of medications.

EXPECTED ACTIONS/OUTCOMES
Identify client expected response to medication.

Evaluate client response to medication.

PHARMACOLOGICAL PAIN MANAGEMENT: Identify client need for pain medication.

Reduction of Risk Potential

DIAGNOSTIC TESTS: Reinforce client teaching about diagnostic tests.

LABORATORY VALUES
Monitor diagnostic or laboratory test results.

Compare client laboratory values to normal laboratory values.

POTENTIAL FOR ALTERATIONS IN BODY SYSTEMS
Identify signs or symptoms of potential prenatal complications.

Perform focused data collection based on client condition.

THERAPEUTIC PROCEDURES: Reinforce client teaching on treatments and procedures.

Physiological Adaptation

ALTERATIONS IN BODY SYSTEMS: Provide care for a client experiencing complications of pregnancy/labor or delivery.

CHAPTER 6

Bleeding During Pregnancy

Vaginal bleeding during pregnancy is always abnormal and must be investigated to determine the cause. It can impair both the outcome of the pregnancy and the mother's life.

Spontaneous abortion

Spontaneous abortion has occurred when a pregnancy ends as the result of natural causes before 20 weeks of gestation (the point of fetal viability) and if a fetus weighs less than 500 g.

Types of abortion are clinically classified according to manifestations and whether the products of conception are partially or completely retained or expulsed. Types of abortions include **threatened**, **inevitable**, **incomplete**, **complete**, and **missed**.

DATA COLLECTION

RISK FACTORS

- Chromosomal abnormalities (account for 25%)
- Maternal illness, such as type 1 diabetes mellitus
- Advanced maternal age
- Premature cervical dilation
- Chronic maternal infections
- Maternal malnutrition
- Trauma or injury
- Anomalies in the fetus or placenta
- Substance use
- Antiphospholipid syndrome

EXPECTED FINDINGS

- Abdominal cramping or pain
- Rupture of membranes
- Dilation of the cervix
- Fever
- Manifestations of hemorrhage (hypotension, tachycardia)

LABORATORY TESTS

Hgb and Hct, if considerable blood loss

Clotting factors monitored for disseminated intravascular coagulopathy (DIC): a complication with retained products of conception

WBC for suspected infection

Serum human chorionic gonadotropin (hCG) levels to confirm pregnancy

DIAGNOSTIC AND THERAPEUTIC PROCEDURES

Ultrasound to determine the presence of a viable or dead fetus, or partial or complete products of conception within the uterine cavity

Examination of the cervix to observe whether it is opened or closed

Dilation and curettage (D&C) to dilate and scrape the uterine walls to remove uterine contents for inevitable and incomplete abortions

Dilation and evacuation (D&E) to dilate and evacuate uterine contents for inevitable and incomplete abortions

Prostaglandins and oxytocin to augment or induce uterine contractions and expulse the products of conception

---

6.1 Causes of bleeding during pregnancy

First trimester

SPONTANEOUS ABORTION: Vaginal bleeding, uterine cramping, and partial or complete expulsion of products of conception

ECTOPIC PREGNANCY: Abrupt unilateral lower-quadrant abdominal pain with or without vaginal bleeding

Second trimester

GESTATIONAL TROPHOBLASTIC DISEASE: Uterine size increasing abnormally fast, abnormally high levels of hCG, nausea and increased emesis, no fetus present on ultrasound, and scant or profuse dark brown or red vaginal bleeding

Third trimester

PLACENTA PREVIA: Painless vaginal bleeding

ABRUPTIO PLACENTAE: Vaginal bleeding, sharp abdominal pain, and tender rigid uterus

VASA PREVIA: Fetal vessels are implanted into the membranes rather than the placenta.

Other causes of bleeding

RECURRENT PREMATURE DILATION OF THE CERVIX: Painless bleeding with cervical dilation leading to fetal expulsion

PRETERM LABOR: Bloody discharge, uterine contractions becoming regular, cervical dilation and effacement

HYDATIDIFORM MOLE: Benign proliferative growth of the placental trophoblast

PATIENT-CENTERED CARE

NURSING CARE

- Perform a pregnancy test.
- Observe color and amount of bleeding (count pads).
- Maintain client on bed rest. Inform client of risk for falls due to sedative medications if prescribed. Qs
- Avoid vaginal exams.
- Assist with an ultrasound.
- Assist with administering medications and blood products as prescribed.
- Determine how much tissue has passed and save passed tissue for examination.
- Assist with termination of pregnancy (D&C, D&E, prostaglandin administration) as indicated.
- Use the lay term "miscarriage" with clients because the medical term "abortion" can be misunderstood.
- Provide client education and emotional support.
- Assist with providing a referral for client and partner to pregnancy loss support groups.

MEDICATIONS

- Analgesics and sedatives
- Prostaglandin, as a vaginal suppository
- Oxytocin
- Broad-spectrum antibiotics, in septic abortion
- $Rh_o(D)$ immune globulin, suppresses immune response of clients who are Rh-negative

CLIENT EDUCATION

- Notify the provider of heavy, bright red vaginal bleeding; elevated temperature; or foul-smelling vaginal discharge.
- A small amount of discharge is normal for 1 to 2 weeks.
- Take prescribed antibiotics.
- Refrain from tub baths, sexual intercourse, or placing anything into the vagina for 2 weeks.
- Discuss grief and loss with the provider before attempting another pregnancy. (6.2)

Ectopic pregnancy

Ectopic pregnancy is the abnormal implantation of a fertilized ovum outside of the uterine cavity usually in the fallopian tube, which can result in a tubal rupture causing a fatal hemorrhage.

Ectopic pregnancy is the second most frequent cause of bleeding in early pregnancy and a leading cause of infertility.

DATA COLLECTION

RISK FACTORS

Any factor that compromises tubal patency (STIs, assisted reproductive technologies, tubal surgery, and contraceptive intrauterine device [IUD])

EXPECTED FINDINGS

- Unilateral stabbing pain and tenderness in the lower-abdominal quadrant
- Menses that is delayed (1 to 2 weeks), lighter than usual, or irregular
- Scant, dark red, or brown vaginal spotting 6 to 8 weeks after last normal menses; red, vaginal bleeding if rupture has occurred
- Referred shoulder pain due to blood in the peritoneal cavity irritating the diaphragm or phrenic nerve after tubal rupture
- Findings of hemorrhage and shock (hypotension, tachycardia, pallor, dizziness) if a large amount of bleeding has occurred

LABORATORY TESTS

Serum levels of progesterone and hCG to help determine whether pregnancy has occurred and whether it is likely to be ectopic

6.2 Spontaneous abortion findings

	CRAMPS	BLEEDING	TISSUE PASSED	CERVICAL OPENING
Threatened	Possible mild cramps	Slight spotting	None	Closed
Inevitable	Mild to severe	Moderate	None	Usually dilated
Incomplete	Severe	Heavy, profuse	Yes	Dilated with tissue in cervical canal or passage of tissue
Complete	Mild	Minimal	Yes	No (cervix closed after tissue passed)
Missed	None	None; spotting	None; prolonged retention of tissue	Closed
Septic	Varies	Varies; malodorous discharge	Varies	Usually dilated
Recurrent	Varies	Varies	Yes	Usually dilated

DIAGNOSTIC AND THERAPEUTIC PROCEDURES

- Transvaginal ultrasound shows an empty uterus.
- Use caution if vaginal and bimanual examination are used.

RAPID TREATMENT

- **Medical management** if rupture has not occurred and tube preservation desired
- **Methotrexate** inhibits cell division and embryo enlargement, dissolving the pregnancy.
- **Salpingostomy** is done to salvage the fallopian tube if not ruptured.
- **Laparoscopic salpingectomy** (removal of the tube) is performed when the tube has ruptured.

PATIENT-CENTERED CARE

NURSING CARE

- Replace fluids and maintain electrolyte balance.
- Provide client education and psychological support.
- Administer medications as prescribed.
- Assist with preparing the client for surgery and postoperative nursing care.
- Provide emotional care and support.
- Assist with providing a referral for client and partner to pregnancy loss support group.
- Obtain serum hCG and progesterone levels, liver and renal function studies, CBC, and type and Rh.

CLIENT EDUCATION

- If taking methotrexate, avoid vitamins containing folic acid to prevent a toxic response to the medication. Qs
- Use protection against sun exposure (photosensitivity).

Gestational trophoblastic disease

Gestational trophoblastic disease (GTD) is the proliferation and degeneration of trophoblastic villi in the placenta that becomes swollen, fluid-filled, and takes on the appearance of grape-like clusters. The embryo fails to develop beyond a primitive state, and these structures are associated with choriocarcinoma, which is a rapidly metastasizing malignancy. Two types of molar growths are identified by chromosomal analysis.

Complete mole

- All genetic material is paternally derived.
- The ovum has no genetic material, or the material is inactive.
- The complete mole contains no fetus, placenta, amniotic membranes, or fluid.
- There is no placenta to receive maternal blood. Hemorrhage into the uterine cavity occurs, and vaginal bleeding results.
- Approximately 20% of complete moles progress toward a choriocarcinoma.

Partial mole

- Genetic material is derived both maternally and paternally.
- A normal ovum is fertilized by two sperm or one sperm in which meiosis or chromosome reduction and division did not occur.
- A partial mole often contains abnormal embryonic or fetal parts, an amniotic sac, and fetal blood, but congenital anomalies are present.
- Approximately 6% of partial moles progress toward a choriocarcinoma.

DATA COLLECTION

RISK FACTORS

- Prior molar pregnancy
- Clients in early teenage years or older than age 40

EXPECTED FINDINGS

Excessive vomiting (hyperemesis gravidarum) due to elevated hCG levels

PHYSICAL FINDINGS

- Rapid uterine growth more than expected for the duration of the pregnancy due to the overproliferation of trophoblastic cells
- Bleeding is often dark brown, resembling prune juice, or bright red that is either scant or profuse and continues for a few days or intermittently for a few weeks and can be accompanied by passage of vesicles.
- Anemia from blood loss
- Clinical findings of preeclampsia that occur prior to 24 weeks of gestation

LABORATORY TESTS

Serum level of hCG is persistently high compared with expected decline after weeks 10 to 12 of pregnancy.

DIAGNOSTIC AND THERAPEUTIC PROCEDURES

- An ultrasound reveals a dense growth with characteristic vesicles but no fetus in utero.
- Suction curettage is done to aspirate and evacuate the mole.
- Post-surgery, Rh-negative clients are given $Rh_o(D)$ immune globulin.
- Following mole evacuation, the client should undergo a baseline pelvic exam and ultrasound scan of the abdomen.
- Serum hCG analysis following molar pregnancy to be done weekly for 3 weeks, then monthly for 6 months up to 1 year to detect GTD.

PATIENT-CENTERED CARE

NURSING CARE

- Measure fundal height.
- Monitor for vaginal bleeding and discharge.
- Monitor for gastrointestinal status and appetite.
- Monitor for manifestations of preeclampsia.
- Administer medications as prescribed.
  - Rho(D) immune globulin to the client who is Rh-negative
  - Chemotherapeutic medications for findings of malignant cells indicating choriocarcinoma
- Advise client to save clots or tissue for evaluation.
- Provide client education and emotional support.

CLIENT EDUCATION

- Consider pregnancy loss support groups referred by the nurse.
- Use reliable contraception as a component of follow-up care. Avoid using an intrauterine device (IUD).
- Follow-up is important due to the increased risk of choriocarcinoma.

Placenta previa

Placenta previa occurs when the placenta abnormally implants in the lower segment of the uterus near or over the cervical os instead of attaching to the fundus. The abnormal implantation results in bleeding during the third trimester of pregnancy as the cervix begins to dilate and efface. (6.3)

Classified into three types dependent on the degree to which the cervical os is covered by the placenta

- **Complete or total:** The cervical os is completely covered by the placental attachment.
- **Incomplete or partial:** The cervical os is only partially covered by the placental attachment.
- **Marginal:** The placenta is attached in the lower uterine segment but does not reach the cervical os.
- **Low-lying:** The exact relationship of the placenta to the internal os has not been determined.

DATA COLLECTION

RISK FACTORS

- Previous placenta previa
- Uterine scarring (previous cesarean birth, curettage, endometritis)
- Maternal age greater than 35 years
- Multifetal gestation
- Multiple gestations
- Smoking

EXPECTED FINDINGS

- Painless, bright red vaginal bleeding during the second or third trimester
- Uterus soft, relaxed, and nontender with normal tone
- Fundal height greater than usually expected for gestational age
- Fetus in a breech, oblique, or transverse position
- Reassuring FHR
- Vital signs within normal limits
- Decreasing urinary output, which can be a better indicator of blood loss

LABORATORY TESTS

- Hgb and Hct for blood loss findings
- CBC
- Blood type and Rh
- Coagulation profile
- Kleihauer-Betke test (used to detect fetal blood in maternal circulation)

DIAGNOSTIC PROCEDURES

- Transabdominal or transvaginal ultrasound for placement of the placenta
- Fetal monitoring for fetal well-being

PATIENT-CENTERED CARE

NURSING CARE

- Monitor for bleeding, leakage, or contractions.
- Obtain fundal height.
- Refrain from performing vaginal exams (can exacerbate bleeding). Qs
- Assist with administering IV fluids, blood products, and medications as prescribed. Corticosteroids, such as betamethasone, promote fetal lung maturation if early delivery is anticipated (cesarean birth).
- Have oxygen equipment available in case of fetal distress.

CLIENT EDUCATION

- Adhere to bed rest.
- Do not insert anything into the vagina because it can worsen bleeding.

Abruptio placentae

Abruptio placentae is the premature separation of the placenta from the uterus, which can be a partial or complete detachment. This separation occurs after 20 weeks of gestation, which is usually in the third trimester. It has significant maternal and fetal morbidity and mortality and is a leading cause of maternal death. (6.4)

Coagulation defect, such as disseminated intravascular coagulopathy (DIC), is often associated with moderate to severe abruption.

DATA COLLECTION

RISK FACTORS

- Maternal hypertension (chronic or gestational)
- Blunt external abdominal trauma (motor-vehicle crash, maternal battering)
- Cocaine use resulting in vasoconstriction
- Previous incidents of abruptio placentae
- Cigarette smoking or other nicotine use
- Premature rupture of membranes
- Multifetal pregnancy

EXPECTED FINDINGS

- Sudden onset of intense localized uterine pain with dark red vaginal bleeding
- Area of uterine tenderness can be localized or diffuse over uterus and boardlike
- Contractions with hypertonicity
- Fetal distress
- Clinical findings of hypovolemic shock

LABORATORY TESTS

- Hgb and Hct decreased
- Coagulation factors decreased
- Clotting defects (disseminated intravascular coagulation)
- Cross and type match for possible blood transfusions
- Kleihauer-Betke test (used to detect fetal blood in maternal circulation)

DIAGNOSTIC PROCEDURES

- Ultrasound for fetal well-being and placental assessment
- Biophysical profile to ascertain fetal well-being

PATIENT-CENTERED CARE

NURSING CARE

- Palpate the uterus for tenderness and tone.
- Assist with monitoring of the fundal height.
- Monitor FHR pattern.
- Immediate birth is the management.
  - Assist with administering IV fluids, blood products, and medications as prescribed.
  - Administer oxygen 8 to 10 L/min via face mask.
  - Monitor maternal vital signs, observing for declining hemodynamic status.
  - Assist with performing continuous fetal monitoring.
  - Monitor urinary output and fluid balance.
- Provide emotional support for the client and family.

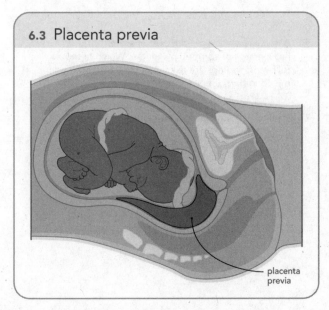

6.3 Placenta previa

placenta previa

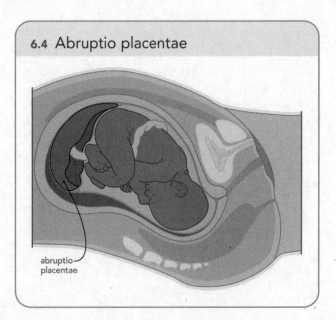

6.4 Abruptio placentae

abruptio placentae

Vasa previa

Vasa previa is a condition when the fetal umbilical vessels implant into the fetal membranes rather than the placenta.

There are variations of vasa previa.
- **Velamentous insertion of the cord:** Cord vessels begin in the branch at the membranes and then course to the placenta.
- **Succenturiate insertion of the cord:** The placenta has divided into two or more lobes and not one mass.
- **Battledore insertion of the cord**
  - A marginal insertion
  - Increased risk of fetal hemorrhage

DATA COLLECTION

DIAGNOSTIC PROCEDURES: Ultrasound for fetal well-being and vessel check

PATIENT-CENTERED CARE

NURSING ACTIONS: Closely monitor the client during labor and delivery for excessive bleeding.

Active Learning Scenario

A nurse is assisting the manager with presenting an educational program on placenta previa for a group of nurses. What should the nurse include in this presentation? Use the ATI Active Learning Template: System Disorder to complete this item.

ALTERATION IN HEALTH (DIAGNOSIS): Describe the three types.

RISK FACTORS: Identify three.

DIAGNOSTIC PROCEDURES: Describe two.

NURSING CARE: Describe a nursing action that is contraindicated.

Application Exercises

1. A nurse in the emergency department is assisting in the care of a client who reports abrupt, sharp, right-sided lower quadrant abdominal pain and bright red vaginal bleeding. The client states, "I missed one menstrual cycle and cannot be pregnant because I have an intrauterine device." The nurse should suspect which of the following?
   A. Missed abortion
   B. Ectopic pregnancy
   C. Severe preeclampsia
   D. Hydatidiform mole

2. A nurse is assisting with the care for a client who is experiencing a ruptured ectopic pregnancy. Which of the following findings is expected with this condition?
   A. No alteration in menses
   B. Transvaginal ultrasound indicating a fetus in the uterus
   C. Blood progesterone greater than the expected reference range
   D. Report of severe shoulder pain

3. A nurse at an antepartum clinic is assisting in the care of a client who is at 4 months of gestation. The client reports continued nausea; vomiting; and scant, prune-colored discharge. The client has experienced no weight loss and has a fundal height larger than expected. Which of the following complications should the nurse suspect?
   A. Hyperemesis gravidarum
   B. Threatened abortion
   C. Hydatidiform mole
   D. Preterm labor

4. A nurse is assisting in the care of a client who is at 32 weeks of gestation and has a placenta previa. The nurse notes that the client is actively bleeding. Which of the following medications should the nurse anticipate that the provider will prescribe?
   A. Betamethasone
   B. Indomethacin
   C. Nifedipine
   D. Methylergonovine

5. A nurse is assisting in the care of a client who has a marginal abruptio placentae. Which of the following findings are risk factors for developing the condition? (Select all that apply.)
   A. Fetal position
   B. Blunt abdominal trauma
   C. Cocaine use
   D. Maternal age
   E. Cigarette smoking

Application Exercises Key

1. B. **CORRECT:** When analyzing cues, the nurse should identify that the client is presenting with manifestations of an ectopic pregnancy, which include unilateral lower quadrant pain with or without bleeding and delayed menses. The use of an intrauterine device (IUD) is also a risk factor associated with this condition. A client who experienced a missed abortion would report brownish discharge and no pain. A client who has severe preeclampsia does not have vaginal bleeding and presents with right upper quadrant epigastric pain. A client who has a hydatidiform mole usually has dark brown vaginal bleeding in the second trimester that is not accompanied by abdominal pain.

   Ⓝ *NCLEX® Connection: Potential for Alterations in Body Systems*

2. D. **CORRECT:** When analyzing cues, the nurse should recognize that a client's report of severe shoulder pain is a finding associated with a ruptured ectopic pregnancy, which is due to the presence of blood in the abdominal cavity that irritates the diaphragm and phrenic nerve. A client experiencing a ruptured ectopic pregnancy has delayed, scant, or irregular menses. A transvaginal ultrasound would indicate an empty uterus in a client who has a ruptured ectopic pregnancy. A blood progesterone level lower than the expected reference range is an indication of ectopic pregnancy.

   Ⓝ *NCLEX® Connection: Potential for Alterations in Body Systems*

3. C. **CORRECT:** When analyzing cues, the nurse should recognize that a client who has a hydatidiform mole exhibits increased fundal height that is inconsistent with the week of gestation and excessive nausea and vomiting due to elevated hCG levels. Scant, dark discharge occurs in the second trimester. A client who is experiencing hyperemesis gravidarum will have weight loss and findings of dehydration. A client who has a threatened abortion would be in the first trimester and report spotting to moderate bleeding with no enlarged uterus. A client who is experiencing preterm labor presents prior to 37 weeks of gestation and is accompanied by pink-stained vaginal discharge and uterine contractions that become more regular.

   Ⓝ *NCLEX® Connection: Potential for Alterations in Body Systems*

4. A. **CORRECT:** When generating solutions, the nurse should anticipate a provider prescription for betamethasone. Betamethasone is a corticosteroid used to promote lung maturity if delivery is anticipated. Indomethacin and nifedipine are indicated for a client who is experiencing preterm labor. Methylergonovine is prescribed for a client who is experiencing postpartum hemorrhage.

   Ⓝ *NCLEX® Connection: Pharmacological Therapies, Expected Actions/Outcomes*

5. B, C, E. **CORRECT:** The nurse should identify the following findings as risk factors for developing an abruptio placentae: blunt abdominal trauma, cocaine use, and cigarette smoking. Fetal position and maternal age are not risk factors for developing an abruptio placentae.

   Ⓝ *NCLEX® Connection: Health Promotion and Maintenance, Health Promotion/Disease Prevention*

Active Learning Scenario Key

Using the ATI Active Learning Template: System Disorder

ALTERATION IN HEALTH (DIAGNOSIS): Types of placenta previa
- Complete or total: Cervical os is covered by the placenta.
- Incomplete or partial: Cervical os is only partially covered by the placenta.
- Marginal: Placenta is attached in the lower uterine segment but does not reach the cervical os.
- Low-lying: The exact relationship of the placenta to the internal os has not been determined.

RISK FACTORS
- Previous placenta previa
- Uterine scarring due to previous cesarean birth, curettage, or endometritis
- Maternal age 35 to 40 years
- Multifetal gestation
- Multiple gestations
- Smoking

DIAGNOSTIC PROCEDURES
- Transabdominal or transvaginal ultrasound
- Fetal monitoring

NURSING CARE: Performing a vaginal exam is contraindicated due to the increased risk of bleeding.

Ⓝ *NCLEX® Connection: Health Promotion and Maintenance, Community Resources*

CHAPTER 7 *Infections*

Maternal infections during pregnancy require prompt identification and treatment by a provider. During pregnancy, the client is at risk for developing infections that can affect the well-being of the fetus. It is important for all clients who are pregnant to get screened routinely during their first prenatal visit and during the third trimester (as needed) for infections. A provider can perform testing during the client's pelvic exam or by obtaining blood, urine, or swab cultures. The initial antepartum screening tests include syphilis, hepatitis, HIV, gonorrhea, and chlamydia. It is recommended that the client have a current Pap smear performed by a provider during pregnancy, which can detect dysplasia and HPV. During the third trimester, the client should receive testing for group B streptococcus (GBS) and retesting (if indicated) for gonorrhea, chlamydia, and HIV. Other infections that could affect pregnancy include COVID-19, TORCH infection, trichomoniasis, BV, HSV, and candidiasis. This chapter will focus on infections as related to clients during pregnancy. Refer to **PN ADULT MEDICAL SURGICAL NURSING CH 57.**

HIV/AIDS

HIV is a retrovirus that attacks and causes destruction of T lymphocytes. It causes immunosuppression in a client. Clients who are severely immunosuppressed develop acquired immunodeficiency syndrome (AIDS). HIV can be transmitted by the birth parent during pregnancy to the fetus through the placenta and postnatally to the newborn/infant through breast milk. The CDC recommends that all clients who are pregnant receive counseling and are offered screening for HIV at their initial prenatal visit and in the third trimester prior to birth (if considered high risk). (Refer to **PN ADULT MEDICAL SURGICAL NURSING CH 78** for more comprehensive information regarding HIV/AIDS.)

Healthy People 2030

Reduce the rate of mother-to-child HIV transmission (increase HIV testing in pregnant clients and those who plan to get pregnant, retest pregnant clients who are in their third trimester if considered high-risk, ensure that clients who have HIV can get treatment, and prevent HIV infections in infancy).

COMPLICATIONS IF UNTREATED

- Preterm birth
- Infants who are low-birth-weight
- Perinatal transmission of HIV to newborn/infant (antepartum, intrapartum, and breastfeeding)

DATA COLLECTION

RISK FACTORS

- IV drug use
- Multiple sexual partners
- History of multiple STIs

EXPECTED FINDINGS

Client may report fatigue, diarrhea, and influenza-like findings.

PHYSICAL EXAMINATION FINDINGS
- Diarrhea and weight loss
- Anemia

LABORATORY/DIAGNOSTIC TESTS

Verify that informed maternal consent is obtained prior to testing. Clients who are pregnant should be informed that HIV testing will be performed as part of a routine prenatal panel; however, clients have the right to refuse. For those who refuse, reinforce with the client the benefits of testing (early detection and management and decreasing harm to fetus). For clients who have no prenatal care, the CDC recommends rapid testing for HIV (blood/urine) prior to delivery.
- Testing begins with an antibody screening test, such as enzyme immunoassay (EIA). Confirmation of positive results is confirmed by Western blot test or immunofluorescence assay.
- Obtain frequent viral load levels and CD4 cell counts throughout pregnancy.

PATIENT-CENTERED CARE

NURSING CARE/CLIENT EDUCATION

ANTEPARTUM: The goals are to keep CD4 cell counts greater than 500 cells/mm³ and to prevent transmission to fetus.
- If the client is HIV positive and taking antiviral medications, they should be informed that they can transmit the infection to the neonate.
- Refer the client if needed for psychosocial support.
- Use standard precautions.
- Discuss HIV and safe sexual relations with the client.

CLIENT EDUCATION: Counseling for nutrition, sleep/rest, exercise, and decreasing stress are recommended for clients who are HIV positive to promote their immune health.
- Instruct the client to take all antiretroviral medications as prescribed.
- Encourage the client to receive immunization against hepatitis B, pneumococcal infection, *Haemophilus influenzae type B*, and viral influenza.
- Encourage use of condoms to minimize exposure if partner is the source of infection.
- Encourage client to receive recommended screenings for other STIs (gonorrhea, chlamydia, syphilis, hepatitis B).
- Review plan for scheduled cesarean birth (prior to onset of labor or ROM) for clients who have a viral load greater than 1,000 copies/mL. (Less than 1,000 copies/mL indicates low risk for transmission.)
- Vaginal birth can be an option for a client who has a viral load of less than 1,000 copies/mL (if membranes have ruptured, labor progresses rapidly, or client refuses cesarean birth).
- Avoid procedures such as amniocentesis due to risk of maternal blood exposure to fetus.
- All states have a reportable diseases list. HIV/AIDS is a commonly reported condition. It is the responsibility of the provider to report cases of these diseases to their local health department.

INTRAPARTUM
- The client may receive IV zidovudine (except those with CD4 less than 1,000 copies and those who received HAART therapy). This should be administered 3 hr prior to scheduled cesarean birth and continued until after the cord is clamped. It is administered intrapartum for vaginal birth and given to the infant for 6 weeks following birth.
- Procedures such as artificial rupture of membranes and episiotomy should be avoided due to the risk of maternal blood exposure.
- Use of internal fetal monitors, fetal scalp electrodes, fetal pH scalp sampling, vacuum extraction, and forceps should be avoided (risk of fetal bleeding). Qs
- Newborn administration of injections and blood testing should not take place until after the first bath is given.

- Wear gloves when caring for the newborn immediately following birth.
- The newborn should be bathed after birth by staff or parents (if rooming-in is desired).
- According to WHO, for a client who has HIV/AIDS, exclusive breastfeeding may not put the infant at risk for HIV, but inconsistent breastfeeding increases the risk for transmitting HIV. Therefore, to decrease the risk of transmission to the newborn/infant, breastfeeding is not recommended for clients who have HIV/AIDS in the U.S.

POSTPARTUM
- Refer birth parent and newborn to a specialist for management of HIV.
- Client should avoid breastfeeding.

THERAPEUTIC MANAGEMENT

Medications

Medication decreases the risk of transmission to the child.

Antiretroviral therapy (ART)
- ART is administered orally and continued throughout pregnancy.
- ART is triple antiretroviral medication therapy that is administered PO (zidovudine [halts maternal/fetal transmission], ritonavir, or indinavir in conjunction with NRTI).
- All HIV-positive clients should be treated with a combination of ART during pregnancy regardless of their CD4 counts and prior to onset of labor or cesarean birth.
- ART can cause bone marrow suppression. Monitor hemoglobin/platelet count and WBCs during pregnancy.

Highly active antiretroviral therapy (HAART)
- INTRAPARTUM: IV zidovudine 3 hr prior to scheduled cesarean section until birth.
- NURSING ACTIONS: Administer zidovudine to the newborn at birth and for 6 weeks following birth.

Chlamydia

Chlamydia is a bacterial infection caused by *Chlamydia trachomatis* and is the most commonly reported STI in American women. The infection can be difficult to diagnose because the client rarely has manifestations. The CDC recommends that all clients who are pregnant receive screening/testing for chlamydia at the first prenatal visit and rescreening in the third trimester (if less than 25 years of age and/or at high risk).

COMPLICATIONS (IF NOT TREATED DURING PREGNANCY)

- Pelvic inflammatory disease (PID)
- Premature rupture of membranes
- Preterm labor
- Postpartum endometritis
- If transmitted to the neonate, it can cause conjunctivitis, ophthalmia neonatorum and pneumonia.

DATA COLLECTION

RISK FACTORS

- Multiple sexual partners
- Unprotected sex

EXPECTED FINDINGS

The client is generally asymptomatic; however, if symptoms are present, the client may report:
- Dysuria
- Urinary frequency
- Spotting or postcoital bleeding
- Vulvar itching
- Gray-white discharge

PHYSICAL EXAMINATION FINDINGS
- Mucopurulent endocervical discharge
- Easily induced endocervical bleeding

LABORATORY TESTS

- Endocervical swab culture of cervical discharge
- Urine culture specimen as alternative

PATIENT-CENTERED CARE

NURSING ACTIONS/CLIENT EDUCATION

- Instruct the client to take the entire prescription as prescribed.
- Identify and treat all exposed sexual partners.
- Clients who are pregnant should be retested within 3-4 weeks after completing the prescribed regimen (test of cure).
- If continued sexual activity is desired, the client should be aware of the sexually transmitted infection status of any sexual partners and use a barrier contraceptive each time they have sex.
- All states have a reportable diseases list. Chlamydia is a commonly reported condition. It is the responsibility of the provider to report cases of these diseases to the local health department.

THERAPEUTIC MANAGEMENT

Medications

Antibiotics: Safe during pregnancy and breastfeeding
- Azithromycin PO single dose (recommended)
- Amoxicillin PO for up to 7 days (alternative)
- Contraindicated during pregnancy: Doxycycline and levofloxacin
- Erythromycin (ointment): Administered to all newborns following birth. This is the medication of choice for ophthalmia neonatorum. This antibiotic is bacteriostatic and bactericidal and thus provides prophylaxis against *Neisseria gonorrhoeae* and *Chlamydia trachomatis*.

Gonorrhea

Neisseria gonorrhoeae is the causative agent of gonorrhea. Gonorrhea is a bacterial infection that is primarily spread by genital-to-genital contact. However, it also can be spread by anal-to-genital or oral-to-genital contact. It can also be transmitted to a newborn during birth. The CDC recommends that all clients who are pregnant receive screening/testing for gonorrhea at the first prenatal visit and rescreening in the third trimester (if less than 25 years of age and/or at high risk).

COMPLICATIONS (IF NOT TREATED DURING PREGNANCY)

- PID
- Salpingitis
- Premature rupture of membranes (PROM)
- Preterm birth
- Chorioamnionitis
- Postpartum sepsis, endometritis
- If transmitted to the neonate, it can cause neonatal sepsis, intrauterine growth restriction (IUGR), and/or ophthalmia neonatorum (which can cause blindness).

DATA COLLECTION

RISK FACTORS

- Multiple sexual partners
- Unprotected sexual practices
- Age less than 25, if sexually active

EXPECTED FINDINGS

Clients often are asymptomatic but can report:
- Dysuria
- Pain in lower abdomen or pelvic area
- Purulent discharge

PHYSICAL EXAMINATION FINDINGS
- Yellowish-green vaginal discharge
- Easily induced endocervical bleeding

LABORATORY TESTS

- Endocervical culture (preferred)
- Urine cultures
- Anal or oral cultures

PATIENT-CENTERED CARE

NURSING ACTIONS/CLIENT EDUCATION

- Provide client education regarding disease transmission.
- Identify and treat all sexual partners.
- The newborn will receive ophthalmic erythromycin following birth. This is the medication of choice for ophthalmia neonatorum. This antibiotic is both bacteriostatic and bactericidal and thus provides prophylaxis against *Neisseria gonorrhoeae* and *Chlamydia trachomatis*.
- Take all medications as prescribed.
- Clients who are pregnant should be retested for gonorrhea within 3 to 4 weeks to determine medication effectiveness (test of cure).
- Adhere to safe sex practices (mutual monogamy; correct, consistent condom use).
- All states have a reportable diseases list. Gonorrhea is a commonly reported condition. It is the responsibility of the provider to report cases of these diseases to the local health department.

THERAPEUTIC MANAGEMENT

Medications

For those who test positive for gonorrhea, the CDC recommends treatment for chlamydia, as well.

Antibiotics

Safe during pregnancy and breastfeeding
- Ceftriaxone IM
- Azithromycin PO single dose (if chlamydia not excluded)
- Erythromycin (ointment): Administered to all newborns following birth. This is the medication of choice for ophthalmia.

Syphilis

Syphilis is an STI caused by the spirochete *Treponema pallidum*. It can have long-term complications if not adequately treated. Syphilis has three stages. It can be transmitted through oral, vaginal, or anal sex, as well as transmitted to an unborn child. Though the rate of congenital syphilis has recently decreased, more cases of congenital syphilis are reported in the U.S. than cases of perinatal HIV infection. The CDC recommends that all clients who are pregnant receive screening/testing for syphilis at the first prenatal visit and rescreening in the third trimester if at high risk (live in areas with high numbers of syphilis cases, were not previously tested, or had a positive test in the first trimester).

Healthy People 2030
- Reduce congenital syphilis.
- Reduce the rate of syphilis.

COMPLICATIONS (IF NOT TREATED DURING PREGNANCY)

- Brain and eye conditions
- Increased risk for developing HIV
- Long-term systemic conditions
- Death
- Transmission to fetus, causing high risk for physical disabilities and death

DATA COLLECTION

RISK FACTORS

- Multiple partners
- Unprotected sexual practices

EXPECTED FINDINGS (RELATED TO STAGE)

Primary stage: The client can notice a chancre, which is a painless papular lesion at the site of infection. Chancres can progress to an ulcerated area. Female report of inguinal lymph node edema can indicate internal lesions (vaginal or cervical).

Secondary stage
- The client can notice skin rashes, such as a reddish-brown maculopapular rash on the palmar surface of the hands and the soles of the feet.
- **Latent phase:** The client does not have any expected findings of syphilis present.

Tertiary stage: Damage to internal organs can occur, for which clients can notice manifestations, including blindness and difficulty coordinating muscle movements.

PHYSICAL EXAMINATION FINDINGS
- **Primary stage:** Provider can observe a chancre in the genital area.
- **Secondary stage:** Provider can observe skin rashes, such as rough, red or reddish-brown spots on the palms of the hands and soles of the feet, and lymphadenopathy.

LABORATORY TESTS

Blood tests: Nontreponemal (VDRL and rapid plasma reagin) and treponemal (enzyme immunoassay, immunoassays)
- Nontreponemal tests are often used for screening, followed by treponemal tests for detecting antibodies specific for syphilis to confirm the diagnosis.
- This sequence of nontreponemal tests followed by treponemal tests is considered the standard for testing.

Microscopic: Dark-field examination of the primary lesion

PATIENT-CENTERED CARE

NURSING ACTIONS/CLIENT EDUCATION

- Abstain from sexual contact until sores have completely healed.
- Partners need to be tested and treated.
- Encourage client to obtain screening/testing for coinfections (chlamydia, gonorrhea, HIV).
- Adhere to safe sex practices.
- All states have a reportable diseases list. Syphilis is a commonly reported condition. It is the responsibility of the provider to report cases of these diseases to the local health department.

THERAPEUTIC MANAGEMENT

Medications

- Benzathine penicillin G IM in a single dose. If the duration of the syphilis is unknown, three doses are recommended. This is safe during pregnancy and breastfeeding.
- If the client has an allergy to penicillin, the CDC recommends desensitization and treatment with penicillin G.
- Contraindicated during pregnancy: Doxycycline or tetracycline orally

Hepatitis

Hepatitis B (HBV) is a virus that is transmitted by contact via blood or sexual intercourse. It can also be transmitted to a fetus during pregnancy. The CDC recommends that all clients who are pregnant receive screening for hepatitis B surface antigen as part of their initial screening tests. (Refer to **PN ADULT MEDICAL SURGICAL NURSING CHAPTER 50** for comprehensive information regarding hepatitis and cirrhosis.)

COMPLICATIONS (IF NOT TREATED DURING PREGNANCY)

Transmission to fetus, causing high risk for physical disabilities and death

DATA COLLECTION

RISK FACTORS

- Multiple sex partners
- Unprotected sexual practices
- Employment in health care (potential for needlesticks)
- Injectable substance abuse
- Recipient of multiple blood transfusions

EXPECTED FINDINGS

The client may report flu-like findings of tiredness, malaise, abdominal discomfort, and anorexia.

LABORATORY TESTS

Blood tests: HBsAg: detects antibodies

PATIENT-CENTERED CARE

NURSING ACTIONS/CLIENT EDUCATION

- Avoid medications that can affect the liver and cause problems.
- Encourage the client to eat a well-balanced diet (high protein, low fat) and drink plenty of fluids (if not contraindicated).
- Explain the condition to the client.
- Inform the client that household members and sexual partners will need immunoprophylaxis.
- Provide education about personal hygiene to prevent exposure (handwashing, no sharing of personal items [razors, toothbrushes]).
- Encourage safe sex practices (consistent and correct condom use).

THERAPEUTIC MANAGEMENT

Nonspecific treatment

Medications

Hepatitis B immune globin (HBV vaccine series with 14 days of recent contact)

Group B streptococcus (GBS)

GBS infection is a bacterial infection that can be passed to a fetus during labor and delivery. GBS is often an expected part of the vaginal flora for nonpregnant clients and present in some who are pregnant.

COMPLICATIONS

- Preterm labor and birth
- Chorioamnionitis
- Infections of the urinary tract
- Maternal sepsis
- Endometritis after birth
- If transmitted to the neonate: pneumonia, respiratory distress syndrome, sepsis, and meningitis

DATA COLLECTION

RISK FACTORS

Maternal

History of positive culture with previous pregnancy

Early-onset neonatal GBS

- Positive GBS culture in current pregnancy
- Prolonged (18 hr or more) rupture of membranes
- Preterm birth
- Low birth weight
- Use of intrauterine fetal monitoring
- Intrapartum maternal fever (38° C [100.4° F] or greater)

LABORATORY DIAGNOSTIC TESTS

Vaginal and rectal cultures are performed at 36 0/7 and up to 37 6/7 weeks of gestation.

PATIENT-CENTERED CARE

NURSING CARE/CLIENT EDUCATION

- Administer intrapartum antibiotic prophylaxis to the following clients to decrease transmission to the neonate.
  - Client who has a GBS-positive screening during current pregnancy
  - Client who has unknown GBS status and is delivering at less than 37 weeks of gestation
  - Client who has maternal fever of 38° C (100.4° F) or greater
  - Client who has rupture of membranes for 18 hr or longer
  - Contraindicated for scheduled cesarean birth or when ROM has not occurred
- Notify labor and delivery nurse of GBS status.
- Educate client about the condition and its management.

THERAPEUTIC MANAGEMENT

Medications

Penicillin G or ampicillin is most often prescribed for GBS.

INTRAPARTUM: Administer penicillin G, initially as IV loading dose (bolus) followed by intermittent IV bolus every 4 hr or administer ampicillin, initially as IV loading dose (bolus) followed by intermittent IV bolus every 4 hr.

Human papilloma virus (HPV)

HPV is the most common STI. There are several strains of the virus. HPV strains 6 and 11 can cause genital warts (Condyloma acuminata). Other strains can affect the cervix and cause dysplasia or cancer. HPV can spread through oral, vaginal, and anal sex (most commonly vaginal or anal routes). During pregnancy, the lesions can expand and cause complications of pregnancy. The CDC recommends that all clients who are pregnant receive a Pap smear to assist with early detection. HPV vaccines are not recommended during pregnancy.

COMPLICATIONS

- Obstruction of birth canal (interfering with fetal descent), which may necessitate cesarean birth (dystocia)
- Cervical cancer

DATA COLLECTION

RISK FACTORS

- Multiple partners
- Unprotected sexual practices

EXPECTED FINDINGS

The client reports lesions/bumps in the genital area that might not itch or hurt, vaginal discharge, dyspareunia, and bleeding after intercourse.

PHYSICAL EXAMINATION FINDINGS

- Small warts or a group of warts in the genital area that can have a cauliflower-like appearance
- Abnormal changes to the cervix that can be detected by a Pap test

LABORATORY/DIAGNOSTIC TESTS OR PROCEDURES

- Pap test with or without HPV co-testing per American Cancer Society and American College of Obstetricians and Gynecologists guidelines
- Genital warts are diagnosed by the provider based on appearance during physical examination.

PATIENT-CENTERED CARE

NURSING ACTIONS/CLIENT EDUCATION

- Therapy may require multiple office visits.
- Consider abstinence or safe sex practices (mutual monogamy; correct, consistent condom use).
- If therapy is deferred until after birth, remember that the lesions are infectious.
- Prepare the client for cesarean birth (depends on the extent of lesions).
- Lesion care: Use oatmeal baths, keep lesions clean and dry, and wear loose-fitting clothing.

THERAPEUTIC MANAGEMENT

Medications

For genital warts and *Condyloma acuminata*:
- Trichloroacetic acid (TCA) or bichloroacetic acid (BCA), which is safe for use during pregnancy and while breastfeeding
- Contraindicated during pregnancy: Podophyllin, podofilox, sinecatechins, imiquimod

Therapeutic procedures

- Cryotherapy (cold therapy that freezes unexpected tissue) is recommended during pregnancy (performed by a provider).
- For a client who has unexpected findings that require further evaluation on their Pap smear, the provider may opt to treat and manage following birth.

Other Infections During Pregnancy

Trichomoniasis

Trichomoniasis is an STI caused by the protozoan parasite *Trichomonas vaginalis*. It is considered the most prevalent nonviral STI. It can be spread penis-to-vagina or vagina-to-vagina. The CDC recommends that all clients with clinical findings of trichomoniasis receive testing.

COMPLICATIONS (IF NOT TREATED DURING PREGNANCY)

- Preterm birth
- PROM
- Increased risk for contracting HIV from a partner who is infected
- PID
- Small for gestational age (neonate)

DATA COLLECTION

EXPECTED FINDINGS

- Yellow-green, frothy vaginal discharge with foul odor
- Dyspareunia and vaginal itching
- Dysuria

PHYSICAL EXAMINATION FINDINGS
- Discharge in the vaginal vault during speculum examination, which can be sampled for microscopy
- Strawberry spots on the cervix (tiny petechiae)
- A cervix that bleeds easily

LABORATORY/DIAGNOSTIC TESTS

- Wet mount saline prep microscopically detects the presence of protozoa-trichomonad(s) and WBCs.
- Cultures, urine specimens (POC, molecular testing, NAAT, rapid tests)
- Pap smear can incidentally detect the presence of trichomonads.

PATIENT-CENTERED CARE

NURSING ACTIONS/CLIENT EDUCATION

- Avoid alcohol while taking this medication and for 3 days after treatment due to the disulfiram-like reaction that occurs (severe nausea, vomiting).
- Take all medication as prescribed.
- Understand the possibility of decreasing effectiveness of oral contraceptives.
- Inform all sexual partners.
- Refrain from sexual intercourse until partner is treated.
- Encourage retesting within 3 months.
- Educate the client regarding safe sex practices (consistent and correct use of condoms, monogamous relationship).

THERAPEUTIC MANAGEMENT

Medications

Metronidazole PO (Although it can cross the placenta and it enters the breast milk, the CDC recommends that it is safe to use during pregnancy and breastfeeding [defer breastfeeding until 12-24 hr after receiving treatment].)

Bacterial vaginosis (BV)

BV management is recommended for all clients who are pregnant and symptomatic. According to the CDC, routine screening is not recommended for asymptomatic clients who are pregnant.

COMPLICATIONS (IF NOT TREATED DURING PREGNANCY)

- Postpartum endometritis
- Increased risk for contracting other STIs (gonorrhea, chlamydia, HIV, trichomoniasis)
- PROM (premature rupture of membranes)
- Preterm birth
- Infections related to amniotic fluid

DATA COLLECTION

EXPECTED FINDINGS

Client may report vaginal pruritus, milky (gray, white) discharge, and fishy odor.

LABORATORY/DIAGNOSTIC TESTS

- Whiff test positive for fishy odor (vaginal secretions with KOH prep)
- Microscopic: Wet mount normal saline positive if clue cells (gram negative rods that stick to epithelial cells) are noted

PATIENT-CENTERED CARE

NURSING ACTIONS/CLIENT EDUCATION

- Avoid alcohol while taking metronidazole due to a disulfiram–like reaction (severe nausea and vomiting).
- Take all medications as prescribed.
- Treatment is not usually indicated for sexual partners.
- Refrain from sexual intercourse, or use condoms consistently and correctly while receiving treatment.
- Adhere to safe sex practices.

THERAPEUTIC MANAGEMENT

Medications

- Metronidazole PO (safe during pregnancy)
- Clindamycin PO (safe during pregnancy and while breastfeeding)
- Contraindicated during pregnancy and while breastfeeding: tinidazole, secnidazole, and intravaginal metronidazole/clindamycin

7.1 Case study

Scenario introduction

A nurse in a local obstetric office has received notification that several clients have positive syphilis screening. The facility is located in a rural community. Four cases of the disease were reported within the facility (population: 60). The nurse has previously discussed the use of condoms to prevent the transmission of sexually transmitted infections (STIs) with the clients, but most of the community's clients are not using condoms for sexual relations.

Scene 1

A nurse in a local obstetric office in the rural community is discussing their concerns with a provider at the facility.

Nurse manager: "Are we using universal precautions when caring for the clients?"

Nurse: "Yes, staff are using universal precautions when caring for clients who have tested positive for syphilis. I would like to recommend that everyone receives education about universal precautions and additional education about caring for clients who have positive test results. All pregnant clients should be screened at the first prenatal visit and rescreened in the third trimester if at high risk (live in areas with high numbers of syphilis cases, were not previously tested, or had positive test in the first trimester)."

Nurse manager: "After speaking with the local health department regarding a high number of syphilis cases within the community, a big concern is that the clients who test positive should be treated immediately and require rescreening in the third trimester. Also, all sexual partners within the past 3 months should be screened for syphilis and other STIs. Only a few can afford to own cars, so most use public transportation to commute between home and job locations."

Scene 2

Several weeks later, the incidence rate in the rural community is 9%, and the incidence in the city is 4%. The nurse and the nurse manager are discussing difficulties with contact tracing in the rural community.

Nurse manager: "What kinds of barriers are you encountering that are making it difficult for us to conduct contact tracing?"

Nurse: "Most clients in the community live at or below the poverty line and do not have internet access. They are not seeing information posted online regarding contact tracing. Also, many do not have phones. About 30% of the population speak English as a second language. Some clients have discussed concerns about confidentiality because it is a small town. Some clients are encouraging others to avoid participating in contact tracing. Additionally, most clients do not have health insurance."

Scenario conclusion

The nurse continues to plan additional actions they can take to support their communities. What are some other interventions related to SDOH that could be helpful in engaging clients during this time?

Case study exercises:

1. What economic factors are social determinants of health for the client that increase the risk for spread of this communicable disease?

2. List some social determinants of health in this community that increase the risk of disease transmission.

3. Name some community partnerships related to SDOH that the community health nurses can explore when assisting clients with obtaining basic supplies.

Candidiasis

Candidiasis, also known as *Vulvovaginal candidiasis* (VVC) or yeast infection, is a fungal infection most often caused by *Candida albicans*, but non-*Candida albicans* infections are possible.

- It is the second most common type of vaginal infection in the U.S.
- All clients who have manifestations should be tested.
- During pregnancy, candidiasis is treated to relieve discomfort and prevent oral thrush in the neonate.

DATA COLLECTION

RISK FACTORS

- Pregnancy
- Diabetes mellitus
- Oral contraceptives
- Recent antibiotic treatment
- Obesity
- Diet high in refined sugars

EXPECTED FINDINGS

Client may report vulvar and vaginal pruritus and/or painful urination due to the excoriation from itching.

PHYSICAL EXAMINATION FINDINGS

- Speculum examination: Thick, creamy, white, cottage cheese–like vaginal discharge
- Vulvar and vaginal erythema and inflammation
- White patches on vaginal walls

LABORATORY/DIAGNOSTIC TESTS

- Sample of discharge used for application to pH paper
- Saline and potassium chloride (KOH) wet mount smear
- pH less than 4.5 (normal pH)
- Wet mount potassium hydroxide prep, which indicates presence of yeast buds, hyphae, pseudohyphae

PATIENT-CENTERED CARE

NURSING ACTIONS/CLIENT EDUCATION

- Avoid tight-fitting clothing, and wear cotton-lined underpants.
- Remove damp clothing as soon as possible.
- Avoid douching.
- Increase dietary intake of yogurt with active cultures.
- If infections are recurrent or frequent, diabetes should be ruled out.

THERAPEUTIC MANAGEMENT

Medications

Topical therapies recommended for use in pregnant clients
- Fluconazole
- Over-the-counter (OTC) treatments, such as clotrimazole, are available to treat candidiasis and are used for 3 to 7 days. However, it is important for the provider to diagnose candidiasis initially.
- Contraindicated during pregnancy: Oral antifungals

COVID-19

COVID-19 is a SARS virus that is caused by a new strain of coronavirus. The CDC and ACOG encourage all clients who are pregnant to get the COVID-19 vaccine. This will prevent the occurrence of the condition. Since COVID-19 is a new condition, research is currently being conducted to provide more information about the condition and its management. Refer to the CDC website to find the latest information about COVID-19 (https://www.cdc.gov/coronavirus/2019-ncov/your-health/about-covid-19.html).

COMPLICATIONS

- Increased risk of maternal and fetal mortality and morbidity (preterm birth, stillbirth)
- Maternal respiratory or cardiovascular conditions, which may necessitate ventilator support or ICU admission
- Hypertension, heavy postpartum bleeding, coagulopathies

DATA COLLECTION

RISK FACTORS

Preexisting condition (obesity, gestational diabetes)

EXPECTED FINDINGS

Client may report cough, shortness of breath, fatigue, sore throat, loss of taste/smell, and congestion.

LABORATORY/DIAGNOSTIC TESTS

- Rapid: Nasal swab specimen (can be performed anywhere [offices, pharmacies] or performed by the client)
- Laboratory: Nasal swab specimens, blood tests
  - Viral tests (antigen, nucleic acid amplification tests [NAATs])
  - PCRs

PATIENT-CENTERED CARE

THERAPEUTIC MANAGEMENT

Refer to the CDC website for more current information.

TORCH infections

TORCH infections are multiple conditions that can affect a client who is pregnant and the fetus in utero. These infections include toxoplasmosis, other infections (e.g., hepatitis), rubella virus, cytomegalovirus, and herpes simplex virus (HSV). These infections can cross the placenta and have teratogenic effects on the fetus. TORCH does not include all the major infections that present risks to the mother and fetus. Screenings for TORCH infections would be as indicated, depending on the client symptoms. There is a TORCH screen immunologic survey used to identify existence of these infections in the mother (to identify fetal risks) or the newborn (detection of antibodies against infections). Refer to the table below for more information. (7.2)

ASSESSMENT

RISK FACTORS

- Toxoplasmosis is caused by a protozoa.
- Toxoplasmosis is caused by consumption of raw or undercooked meat or handling cat feces.
- Other infections can include hepatitis A and B, syphilis, mumps, parvovirus B19, and varicella-zoster. These are some of the most common and can be associated with congenital anomalies.
- Rubella (German measles) is contracted through children who have rashes or neonates who are born to clients who had rubella during pregnancy.
- Cytomegalovirus (member of herpes virus family) is transmitted by droplet infection from person to person, through semen, cervical and vaginal secretions, breast milk, placental tissue, urine, feces, and blood. A latent virus can be reactivated and cause disease to the fetus in utero or during passage through the birth canal.
- HSV is spread by direct contact with oral or genital lesions. Transmission to the fetus is greatest during vaginal birth if the client has active lesions. The CDC recommends initiating suppressive therapy at 36 weeks of gestation to reduce frequency of cesarean delivery.

EXPECTED FINDINGS

Toxoplasmosis
- Often asymptomatic
- Manifestations are similar to influenza or lymphadenopathy, (malaise, muscle aches, and flu-like manifestations

Rubella: Joint and muscle pain, rash, and fever

Cytomegalovirus: manifestations or mononucleosis-like manifestations

HSV
- Client may report multiple painful blisters on genital area, itching, fever, malaise, and tender lymph nodes
- Lesions that appear as vesicles then pustules, and ulcerate and form crusts

LABORATORY AND DIAGNOSTIC TESTS

HSV: Obtain cultures from lesions

PATIENT-CENTERED CARE

CLIENT EDUCATION

- Discuss safe sexual relations with client.
- Provide client with emotional support.

Toxoplasmosis
- Client may experience immunity after first incident.
- Adhere to prevention practices, including correct hand hygiene and cooking meat properly. Avoid contact with contaminated cat litter.

Rubella: For rubella, immunization of clients who are pregnant is contraindicated because rubella infection can develop. These clients should avoid crowds and young children. Clients who have low titers prior to pregnancy should receive immunizations.

Cytomegalovirus
- Reinforce with client about condition
- Encourage client to use proper handwashing to prevent exposure by frequent hand hygiene before eating, and after handling newborn diapers and toys.

HSV
- A cesarean birth is recommended for all clients in labor who have active genital herpes lesions or early findings of impending outbreak (vulvar pain, itching.)
- Refrain from sexual intercourse during 3rd trimester with partners known or suspected of having HSV
- Routine screening for HSV is not recommended
- Prior to birth, ask client about history of HSV

MEDICATIONS

Toxoplasmosis: Treatment of toxoplasmosis includes sulfonamides or a combination of pyrimethamine and sulfadiazine (potentially harmful to the fetus, but parasitic treatment is essential).

Rubella: Rubella vaccination is received postpartum because of fetus in utero. Clients should avoid pregnancy for at least 1 month after receiving the vaccine.

HSV
- Acyclovir PO (IV if severe)
- Valacyclovir PO

Application Exercises

1. A nurse is assisting with the care for a client who is in labor and has HIV. Which of the following therapeutic interventions should the nurse identify as contraindicated for this client? (Select all that apply.)

   A. Vacuum extractor

   B. Oxytocin infusion

   C. Forceps

   D. Cesarean birth

   E. Internal fetal monitoring

2. A nurse is assisting with the care for a client who is at 32 weeks of gestation and tested positive for gonorrhea and chlamydia. Which of the following medications should the nurse anticipate that the provider will prescribe? (Select all that apply.)

   A. Azithromycin

   B. Metronidazole

   C. Zidovudine

   D. Doxycycline

   E. Ceftriaxone

3. A nurse is assisting with providing care for a client who is pregnant and has *Condyloma acuminata*. Which of the following therapeutic procedures should the nurse anticipate the provider performing?

   A. Cauterization

   B. Cryotherapy

   C. Cervical ablation

   D. Darkfield microscopy

4. A nurse is discussing maternal conditions and the appropriate medications to administer with a newly licensed nurse. Match the maternal conditions below with the anticipated prescribed medications.

A. Group B streptococcus	1. Acyclovir
B. Candidiasis	2. Antiretroviral therapy (ART)
C. Trichomoniasis	3. Azithromycin
D. Chlamydia	4. Metronidazole
E. HIV	5. Clotrimazole
F. Genital herpes	6. Penicillin G

5. A nurse in an antepartum clinic is collecting data from a client who has a TORCH infection. Which of the following findings should the nurse expect? (Select all that apply.)

   A. Joint pain

   B. Malaise

   C. Rash

   D. Urinary frequency

   E. Tender lymph nodes

Active Learning Scenario

A nurse is contributing to the plan of care for a client who is pregnant and positive for group B streptococcus beta-hemolytic. Use the ATI Active Learning Template: System Disorder to complete this item.

LABORATORY TESTS: Describe the test and when it is performed.

RISK FACTORS: Describe two maternal risk factors and three fetal risk factors.

MEDICATIONS: Describe three clients who should receive intrapartum antibiotic prophylaxis.

Active Learning Scenario Key

Using the ATI Active Learning Template: System Disorder

LABORATORY TESTS: Vaginal and rectal cultures are performed beginning at 36 0/7 and up to 37 6/7 weeks of gestation to detect for the presence of group B streptococcus prior to labor.

RISK FACTORS

Maternal: Maternal age less than 20 years

Fetal
- Positive GBS culture in current pregnancy
- Prolonged (18 hr or more) rupture of membranes
- Preterm delivery
- Low birth weight
- Use of intrauterine fetal monitoring
- Intrapartum maternal fever (38° C [100.4° F] or greater)

Medications
- Clients to be considered for antibiotic prophylaxis
- Client who has GBS bacteriuria during current pregnancy
- Client who has a GBS-positive screen during current pregnancy
- Client who has unknown GBS status who is delivering at less than 37 weeks of gestation
- Client who has maternal fever of 38° C (100.4° F)
- Client who has rupture of membranes for 18 hr or longer

Ⓝ *NCLEX® Connection: Reduction of Risk Potential, Potential for Complications from Surgical Procedures and Health Alterations*

Case Study Exercises Key

1. When analyzing cues, the nurse should recognize that inability to afford condoms for sexual relations and the need to use public transportation are economic factors that increase the risk for spreading a communicable disease.

2. When analyzing cues, the nurse recognizes that factors related to economic stability, including poverty level, lack of health insurance, and living in a rural area, lead to less health-seeking behaviors and increase the risk of disease transmission. The nurse recognizes that factors related to health care access and quality, including language barriers, increase the risk of disease transmission. The nurse recognizes that factors related to social and cultural context, including concerns about confidentiality and avoidance of contact tracing, increase the risk of disease transmission.

3. When generating solutions, the nurse recognizes that possible community partnerships include assisting clients with obtaining public transportation and asking for volunteers within the community who can assist residents who are unable to obtain prescriptions.

Application Exercises Key

1. **A, C, E. CORRECT:** The use of a vacuum extractor should be avoided for a client who is HIV positive due to risk of exposing the fetus to maternal blood. The use of forceps during birth should be avoided due to the risk of fetal bleeding. Internal fetal monitoring should be avoided due to the risk of fetal bleeding. Oxytocin infusion is not contraindicated for this client. Cesarean birth is not contraindicated for this client.

Ⓝ *NCLEX® Connection: Health Promotion and Maintenance, Ante-/Intra-/Postpartum and Newborn Care*

2. **A, E. CORRECT:** When analyzing cues, the nurse should anticipate a provider prescription for azithromycin and ceftriaxone, which are medications that are safe to administer during pregnancy to manage gonorrhea and chlamydia. Ceftriaxone would manage gonorrhea and azithromycin would manage chlamydia. Doxycycline is used to manage chlamydia infections; however, it contraindicated to administer to a client who is pregnant. Metronidazole is used to manage infections, such as trichomoniasis and bacterial vaginosis, zidovudine is used to manage HIV, and fluconazole is used to manage candidiasis.

Ⓝ *NCLEX® Connection: Pharmacological Therapies, Adverse Effects/Contraindications/Side Effects/Interactions*

3. **B. CORRECT:** Cryotherapy is the application of cold therapy to freeze unexpected tissue. This procedure is safe during pregnancy and is recommended for the management of HPV. Cervical ablation is a procedure that can destroy cervical tissue and is not recommend during pregnancy or for management of HPV. Cauterization is a procedure that can burn blood vessels and tissue. Darkfield microscopy is a diagnostic procedure used to determine the presence of lesions related to syphilis.

Ⓝ *NCLEX® Connection: Physiological Adaptation, Alterations in Body System*

4. **A, 6; B, 5; C, 4; D, 3; E, 2; F, 1**

Genital herpes is treated with acyclovir. ART is used as one of the medications for all HIV positive infected clients and should be used with a combination of other medications for treatment of the infection. It is given orally and should be given as soon as possible throughout pregnancy. Chlamydia is a bacterial infection, which is treated during pregnancy with azithromycin or amoxicillin. Trichomoniasis is a sexually transmitted infection, which is caused by the protozoan parasite *Trichomoniasis vaginalis* and is treated with oral metronidazole. However, it cannot be administered during the first trimester due to the teratogenic effects on the fetus. Candidiasis is also known as a yeast infection. It is a fungal infection which is mostly caused by *Candida albicans*. It is treatment with an over-the-counter topical medication, which is clotrimazole. Oral medication cannot be prescribed to pregnant or lactating clients. Group B streptococcus is treated with IV penicillin G. The nurse should administer intrapartum antibiotic prophylaxis to clients to decrease transmission to the neonate.

Ⓝ *NCLEX® Connection: Health Promotion and Maintenance, Ante-/Intra-/Postpartum and Newborn Care*

5. **A, B, C, E. CORRECT:** TORCH infections can present as the following: flu-like in presentation, such as joint pain, malaise, and tender lymph nodes. The client also can have a rash. TORCH infections do not include urinary tract infections.

Ⓝ *NCLEX® Connection: Physiological Adaptation, Alterations in Body System*

CHAPTER 8 *Medical Conditions*

Unexpected medical conditions can occur during pregnancy. Awareness, early detection, and interventions are crucial components to ensure fetal well-being and maternal health.

Unexpected medical conditions include cervical insufficiency, hyperemesis gravidarum, anemia, gestational diabetes mellitus, and gestational hypertension.

Cervical insufficiency (premature cervical dilatation)

Cervical insufficiency is a variable condition whereby expulsion of the products of conception occurs. It is thought to be related to tissue changes and alterations in the length of the cervix.

DATA COLLECTION

RISK FACTORS

- History of cervical trauma (cervical tears from previous deliveries, excessive dilations, curettage for biopsy, and surgical procedures involving the cervix), short labors, pregnancy loss in early gestation, or advanced cervical dilation at earlier weeks of gestation
- In utero exposure to diethylstilbestrol, ingested by the client during pregnancy
- Congenital structural defects of the uterus or cervix

EXPECTED FINDINGS

Increase in pelvic pressure or urge to push

PHYSICAL FINDINGS

- Pink-stained vaginal discharge or bleeding
- Possible gush of fluid (rupture of membranes)
- Uterine contractions with the expulsion of the fetus
- Postoperative (cerclage) monitoring for uterine contractions, rupture of membranes, and manifestations of infection

DIAGNOSTIC AND THERAPEUTIC PROCEDURES

- An **ultrasound** showing a short cervix (less than 25 mm in length), presence of cervical funneling (beaking), or effacement of the cervical os indicates reduced cervical competence.
- **Prophylactic cervical cerclage** is the surgical reinforcement of the cervix with a heavy ligature that is placed submucosally around the cervix to strengthen it and prevent premature cervical dilation. Best results occur if this is done at 12 to 14 weeks of gestation. The cerclage is removed at 36 to 38 weeks of gestation or when spontaneous labor occurs.

PATIENT-CENTERED CARE

NURSING CARE

- Monitor the client's support systems and availability of assistance if activity restrictions or bed rest is prescribed.
- Monitor vaginal discharge.
- Monitor client reports of pressure and contractions.
- Check vital signs.

CLIENT EDUCATION

DISCHARGE INSTRUCTIONS

- Adhere to activity restriction or bed rest.
- Encourage hydration to promote a relaxed uterus. (Dehydration stimulates uterine contractions.)
- Avoid intercourse.
- Monitor for cervical/uterine changes.
- Cervical cerclage might be required (indicated for clients who are experiencing singleton pregnancy), often placed at 12 to 14 weeks gestation and removed at 36 to 38 weeks of gestation.

NURSING ACTIONS

- Reinforce with the client to have follow-up for observation and supervision.
- Anticipate the removal of the cerclage between 36 and 38 weeks of gestation.
- Inform client about iron-deficiency anemia.

Hyperemesis gravidarum

- Hyperemesis gravidarum is excessive nausea and vomiting (possibly related to elevated hCG levels) that is prolonged throughout the pregnancy or that is excessive and causes weight loss, dehydration, nutritional deficiencies, electrolyte imbalances, and ketonuria.
- There is a risk to the fetus for intrauterine growth restriction, small for gestational age, or preterm birth if the condition persists.

DATA COLLECTION

RISK FACTORS

- Maternal age younger than 30 years
- Multifetal gestation
- Gestational trophoblastic disease
- Psychosocial issues and high levels of emotional stress
- Clinical hyperthyroid disorders
- Diabetes
- Gastrointestinal disorders
- Family history of hyperemesis

EXPECTED FINDINGS

PHYSICAL FINDINGS
- Excessive vomiting for prolonged periods
- Dehydration with possible electrolyte imbalance
- Weight loss
- Increased pulse rate
- Decreased blood pressure
- Poor skin turgor and dry mucous membranes

LABORATORY TESTS

- **Urinalysis** for ketones and acetones (breakdown of protein and fat)
  - The most important laboratory test is positive ketonuria.
  - Elevated urine specific gravity
- **Chemistry profile** revealing electrolyte imbalances
  - Sodium, potassium, and chloride reduced from low intake
  - Metabolic acidosis (secondary to starvation)
  - Metabolic alkalosis due to excessive vomiting
  - Elevated liver enzymes
  - Bilirubin level
- **Thyroid test** indicating hyperthyroidism
- **Complete blood count (CBC):** Elevated Hct concentration because inability to retain fluid results in hemoconcentration

PATIENT-CENTERED CARE

NURSING CARE

- Monitor I&O.
- Evaluate skin turgor and mucous membranes.
- Monitor vital signs.
- Monitor weight.
- Have the client remain NPO until vomiting stops.

MEDICATIONS

- Give IV lactated Ringer's for hydration.
- Give pyridoxine (vitamin B6) and other vitamin supplements as tolerated. American College of Obstetricians and Gynecologists recommends the use of pyridoxine alone or in combination with doxylamine as the initial medication management because these medications are considered both safe and effective.
- Use antiemetic medications (metoclopramide) cautiously for uncontrollable nausea and vomiting.
- Use corticosteroids to treat refractory hyperemesis gravidarum.

CLIENT EDUCATION

DISCHARGE INSTRUCTIONS
- Advance to a diet of clear liquids and bland foods once the vomiting has stopped.
- Advance the client's diet as tolerated, with frequent, small meals. Start with dry toast, crackers, or cereal; then move to a soft diet; and finally to a normal diet as tolerated. Q EBP
- In severe cases, enteral nutrition per feeding tube or total parental nutrition can be considered.

Iron-deficiency anemia

Iron-deficiency anemia occurs during pregnancy due to inadequacy in maternal iron stores and consumption of insufficient amounts of dietary iron.

DATA COLLECTION

RISK FACTORS

- Less than 2 years between pregnancies
- Heavy menses
- Diet low in iron
- Unhealthy weight loss programs

EXPECTED FINDINGS

- Fatigue and weakness
- Craving unusual food (pica)

LABORATORY TESTS

- **Hgb** less than 11 mg/dL in the first and third trimesters and less than 10.5 mg/dL in the second trimester
- **Hct** less than 33.0%
- **Blood ferritin** less than 12 mcg/L in presence of low Hgb

PATIENT-CENTERED CARE

NURSING CARE

- The recommended iron intake for pregnant clients is 27 mg/day. Prenatal vitamins typically contain 30 mg iron. If maternal iron deficiency anemia is present, increased dosages of 60 to 120 mg/day can be required.
- Increase dietary intake of foods rich in iron (legumes, dried fruit, dark green leafy vegetables, and meat).
- Educate the client about ways to minimize gastrointestinal adverse effects.

MEDICATIONS

Ferrous sulfate iron supplements

CLIENT EDUCATION
- Take the supplement on an empty stomach and take with orange juice to increase absorption.
- Adhere to a diet rich in vitamin C–containing foods to increase absorption.
- Increase fiber and fluid intake in diet to assist with discomforts of constipation.

Parenteral iron therapy

For pregnant clients who cannot tolerate oral iron. Severe anemic clients can receive blood transfusions.

Gestational diabetes mellitus

- Gestational diabetes mellitus (GDM) is an impaired tolerance to glucose with the first onset or recognition during pregnancy. The ideal blood glucose level during pregnancy should range between 60 and 99 mg/dL before meals or fasting and less than or equal to 120 mg/dL 2 hr after meals.
- Findings of diabetes mellitus can disappear a few weeks following birth. However, approximately 50% of clients will develop type II diabetes mellitus later in life.

INCREASED RISKS TO FETUS
- **Macrosomia,** birth trauma, electrolyte imbalances, and neonatal hypoglycemia
- **Infections** (urinary and vaginal), related to increased glucose in the urine and decreased resistance because of altered carbohydrate metabolism
- **Hydramnios,** which can cause overdistention of the uterus, placental abruption, preterm labor, and postpartum hemorrhage

- **Ketoacidosis** from diabetogenic effect of pregnancy (increased insulin resistance), untreated hyperglycemia, or inappropriate insulin dosing
- **Hypoglycemia**, caused by overdosing in insulin, skipped or late meals, or increased exercise
- **Hyperglycemia**, which can cause excessive fetal growth (macrosomia)

DATA COLLECTION

RISK FACTORS

- Obesity
- Hypertension
- Glycosuria
- Maternal age older than 25 years
- Family history of diabetes mellitus
- Previous birth of an infant who was large or stillborn

EXPECTED FINDINGS

Hypoglycemia: nervousness, headache, weakness, irritability, hunger, blurred vision

Hyperglycemia: polydipsia; polyphagia; polyuria; nausea; abdominal pain; flushed, dry skin; fruity breath

PHYSICAL FINDINGS
- Hypoglycemia
- Shaking
- Clammy, pale skin
- Shallow respirations
- Rapid pulse
- Hyperglycemia
- Vomiting
- Excess weight gain during pregnancy

LABORATORY TESTS

- **Glucose screening test/1-hr glucose tolerance test:** 50 g oral glucose load, followed by plasma glucose analysis 1 hr later performed at 24 to 28 weeks of gestation; fasting not necessary; a positive blood glucose screening is 130 to 140 mg/dL or greater; additional testing with a 3-hr oral glucose tolerance test (OGTT) is indicated Q EBP
- **Oral glucose tolerance test** following overnight fasting, avoidance of caffeine, and abstinence from smoking for 12 hr prior to testing; a fasting glucose is obtained, a 100 g glucose load is given, and serum glucose levels are determined at 1, 2, and 3 hr following glucose ingestion
- **Presence of ketones in urine** to determine severity of ketoacidosis

DIAGNOSTIC PROCEDURES

- Biophysical profile to ascertain fetal well-being if nonstress test is nonreactive
- Amniocentesis with amniotic fluid phosphatidylglycerol measured to determine fetal lung maturity
- Nonstress test to monitor fetal well-being

PATIENT-CENTERED CARE

NURSING CARE

- Monitor the client's blood glucose.
- Monitor the fetus.

MEDICATIONS

In contrast to clients who have type I diabetes mellitus, clients who have GDM are managed initially with diet and exercise alone. If glucose levels are persistently high, insulin is begun.

Oral hypoglycemic therapy is an alternative to insulin in clients who have GDM who require medication in addition to diet for blood glucose control. Most oral hypoglycemic agents are contraindicated for gestational diabetes mellitus, but there is limited use of glyburide. The provider will need to make the determination if these medications can be used.

CLIENT EDUCATION

- Perform daily kick counts.
- Adhere to the appropriate diet, including standard diabetic diet and restricted carbohydrate intake. Dietary counseling by a registered dietitian should occur.
- Exercise.
- Perform self-administration of insulin.
- Understand the need for postpartum laboratory testing to include OGTT and blood glucose levels.

Gestational hypertension

- Hypertensive disease in pregnancy is divided into clinical subsets of the disease based on end-organ effects and progresses along a continuum from gestational hypertension, preeclampsia without severe features, preeclampsia with severe features, and eclampsia.
- Vasospasm contributing to poor tissue perfusion is the underlying mechanism for the manifestations of pregnancy hypertensive disorders.
- Gestational hypertensive disease and chronic hypertension can occur simultaneously.
- Gestational hypertensive diseases are associated with placental abruption, kidney failure, hepatic rupture, preterm birth, and fetal and maternal death.

Gestational hypertension (GH), which begins after the 20th week of pregnancy, describes hypertensive disorders of pregnancy whereby the client has an elevated blood pressure at 140/90 mm Hg or greater recorded on two different occasions, at least 4 hr apart. There is no proteinuria. The presence of edema is no longer considered in the definition of hypertensive disease of pregnancy. Blood pressure returns to baseline by 12 weeks postpartum.

Preeclampsia: Traditionally, preeclampsia has been diagnosed when proteinuria occurs with GH. However, current research indicates that clients who have preeclampsia may not exhibit proteinuria. Therefore, the diagnosis of preeclampsia can be made in the absence of this finding. Report of headaches might occur along with episodes of irritability. Edema can be present.

Severe preeclampsia consists of blood pressure that is 160/110 mm Hg or greater, proteinuria greater than 3+, oliguria, elevated blood creatinine greater than 1.1 mg/dL, cerebral or visual disturbances (headache and blurred vision), hyperreflexia with possible ankle clonus, pulmonary or cardiac involvement, extensive peripheral edema, hepatic dysfunction, epigastric and right upper-quadrant pain, and thrombocytopenia.

Eclampsia is severe preeclampsia manifestations with the onset of seizure activity or coma. Eclampsia is usually preceded by headache, severe epigastric pain, hyperreflexia, and hemoconcentrations, which are warning manifestations of probable convulsions.

HELLP syndrome is a variant of GH in which hematologic conditions coexist with severe preeclampsia involving hepatic dysfunction. HELLP syndrome is diagnosed by laboratory tests, not clinically.
- **H: Hemolysis** resulting in anemia and jaundice
- **EL: Elevated liver enzymes** resulting in elevated alanine aminotransferase (ALT) or aspartate transaminase (AST), epigastric pain, and nausea and vomiting
- **LP: Low platelets** (less than 100,000/mm3), resulting in thrombocytopenia, abnormal bleeding and clotting time, bleeding gums, petechiae, and possibly disseminated intravascular coagulopathy

DATA COLLECTION

RISK FACTORS

No single profile identifies risks for gestational hypertensive disorders, but some high risks include the following.
- Maternal age younger than 19 or older than 40 years
- First pregnancy
- Extreme obesity
- Multifetal gestation
- Chronic renal disease
- Chronic hypertension
- Familiar history of preeclampsia
- Diabetes mellitus
- Rheumatoid arthritis
- Systemic lupus erythematosus

EXPECTED FINDINGS

- Severe continuous headache
- Nausea
- Blurring of vision
- Flashes of lights or dots before the eyes

PHYSICAL FINDINGS

- Hypertension
- Proteinuria
- Periorbital, facial, hand, and abdominal edema
- Pitting edema of lower extremities
- Vomiting
- Oliguria
- Hyperreflexia
- Scotoma
- Epigastric pain
- Right upper quadrant pain
- Dyspnea
- Diminished breath sounds
- Seizures
- Jaundice
- Manifestations of progression of hypertensive disease with indications of worsening liver involvement, kidney failure, worsening hypertension, cerebral involvement, and developing coagulopathies

LABORATORY FINDINGS

- Elevated liver enzymes (LDH, AST)
- Increased creatinine
- Increased plasma uric acid
- Thrombocytopenia
- Hgb (decreased in HELLP, increased in preeclampsia)
- Hyperbilirubinemia

LABORATORY TESTS

- Liver enzymes
- Blood creatinine, BUN, uric acid
- CBC
- Clotting studies
- Chemistry profile

DIAGNOSTIC PROCEDURES

- Dipstick testing of urine for proteinuria
- 24-hr urine collection for protein and creatinine clearance
- Nonstress test, contraction stress test, biophysical profile, and serial ultrasounds to monitor fetal status
- Doppler blood flow analysis to monitor fetal well-being
- Daily kick counts

PATIENT-CENTERED CARE

NURSING CARE

- Monitor level of consciousness.
- Obtain pulse oximetry.
- Monitor urine output.
- Obtain daily weights.
- Monitor vital signs with careful attention to blood pressure measurement (using proper size cuff, not talking to client during measurement).
- Encourage lateral positioning.
- Assist with obtaining NST and daily kick counts.
- Reinforce instructions for the client to monitor I&O.

MEDICATIONS

It is recommended that daily low dose aspirin therapy be initiated late in the first trimester for clients who have a history of early onset preeclampsia.

Antihypertensive medications

- Methyldopa
- Nifedipine
- Hydralazine
- Labetalol

CLIENT EDUCATION: Avoid ACE inhibitors and angiotensin II receptor blockers.

Anticonvulsant medications: Magnesium sulfate

Medication of choice for prophylaxis or treatment to depress the CNS and prevent seizures in the client who has eclampsia and severe preeclampsia

NURSING ACTIONS

- Use an infusion control device to maintain a regular flow rate.
- Monitor blood pressure, pulse, respiratory rate, deep-tendon reflexes, level of consciousness, urinary output (indwelling urinary catheter for accuracy), presence of headache, visual disturbances, epigastric pain, uterine contractions, and fetal heart rate and activity.
- Monitor for manifestations of magnesium sulfate toxicity. Qs
  - Absence of patellar deep tendon reflexes
  - Urine output less than 25-30 mL/hr
  - Respirations less than 12/min
  - Decreased level of consciousness
  - Cardiac dysrhythmias
- If magnesium toxicity is suspected:
  - Notify the RN.
  - Immediately discontinue infusion.
  - Administer antidote calcium gluconate or calcium chloride. Qs
  - Assist with preparing for actions to prevent respiratory or cardiac arrest.

CLIENT EDUCATION: There can be initial feelings of flushing, heat, sedation, diaphoresis, and burning at IV site with the magnesium sulfate bolus.

CLIENT EDUCATION

DISCHARGE INSTRUCTIONS

- Remain on bed rest and in the side-lying position.
- Perform diversional activities (TV, visits from family or friends, gentle exercise).
- Avoid foods that are high in sodium.
- Avoid alcohol and tobacco, and limit caffeine intake.
- Drink six to eight 8-ounce glasses of water per day.
- Maintain a dark, quiet environment to avoid stimuli that can precipitate a seizure.
- Maintain a patent airway in the event of a seizure.
- Take antihypertensive medications as prescribed.

Application Exercises

1. A nurse is caring for a client who is at 14 weeks of gestation and has hyperemesis gravidarum. The nurse should identify that which of the following are risk factors for the client? (Select all that apply.)

   A. Diabetes

   B. Multifetal pregnancy

   C. Maternal age greater than 40

   D. Gestational trophoblastic disease

   E. Oligohydramnios

2. A nurse is discussing with a newly licensed nurse two conditions, gestational diabetes mellitus and gestational hypertension. Sort the following risk factors that the nurse should include in the teaching for each condition.

   A. Maternal age older than 25 years

   B. Maternal older than 40 years

   C. Rheumatoid arthritis

   D. Previous birth of an infant who was large or stillborn

   E. Chronic renal disease

3. A nursing is assisting with the care of a client who is receiving IV magnesium sulfate. What medication should the nurse anticipate administering if magnesium sulfate toxicity is suspected?

4. A nursing is assisting with the care of a client who has severe preeclampsia and is receiving IV magnesium sulfate. Which of the following findings should the nurse identify and report as magnesium sulfate toxicity?

   A. Respirations less than 12/min

   B. Urinary output less than 25 mL/hr

   C. Hyperreflexic deep-tendon reflexes

   D. Decreased level of consciousness

   E. Flushing and sweating

Active Learning Scenario

A nurse is reinforcing preprocedure teaching with a client who is at 20 weeks of gestation about prophylactic cervical cerclage. What information should the nurse include? Use the ATI Active Learning Template: Therapeutic Procedure to complete this item.

DESCRIPTION OF PROCEDURE

POTENTIAL COMPLICATIONS: Identify two.

CLIENT EDUCATION: Describe at least four instructions to give the client.

Application Exercises Key

1. A, B, D. **CORRECT:** Diabetes is a risk factor for hyperemesis gravidarum. Multifetal pregnancy is a risk factor for hyperemesis gravidarum. Maternal age less than 30 is a risk factor for hyperemesis gravidarum. Gestational trophoblastic disease is a risk factor for hyperemesis gravidarum. Oligohydramnios is not a risk factor for hyperemesis gravidarum.

   Ⓝ NCLEX Connection: Physiological Adaptation, Alterations in Body Systems

2. **GESTATIONAL HYPERTENSION:** B, C, E; **GESTATIONAL DIABETES MELLITUS:** A, D

   The nurse should teach the newly licensed nurse about the risk factors for clients who have gestational hypertension and gestational diabetes mellitus. Some risk factors for gestational hypertension include maternal age younger than 19 and older than 40 years, rheumatoid arthritis, and first pregnancy. Gestational diabetes mellitus has some of the following as risk factors for the condition: maternal age older than 25 years and a previous birth of an infant who was large or stillborn.

   Ⓝ NCLEX Connection: Health Promotion and Maintenance, Health Promotion/Disease Prevention

3. Calcium gluconate is the antidote for magnesium sulfate and should be readily available for clients who are receiving magnesium sulfate IV.

   Ⓝ NCLEX Connection: Pharmacological Therapies, Expected Actions/Outcomes

4. A, B, D. **CORRECT:** A respiratory rate less than 12/min is a manifestation of magnesium sulfate toxicity. Urinary output less than 25 mL/hr is a manifestation of magnesium sulfate toxicity. The absence of patellar deep-tendon reflexes is a manifestation of magnesium sulfate toxicity. Decreased level of consciousness is a manifestation of magnesium sulfate toxicity. Flushing and sweating are adverse effects of magnesium sulfate but are not manifestations of toxicity.

   Ⓝ NCLEX Connection: Pharmacological Therapies, Expected Actions/Outcomes

Active Learning Scenario Key

Using the ATI Active Learning Template: Therapeutic Procedure

DESCRIPTION OF PROCEDURE: Surgical reinforcement of the cervix with a heavy ligature (suture) that is placed submucosally around the cervix to strengthen it and prevent premature cervical dilation

POTENTIAL COMPLICATIONS
- Uterine contractions
- Rupture of membranes
- Infection

CLIENT EDUCATION
- Remain on activity restrictions/bed rest as prescribed.
- Increase hydration to promote a relaxed uterus.
- Refrain from sexual intercourse.
- Findings to report to the provider include preterm labor, rupture of membranes, manifestations of infection, strong contractions less than 5 min apart, perineal pressure, and the urge to push.
- Plan for removal of the cerclage between 36 and 38 weeks of gestation.

Ⓝ NCLEX® Connection: Reduction of Risk Potential, Potential for Complications From Surgical Procedures and Health Alterations

CHAPTER 9 *Early Onset of Labor*

Understanding the importance of identifying the onset of early labor in a client who is pregnant is crucial for maternal and fetal well-being. This chapter includes preterm labor, prelabor rupture of membranes, and preterm prelabor rupture of membranes.

Preterm labor

Preterm labor is uterine contractions and cervical changes that occur between 20 and 36 weeks and 6 days of gestation. Preterm labor can be categorized as very preterm (less than 32 weeks of gestation), moderately preterm (32 to 34 weeks of gestation), and late preterm (34 to 36 weeks of gestation). Shorter gestation is associated with increased neonatal risks.

DATA COLLECTION

RISK FACTORS

- Infections of the urinary tract or vagina, HIV, active herpes infection, or chorioamnionitis (infection of the amniotic sac)
- Previous preterm birth
- Multifetal pregnancy
- Smoking
- Substance use
- Violence or abuse
- Lack of prenatal care
- Uterine abnormalities
- Low prepregnancy weight
- Advanced maternal age

EXPECTED FINDINGS

- Uterine contractions
- Pressure in the pelvis and menstrual-like cramping
- Persistent low backache
- Gastrointestinal cramping, sometimes with diarrhea
- Urinary frequency
- Vaginal discharge

PHYSICAL FINDINGS

- Increase, change, odor, or blood in vaginal discharge
- Change in cervical dilation
- Regular uterine contractions with a frequency of every 10 min or greater, lasting 1 hr or longer
- Prelabor rupture of membranes
- Discomfort (dull lower abdominal pain or back pain, pelvic pressure or heaviness)

LABORATORY TESTS

- Fetal fibronectin (fFN)
- Cervical cultures
- CBC
- Urinalysis

DIAGNOSTIC PROCEDURES

- fFN: Swabs of vaginal secretions are collected to determine the presence of fFN. This protein can be expected during early and late pregnancy, but presence between 24 weeks and 34 weeks 6 days can indicate inflammation, which increases risk for preterm labor within the next 2 weeks. fFN testing combined with cervical measurements is the best way to determine risk for preterm labor.
- Ultrasound: To determine the measurement of the endocervical length. Cervical shortening occurs before uterine activity (contractions), so this can be a predictor of risk in conjunction with other findings. Cervical length greater than 30 mm indicates low risk of preterm labor.
- Cervical cultures: To check for presence of infectious organisms. Culture and sensitivity results guide prescription of an appropriate antibiotic, if indicated.
- Biophysical profile and/or a nonstress test: To provide information about the fetal well-being

PATIENT-CENTERED CARE

NURSING CARE

Assisting with the care of a client who is in preterm labor includes focusing on stopping uterine contractions.

Activity restriction

- Usually modified bed rest with bathroom privileges. Encourage the client to engage in activities that can be completed in bed or on the couch. Strict bed rest can have adverse effects. Q EBP
- Encourage the client to rest in the left lateral position to increase blood flow to the uterus and decrease uterine activity. Q EBP
- Tell the client to avoid sexual intercourse.

Ensuring hydration: Dehydration stimulates the pituitary gland to secrete an antidiuretic hormone and oxytocin. Preventing dehydration prevents the release of oxytocin, which stimulates uterine contractions.

Identifying and treating an infection

- Have the client report any vaginal discharge, noting amount, color, consistency, and odor.
- Monitor vital signs and temperature.

Chorioamnionitis should be suspected with the occurrence of elevated temperature and tachycardia.

Monitor FHR and contraction pattern

Fetal tachycardia, which is a prolonged increase in the FHR greater than 160/min can indicate infection, is frequently associated with preterm labor.

MEDICATIONS

Nifedipine

CLASSIFICATION AND THERAPEUTIC INTENT: A calcium channel blocker that is used to suppress contractions by inhibiting calcium from entering smooth muscles

NURSING ACTIONS
- Monitor for headache, flushing, dizziness, and nausea. These usually are related to orthostatic hypotension that occurs with administration.
- Should not be administered concurrently with magnesium sulfate, or with or immediately following a beta₂-adrenergic agonist Qs

CLIENT EDUCATION Qs
- Slowly change positions from supine to upright, and sit until dizziness disappears.
- Maintain adequate hydration to counter hypotension.

Magnesium sulfate

CLASSIFICATION AND THERAPEUTIC INTENT: A commonly used tocolytic that is a central nervous system depressant and relaxes smooth muscles, thus inhibiting uterine activity by suppressing contractions. Magnesium sulfate reduces the severity and risk of fetal neuroprotection in surviving infants if administered when birth is anticipated before 32 weeks' gestation.

NURSING ACTIONS
- Contraindications for tocolysis include active vaginal bleeding, dilation of the cervix greater than 6 cm, chorioamnionitis, greater than 34 weeks of gestation, and acute fetal distress. Do not use concurrently with nifedipine. Do not give to clients who have myasthenia gravis.
- Monitor the client closely. Discontinue tocolytic therapy immediately if the client exhibits manifestations of pulmonary edema, which include chest pain, shortness of breath, respiratory distress, audible wheezing and crackles, and a productive cough containing blood-tinged sputum.
- Monitor for adverse effects (hot flashes, diaphoresis, burning at IV site, nausea, vomiting, drowsiness, blurred vision, headache, nonreactive nonstress test, reduced fetal heart rate variability).
- Monitor for magnesium sulfate toxicity and discontinue for any of the following adverse effects: loss of deep tendon reflexes, urinary output less than 30 mL/hr, respirations less than 12/min, pulmonary edema, severe hypotension, or chest pain. Qs
- Administer calcium gluconate or calcium chloride as an antidote for magnesium sulfate toxicity.

CLIENT EDUCATION: Notify the nurse of blurred vision, headache, nausea, vomiting, or difficulty breathing.

Terbutaline

CLASSIFICATION AND THERAPEUTIC INTENT: A beta₂-adrenergic agonist that is used as a tocolytic that relaxes smooth muscles and inhibits uterine activity

NURSING ACTIONS
- Collect data for history of cardiac disease, pregestational or gestational diabetes, preeclampsia with severe features of eclampsia, severe gestational hypertension, hyperthyroidism, or significant hemorrhage. If the client has any of these, the medication should not be administered.
- Monitor for chest discomfort, palpitations, dysrhythmia, tachycardia, tremors, nervousness, vomiting, hypokalemia, hyperglycemia, and hypotension.
- Notify the RN of heart rate greater than 130/min, chest pain, cardiac arrhythmias, myocardial infarction, blood pressure less than 90/60 mm Hg, or pulmonary edema.
- Administer 0.25 mg subcutaneously every 4 hr, for up to 24 hr.
- Discontinue if the client can't tolerate adverse effects.

Betamethasone

CLASSIFICATION AND THERAPEUTIC INTENT: A glucocorticoid that requires 24 hr to be effective. The therapeutic action is to enhance fetal lung maturity and surfactant production in fetuses between 24 and 34 weeks of gestation.

NURSING ACTIONS
- Administer betamethasone 12 mg IM for two doses 24 hr apart.
- Administer deep IM using the ventral gluteal or vastus lateralis muscle at least 24 hr prior to birth.
- Monitor for maternal hyperglycemia.

CLIENT EDUCATION: Report findings of pulmonary edema (chest pain, shortness of breath, and crackles).

Prelabor rupture of membranes and preterm prelabor rupture of membranes

Prelabor rupture of membranes (PROM) is the spontaneous rupture of the amniotic membranes prior to the onset of true labor.

Preterm prelabor rupture of membranes (preterm PROM) is the prelabor spontaneous rupture of membranes after 20 weeks of gestation and prior to 37 weeks of gestation.

DATA COLLECTION

RISK FACTORS
- Infection
- Prior preterm birth
- Shortening of the cervix
- Second/third trimester bleeding

- Pulmonary or connective tissue disorders
- Low BMI
- Copper or ascorbic acid deficiencies
- Tobacco or substance use

EXPECTED FINDINGS

Client reports a gush or leakage of clear fluid from the vagina.

PHYSICAL FINDINGS: Presence of clear fluid

Monitor for a prolapsed umbilical cord. Qs
- Abrupt FHR variable or prolonged deceleration
- Visible or palpable cord at the introitus

LABORATORY TESTS

A positive nitrazine paper test (blue, pH 6.5 to 7.5) or positive ferning test is conducted on amniotic fluid to verify rupture of membranes.

PATIENT-CENTERED CARE

NURSING CARE

Nursing management depends on gestational duration, if there is evidence of infection, or an indication of fetal or maternal compromise. The nurse can assist the RN with the following.
- Prepare for birth if indicated.
- Obtain vaginal/rectal cultures for streptococcus beta-hemolytic.
- Obtain vaginal cultures for chlamydia and Neisseria gonorrhoeae.
- Limit vaginal exams.
- Provide reassurance to reduce anxiety.
- Check vital signs every 2 hr. Notify the provider of a temperature greater than 38° C (100.4° F).
- Monitor FHR and uterine contractions.
- Encourage hydration.
- Obtain a CBC.
- Anticipate a prescription for 7-day course of broad spectrum antibiotics.

CLIENT EDUCATION
- Perform daily fetal kick counts and notify the nurse of uterine contractions.
- Adhere to bed rest with bathroom privileges.

MEDICATIONS

Ampicillin

CLASSIFICATION AND THERAPEUTIC INTENT: Ampicillin is an antibiotic used to treat infection. It is commonly used to treat chorioamnionitis.

NURSING ACTIONS: Obtain vaginal, urine, and blood cultures prior to administration of antibiotic.

9.1 Case study

Scenario introduction

A nurse is discussing with a newly licensed nurse the administration of betamethasone for a client who is at 32 weeks of gestation and experiencing preterm labor. Include the information the nurse should provide to the newly licensed nurse to include the therapeutic intent and nursing actions.

Scene 1

Nurse Charlie: "Sam, Dr. Wong prescribed betamethasone to the client you are caring for. It is important to understand the therapeutic intent and appropriate nursing inventions prior to medication administration. Do you understand the findings you should report to the provider if the client develops complications related to the medication?"

Newly licensed nurse Sam: "Yes, Charlie. I should report chest pain, shortness of breath, and crackles. Those are findings of pulmonary edema, which could be a complication of betamethasone."

Scene 2

Newly Licensed Nurse Sam: "I have prepared the medication, and I have a medication information sheet that I plan to discuss with the client and their support person so they understand the medication regimen."

Nurse Charlie: "Sounds good. Let me know if you have any questions I need to address before you administer the medication."

Scene 3

Newly Licensed Nurse Sam (enters the client's room.): "Good afternoon. I have a medication called betamethasone your provider has prescribed that I am going to discuss with your prior to giving it. Also, here is an information sheet with additional information regarding the medication. Let me know if you have any questions."

Scenario conclusion

Newly Licensed Nurse Sam: "Betamethasone is a glucocorticoid that requires 24 hours to be effective. It helps to stimulate fetal lung maturity in fetuses who are between 24 and 34 weeks of gestation. I am going to administer one IM injection now of 12 mg and then in 24 hours you will get another dose. I will need to monitor your blood glucose level to make sure it is not elevated. Do you have any questions or concerns regarding the medication?"

Betamethasone

CLASSIFICATION AND THERAPEUTIC INTENT
- Betamethasone is a glucocorticoid administered IM in two injections, 24 hr apart, and requires 24 hr to be effective. The therapeutic action is to enhance fetal lung maturity and surfactant production.
- A single dose is given with PROM at 24 to 34 weeks of gestation to reduce the risk of perinatal mortality, respiratory distress syndrome, and other morbidities.
- Betamethasone is given to PROM and preterm PROM clients between 24 and 34 weeks of gestation to reduce the risk of distress syndrome.

COMPLICATIONS

Infection

Infection, particularly chorioamnionitis, is the most common complication of preterm PROM.

Other complications

Placental abruption, umbilical cord compression or prolapse, fetal pulmonary hypoplasia, and death

CLIENT EDUCATION

- Depending on gestational age, treatment is conservative, and hospitalization can prolong pregnancy while monitoring for risk factors (infection, vaginal bleeding, fetal complications).
- Adhere to limited activity with bathroom privileges.
- Hydrate.
- Conduct a self-assessment for uterine contractions.
- Record daily kick counts for fetal movement.
- Monitor for foul-smelling vaginal discharge.
- Refrain from inserting anything into the vagina.
- Abstain from intercourse.
- Avoid tub baths.
- Wipe the perineal area from front to back after voiding and fecal elimination.
- Take temperature every 4 hr when awake and report a temperature that is greater than 38° C (100° F).

Active Learning Scenario

A nurse in the prenatal clinic is assisting the nurse manager with providing education to the staff nurses about preterm labor. What should the nurse suggest to include in the discussion? Use the ATI Active Learning Template: System Disorder to complete this item.

ALTERATION IN HEALTH (DIAGNOSIS)

EXPECTED FINDINGS: Describe at least six manifestations.

DIAGNOSTIC PROCEDURES: Describe at least three.

Application Exercises

1. A nurse is assisting with the care for a client who reports manifestations of preterm labor. Which of the following findings are risk factors of this condition? (Select all that apply.)

   A. Urinary tract infection

   B. Multifetal pregnancy

   C. Maternal age < 20

   D. Substance use disorder

   E. Uterine abnormalities

2. A nurse is assisting with the care for a client who has a prescription for magnesium sulfate. The nurse should recognize that which of the following are contraindications for use of this medication? (Select all that apply.)

   A. Fetal distress

   B. Preterm labor

   C. Vaginal bleeding

   D. Gestational diabetes mellitus

   E. Severe gestational hypertension

3. A nurse is assisting with providing care for a client who is in preterm labor at 32 weeks of gestation. What medication should the nurse anticipate the provider will prescribe to hasten fetal lung maturity?

Active Learning Scenario Key

Using the ATI Active Learning Template: System Disorder

ALTERATION IN HEALTH (DIAGNOSIS): Uterine contractions and cervical changes that occur between 20 and 37 weeks of gestation

EXPECTED FINDINGS
- Persistent low backache
- Pressure in the pelvis and cramping
- Gastrointestinal cramping, sometimes with diarrhea
- Urinary frequency
- Vaginal discharge
- Increase, change, or blood in vaginal discharge
- Change in cervical dilation
- Regular uterine contractions with a frequency of every 10 min or greater, lasting 1 hr or longer
- Premature rupture of membranes

DIAGNOSTIC PROCEDURES
- Test for fetal fibronectin
- Ultrasound to measure endocervical length
- Cervical culture to detect presence of infectious organisms
- Biophysical profile
- Nonstress test
- Home uterine activity monitoring for uterine contractions

Ⓝ *NCLEX® Connection: Health Promotion and Maintenance, Community Resources*

Application Exercises Key

1. A, B, D, E. **CORRECT:** A nurse should identify the following findings as manifestations of preterm labor: multifetal pregnancy, substance use disorder, urinary tract infection, and uterine abnormalities. Advanced maternal age is a risk factor for preterm labor.

Ⓝ *NCLEX Connection: Health Promotion and Maintenance, Health Promotion/Disease Prevention*

2. A, C. **CORRECT:** The nurse should identify the following findings as contraindications for magnesium sulfate therapy: acute fetal distress and vaginal bleeding. Preterm labor is an indication for use of magnesium sulfate. Gestational diabetes mellitus is a complication, not a contraindication, for magnesium sulfate therapy. Severe gestational hypertension is an indication for the use of magnesium sulfate.

Ⓝ *NCLEX Connection: Pharmacological Therapies, Adverse Effects/Contraindications/Side Effects/Interactions*

3. Betamethasone is a glucocorticoid given to clients in preterm labor to hasten surfactant production.

Ⓝ *NCLEX Connection: Pharmacological Therapies, Expected Actions/Outcomes*

NCLEX® Connections

When reviewing the following chapters, keep in mind the relevant topics and tasks of the NCLEX outline.

Health Promotion and Maintenance

ANTE-/INTRA-/POSTPARTUM AND NEWBORN CARE
Assist with monitoring a client in labor.

Assist with fetal heart monitoring for the antepartum client.

DATA COLLECTION TECHNIQUES: Prepare client for physical examination.

Basic Care and Comfort

NONPHARMACOLOGICAL COMFORT INTERVENTIONS: Provide nonpharmacological measures for pain relief.

Pharmacological Therapies

ADVERSE EFFECTS/CONTRAINDICATIONS/SIDE EFFECTS/ INTERACTIONS
Monitor and document client side effects to medications.

Identify a contraindication to the administration of a prescribed or over-the-counter medication to the client.

MEDICATION ADMINISTRATION: Reinforce client teaching on client self-administration of medications.

PN MATERNAL NEWBORN NURSING

ALTERATIONS IN BODY SYSTEMS
Provide care for a client experiencing complications of pregnancy/labor or delivery.

Notify the primary health care provider of a change in client status.

MEDICAL EMERGENCIES: Respond and intervene to a client life-threatening situation.

UNEXPECTED RESPONSE TO THERAPIES
Recognize and report change in client condition.

Intervene in response to client unexpected negative response to therapy.

CHAPTER 10

CHAPTER 10 *Nursing Care of the Client in Labor*

An intrapartum nurse should assist with the care for three clients during each labor and delivery: the fetus, mother, and family unit.

DATA COLLECTION

An intrapartum nurse should collect data on maternal and fetal well-being during labor, the progress of labor, and psychosocial and cultural factors that affect labor. Qpcc

PHYSIOLOGIC CHANGES PRECEDING LABOR (PREMONITORY SIGNS)

Backache: Constant low, dull backache caused by pelvic muscle relaxation

Weight loss: 0.5 to 1.5 kg (1 to 3.5 lb) weight loss

Lightening: Fetal head descends into true pelvis about 14 days before labor; feeling that the fetus has "dropped"; easier breathing, but more pressure on bladder, resulting in urinary frequency; more pronounced in clients who are primigravida.

Contractions: Begin with irregular uterine contractions (Braxton Hicks) that eventually progress in strength and regularity

Increased vaginal discharge or bloody show: Expulsion of the cervical mucus plug may occur. Brownish or blood-tinged mucus plug resulting from the onset of cervical dilation and effacement.

Energy burst: Sometimes called "nesting" response

Gastrointestinal changes: Less common; include nausea, vomiting, and indigestion

Cervical ripening: Cervix becomes soft (opens) and partially effaced and can begin to dilate.

Rupture of membranes: Spontaneous rupture of membranes can initiate labor or can occur anytime during labor.
- Labor usually occurs within 24 hr of the rupture of membranes.
- Prolonged rupture of membranes greater than 24 hr before birth of fetus can lead to an infection
- Immediately following the rupture of membranes, a nurse should check the FHR for abrupt decelerations, which are indicative of fetal distress, to rule out umbilical cord prolapse. Qs

---

10.1 Stages of labor

FIRST STAGE		SECOND STAGE	THIRD STAGE	FOURTH STAGE
LATENT PHASE *0 CM – 5 CM*	*ACTIVE PHASE* *6 CM – 10 CM*			
Onset of labor				
Contractions • Irregular, mild to moderate • Frequency: 5 to 30 min • Duration: 30 to 45 seconds	Contractions • More regular, moderate to strong • Frequency: 3 to 5 min • Duration: 40 to 90 seconds Complete dilation	Full dilation Pushing and fetal descent Birth of the newborn	Delivery of placenta	Maternal stabilization of vital signs
MATERNAL CHARACTERISTICS Scant amount of brownish discharge, pale pink mucus, or mucus plug. Talkative or calm. Thoughts are focused on labor, self, and baby. Ability to talk and walk through most contractions. Easily follows directions. Can be apprehensive.	Becomes more serious. Feelings of helplessness, anxiety, apprehension, and attention are more of an inward focus. Pain may be more severe and may feel out of control, irritable, and doubt ability to continue. Can have nausea and vomiting, urge to push, increased rectal pain and feelings of needing to have a bowel movement. Increased blood show. Most difficult part of labor.	Pushing results in birth of newborn	Placental separation and expulsion Schultze presentation: shiny fetal surface of placenta emerges first Duncan presentation: dull maternal surface of placenta emerges first	Achievement of vital sign homeostasis

---

Evaluation of amniotic fluid: Completed once the membranes rupture
- Amniotic fluid should be watery, clear, and have a slightly yellow tinge.
- Odor should not be foul.
- Volume is between 700 and 1,000 mL.
- Use nitrazine paper to confirm that amniotic fluid is present.
  - **Amniotic fluid is alkaline:** Nitrazine paper is deep blue, indicating pH of 6.5 to 7.5.
  - **Urine is slightly acidic:** Nitrazine paper remains yellow.

Psychological response

Maternal stress, tension, and anxiety can produce physiological changes that impair the progress of labor.

PATIENT-CENTERED CARE

FIRST STAGE

Lasts from onset of regular uterine contractions to full effacement and dilation of cervix (longer than second and third stages combined) preprocedure

NURSING ACTIONS
- **Leopold maneuvers:** Abdominal palpation of the fetal presenting part, lie, attitude, descent, and the probable location where fetal heart tones can be best auscultated on the client's abdomen
- **External electronic monitoring (tocotransducer):** Separate transducer applied to the maternal abdomen over the fundus that measures uterine activity
  - Displays uterine contraction patterns
  - Easily applied by the nurse but must be repositioned with maternal movement to ensure proper placement
- **External fetal monitoring (EFM):** Transducer applied to the abdomen of the client to monitor FHR patterns during labor and birth

10.2 Findings in the first stage

	LATENT/EARLY	ACTIVE PHASE
Blood pressure, pulse, and respiration measurements	Every 30 to 60 min	Every 15 to 30 min
*Temperature**	Every 2 to 4 hr	Every 2 to 4 hr
Contraction monitoring	Every 30 to 60 min	Every 15 to 30 min
FHR monitoring (expected range 110 to 160/min)	Every 30 to 60 min	Every 15 to 30 min

*Temperature is checked every 4 hr until membranes rupture and then every 2 hr

Laboratory analysis

- **Group B streptococcus:** Culture is obtained if results are not available from antepartal screening. If positive, an intravenous prophylactic antibiotic is prescribed. Qs
- **Urinalysis**: Clean-catch urine sample obtained to check the client for:
  - Dehydration via specific gravity
  - Ketonuria (impaired nutrition or uncontrolled glucose)
  - Proteinuria, which can be indicative of gestational hypertension or preeclampsia
  - Glucosuria, which can be indicative of gestational diabetes
  - Urinary tract infection (UTI) via bacterial count (more common in clients who have diabetes mellitus)
  - Universal drug screening
- **Blood tests**
  - CBC level
  - ABO typing and Rh-factor
  - If a client has no prenatal care, all initial laboratory tests that should have been obtained during prenatal care should be drawn.

CLIENT EDUCATION: The health care team will update the client regarding the labor and birth process. The client should ask questions about any procedure or information they do not understand.

INTRAPROCEDURE

NURSING ACTIONS
- **Check maternal vital signs** per agency protocol. Check maternal temperature every 2 hr if membranes are ruptured.
- **Monitor FHR** to determine fetal well-being. This can be performed by use of EFM or spiral electrode that is applied to the fetal scalp by a registered nurse trained in the procedure or the provider. Prior to electrode placement, cervical dilation and rupture of membranes must occur.
- **Monitor uterine labor contraction characteristics** by palpation (placing a hand over the fundus to check contraction frequency, duration, and intensity) or by the use of external or internal monitoring.
- The frequency, duration, and strength (intensity) of the uterine contractions cause fetal descent and cervical dilation.
  - **Frequency:** Established from the beginning of one contraction to the beginning of the next
  - **Duration:** Time between the beginning of a contraction to the end of that same contraction
  - **Intensity:** Strength of the contraction at its peak, described as mild (slightly tense, like pressing finger to tip of nose), moderate (firm, like pressing finger to chin), or strong (rigid, like pressing finger to forehead)
  - **Resting tone of uterine contractions:** Tone of the uterine muscle in between contractions. A prolonged contraction duration (greater than 90 seconds) or too frequent contractions (more than five in a 10-min period) without sufficient time for uterine relaxation (less than 30 seconds) in between can reduce blood flow to the placenta. This can result in fetal hypoxia and decreased FHR. Qs

- **Intrauterine pressure catheter:** Insertion of a sterile solid or fluid-filled intrauterine pressure catheter by the provider or a qualified nurse inside the uterus to measure intrauterine pressure
  - Displays uterine contraction patterns on monitor
  - Requires the membranes to be ruptured and the cervix to be sufficiently dilated
- **Vaginal examination:** Performed digitally by the provider or qualified nurse to check for the following
  - Cervical dilation (stretching of cervical os adequate to allow fetal passage) and effacement (cervical thinning and shortening) (10.4)
  - Descent of the fetus through the birth canal as measured by fetal station in centimeters
  - Fetal position, presenting part, and lie
  - Membranes that are intact or ruptured
- Cervical dilation is the single most important indicator of the progress of labor.

SECOND STAGE

Lasts from the time the cervix is fully dilated to the birth of the fetus

DATA COLLECTION AND NURSING INTERVENTIONS
Begins with complete dilation and effacement
- Blood pressure, pulse, and respiration measurements every 5 to 30 min
- Uterine contractions
- Pushing efforts by client
- Increase in bloody show
- Assist in positioning the client for effective pushing.
- Assist in partner involvement with pushing efforts and in encouraging bearing-down efforts during contractions.
- Promote rest between contractions.
- FHR every 5 to 15 min (depending on fetal risk status) and immediately following birth

---

10.3 Contraction pattern

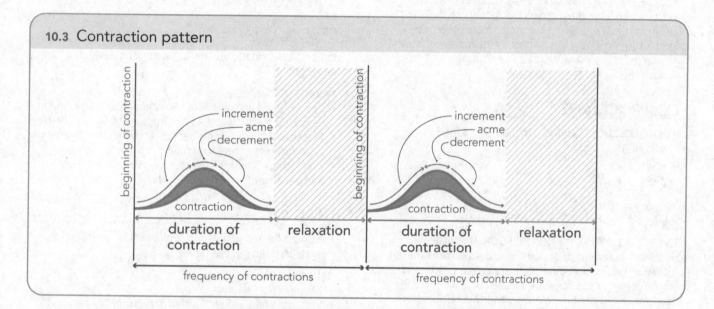

10.4 Characteristics of true vs. false labor

	TRUE LABOR	FALSE LABOR
CONTRACTIONS	Can begin irregularly, but become regular in frequency Stronger, last longer, and are more frequent Felt in lower back, radiating to abdomen Walking can increase contraction intensity Continue despite comfort measures	Painless, irregular frequency, and intermittent Decrease in frequency, duration, and intensity with walking or position changes Felt in lower back or abdomen above umbilicus Often stop with sleep or comfort measures (oral hydration, emptying of the bladder)
CERVIX (ASSESSED BY VAGINAL EXAM)	Progressive change in dilation and effacement Moves to anterior position Bloody show True labor leads to cervical dilation and effacement	No significant change in dilation or effacement Often remains in posterior position No significant bloody show
FETUS	Presenting part engages in pelvis	Presenting part is not engaged in pelvis

THIRD STAGE

Lasts from the birth of the fetus until the placenta is delivered

DATA COLLECTION
- Blood pressure, pulse, and respiration measurements every 15 min
- Assignment of 1 and 5 min Apgar scores to the newborn by a registered nurse or provider

NURSING ACTIONS
- The registered nurse will administer oxytocics as prescribed to stimulate the uterus to contract and thus prevent hemorrhage.
- Administer analgesics.
- Gently cleanse the perineal area with warm water and apply a perineal pad or ice pack to the perineum.
- Promote baby-friendly activities between the family and the newborn, which facilitates the release of endogenous maternal oxytocin. Examples of such activities include introducing the parents to the newborn and facilitating the attachment process by promoting skin-to-skin contact immediately following the birth. Allow private time and encourage breastfeeding. Qтс

POSTPROCEDURE

DATA COLLECTION DURING THE FOURTH STAGE
- Maternal vital signs
- Fundus
- Lochia
- Perineum
- Urinary output
- Maternal/newborn baby-friendly activities

NURSING ACTIONS DURING THE FOURTH STAGE
- American Academy of Pediatrics and American College of Obstetricians and Gynecologists recommends that blood pressure and pulse be checked at least every 15 min for the first 2 hr after birth and that temperature be checked every 4 hr for the first 8 hr after birth and then at least every 8 hr.
- Check fundus and lochia every 15 min for the first hour and then according to facility protocol.
- Massage the uterine fundus and/or administer oxytocics as prescribed to maintain uterine tone to prevent hemorrhage. Qs
- Check the client's perineum, and provide comfort measures as indicated.
- Encourage voiding to prevent bladder distention.
- Promote an opportunity for maternal/newborn bonding.
- Offer assistance with breastfeeding, and provide reassurance.

CLIENT EDUCATION: Notify the nurse of increased vaginal bleeding or passage of blood clots.

Pain management

Pain is a subjective and individual experience, and each client's response to the pain of labor is unique. Safety for the mother and fetus must be the first consideration of the nurse when assisting with planning pain management measures. Qs

SOURCES OF PAIN DURING LABOR

FIRST STAGE

Internal visceral pain that can be felt as back and leg pain

PAIN CAUSES
- Dilation, effacement, and stretching of the cervix
- Distention of the lower segment of the uterus
- Contractions of the uterus with resultant uterine ischemia

SECOND STAGE

Pain that is somatic and occurs with fetal descent and expulsion

PAIN CAUSES
- Pressure and distention of the vagina and the perineum, described by the client as burning, splitting, and tearing
- Pressure and pulling on the pelvic structures (ligaments, fallopian tubes, ovaries, bladder, and peritoneum)
- Lacerations of soft tissues (cervix, vagina, and perineum)

THIRD STAGE

Pain with the expulsion of the placenta is similar to pain experienced during the first stage.

PAIN CAUSES
- Uterine contractions
- Pressure and pulling of pelvic structures

FOURTH STAGE

Pain is caused by distention and stretching of the vagina and perineum incurred during the second stage with a splitting, burning, and tearing sensation.

DATA COLLECTION

- Pain level cannot always be evaluated by monitoring the outward expressions of a client. Data collection for the client's pain can require persistent questioning and observations by the nurse. Cultural beliefs and behaviors of clients during labor and birth can affect the client's pain management.
- Anxiety and fear are associated with pain. As fear and anxiety increase, muscle tension increases, and thus the experience of pain increases, becoming a cycle of pain. Fear, tension, and pain slow the progression of labor.

- Check beliefs and expectations related to discomfort, pain relief, and birth plans regarding pain relief methods for clients in labor.
- Monitor level, quality, frequency, duration, intensity, and location of pain through verbal and nonverbal cues. Use an appropriate pain scale allowing the client to indicate the severity of their pain on a scale of 0 to 10, with 10 representing the most severe pain.
- **Indications of pain**
  - Behavioral manifestations (crying, moaning, screaming, gesturing, writhing, avoidance, withdrawal, inability to follow instructions)
  - Increasing blood pressure, tachycardia, and hyperventilation
  - Nausea and vomiting with an increase in gastric acidity
- Help the client maintain the proper position during administration of pharmacological interventions. Assist the client with positioning for comfort during labor and birth, and follow pharmacological interventions.
- Provide client safety after any pharmacological intervention by putting the bed in a low position, maintaining side rails in the up position, placing the call light within the client's reach, and reinforcing with the client and their partner to call for assistance if they need to leave the bed or ambulate. Qs
- Evaluate the client's response to pain relief methods used (verbal report that pain is relieved or being relieved, appears relaxed between contractions).

NONPHARMACOLOGICAL PAIN MANAGEMENT

Nonpharmacological pain management measures reduce anxiety, fear, and tension, which are major contributing factors to pain in labor.

GATE-CONTROL THEORY OF PAIN

- Based on the concept that the sensory nerve pathways that pain sensations use to travel to the brain will allow only a limited number of sensations to travel at any given time. By sending alternate signals through these pathways, the pain signals can be blocked from ascending the neurologic pathway and inhibit the brain's perception and sensation of pain.
- Assists in the understanding of how nonpharmacological pain techniques can work to relieve pain

INTERVENTIONS

Cognitive strategies

- Childbirth education
- Childbirth preparation methods (Lamaze, patterned breathing exercises) promote relaxation and pain management.
- Doulas can assist clients using methods for nonpharmacological pain management.

- Nursing implications include monitoring for findings of hyperventilation (caused by low blood levels of PCO_2 from blowing off too much CO2), such as lightheadedness and tingling of the fingers. If this occurs, have the client breathe into a paper bag or their cupped hands.
- Hypnosis
- Biofeedback

Sensory stimulation strategies

Based on the gate-control theory to promote relaxation and pain relief
- Aromatherapy
- Breathing techniques
- Imagery
- Music
- Use of focal points
- Subdued lighting

Cutaneous stimulation strategies

Based on the gate-control theory to promote relaxation and pain relief
- Therapeutic touch and massage: back rubs and massage
- Walking
- Rocking
- Effleurage: Light, gentle circular stroking of the client's abdomen with the fingertips in rhythm with breathing during contractions
- Sacral counterpressure: Consistent pressure is applied by the support person using the heel of the hand or fist against the client's sacral area to counteract pain in the lower back
- Application of heat or cold
- Transcutaneous electrical nerve stimulation (TENS) therapy
- Hydrotherapy (whirlpool or shower) increases maternal endorphin levels.
- Acupressure
- Frequent maternal position changes to promote relaxation and pain relief.
  - Semi-sitting
  - Squatting
  - Kneeling
  - Kneeling and rocking back and forth
  - Supine position only with the placement of a wedge under one of the client's hips to tilt the uterus and avoid supine hypotension syndrome

CLIENT EDUCATION: Use techniques to promote pain management (patterned breathing, progressive relaxation exercises).

PHARMACOLOGICAL PAIN MANAGEMENT

Includes analgesia and local/regional analgesics. To avoid slowing the progress of labor, prior to administering analgesic medications, the nurse should verify that labor is well-established by performing a vaginal exam and evaluating uterine contraction pattern. Q_{EBP}

Alleviates pain sensations or raises the threshold for pain perception. Also, the registered nurse should conduct a fall safety risk assessment for clients who request pain management interventions during labor and birth, which increases the risk for falls.

ANALGESIA

Sedatives (barbiturates)

Sedatives (secobarbital, pentobarbital, phenobarbital) are not typically used during birth, but they can be used during the early or latent phase of labor to relieve anxiety and induce sleep.

ADVERSE EFFECTS
- Neonate respiratory depression secondary to the medication crossing the placenta and affecting the fetus. These medications should not be administered if birth is anticipated within 12 to 24 hr. Q_{EBP}
- Unsteady ambulation of the client
- Inhibition of the mother's ability to cope with the pain of labor. Sedatives should not be given if the client is experiencing pain because apprehension can increase and cause the client to become hyperactive and disoriented.

CLIENT EDUCATION
- The medication will cause drowsiness.
- Request assistance with ambulation.

NURSING ACTIONS
- Dim the lights, and provide a quiet atmosphere.
- Provide safety for the client by lowering the position of the bed and elevating the side rails.
- Assist the mother to cope with labor. Q_S
- Monitor the neonate for respiratory depression.

Opioid analgesics

Opioid analgesics (meperidine hydrochloride, fentanyl, butorphanol, nalbuphine) act in the CNS to decrease the perception of pain without the loss of consciousness. The client can receive opioid analgesics IM or IV, but the IV route is recommended during labor because the action is quicker. These are usually given during the early part of active labor.

Butorphanol and nalbuphine provide pain relief without causing significant respiratory depression in the mother or fetus. Both IM and IV routes are used.

ADVERSE EFFECTS
- Respiratory depression in the neonate if mother medicated too close to time of birth
- Reduction of gastric emptying; increased risk for nausea and emesis
- Increased risk for aspiration of food or fluids in the stomach
- Bladder and bowel elimination can be inhibited.
- Sedation
- Altered mental status
- Tachycardia
- Hypotension
- Decreased FHR variability
- Allergic reaction

NURSING ACTIONS
- Prior to administering analgesic medication, the RN would verify that labor is well-established by performing a vaginal exam by a qualified nurse.
- Administer antiemetics as prescribed.
- Monitor maternal vital signs, uterine contraction pattern, and continuous FHR monitoring. Check maternal vital signs and fetal heart rate and pattern and documented before and after administration of opioids for pain relief.
- Monitor for adverse reactions (difficulty breathing) and be prepared to administer antidotes whenever medications are administered.

Naloxone, an opioid antagonist, should be readily available for reversal of opioid-induced respiratory depression. Q_S

CLIENT EDUCATION
- The medication will cause drowsiness.
- Request assistance with ambulation.

Metoclopramide

Can control nausea and anxiety. It does not relieve pain and is used as an adjunct with opioids.

ADVERSE EFFECTS: Dry mouth and sedation

NURSING ACTIONS
- Provide ice chips or mouth swabs.
- Provide safety measures for the client.
- Anesthesia used in childbirth includes regional blocks, nitrous oxide, and general anesthesia.
- Nitrous oxide is an inhaled anesthetic that can be used for labor analgesia. The client uses inhaled nitrous oxide intermittently for pain. However, it does not eliminate the uterine contraction pain but does decrease the client's perception of the pain. An advantage of nitrous oxide is that it has a rapid onset and quickly clears the body by exhalation and does not accumulate in fetal or maternal tissues. Also, the client self-administers the nitrous while they are alert and awake. An adverse effect is dizziness and nausea.

Epidural and spinal regional analgesia

Consists of using analgesics, such as fentanyl and sufentanil, which are short-acting opioids that are administered as a motor block into the epidural or intrathecal space without anesthesia. These opioids produce regional analgesia, providing rapid pain relief while still allowing the client to sense contractions and maintain the ability to bear down.

ADVERSE EFFECTS

- Decreased gastric emptying resulting in nausea and vomiting
- Inhibition of bowel and bladder elimination sensations
- Bradycardia or tachycardia
- Hypotension
- Respiratory depression
- Allergic reaction and pruritus
- Elevated temperature

NURSING ACTIONS

- Provide safety precautions, such as putting side rails up on the client's bed. The client can experience dizziness and sedation, which increases maternal risk for injury. Qs
- Monitor for nausea and emesis, and administer antiemetics as prescribed.
- Monitor maternal vital signs per facility protocol.
- Monitor for allergic reaction.
- Continue FHR pattern monitoring.

PHARMACOLOGICAL ANESTHESIA

- Pharmacological anesthesia eliminates pain perceptions by interrupting the nerve impulses to the brain.
- Anesthesia used in childbirth includes regional blocks and general anesthesia.

Regional blocks

Regional blocks are most commonly used and consist of pudendal, epidural, spinal, and paracervical nerve block.

Pudendal block: Consists of a local anesthetic (lidocaine, bupivacaine) administered transvaginally into the space in front of the pudendal nerve. This type of block has no maternal or fetal systemic effects, but it does provide local anesthesia to the perineum, vulva, and rectal areas during delivery, episiotomy, and episiotomy repair. It is administered during the late second stage of labor 10 to 20 min before delivery, providing analgesia prior to spontaneous expulsion of the fetus or forceps-assisted or vacuum-assisted birth. It is suitable during the second and third stages of labor and for repair of episiotomy and lacerations.

ADVERSE EFFECTS: Compromise of maternal bearing-down reflex

NURSING ACTIONS

- Instruct the client about the method.
- Coach the client about when to bear down.

Epidural block: Consists of a local anesthetic, bupivacaine, along with an analgesic, morphine or fentanyl, injected into the epidural space at the level of the fourth or fifth vertebrae. This eliminates pain from the level of the umbilicus to the thighs, relieving the discomfort of uterine contractions, fetal descent, and stretching of the perineum. However, this might not remove pressure sensations. Continuous infusion or intermittent injections can be administered through an indwelling epidural catheter. Patient-controlled epidural analgesia is a technique for labor analgesia and is a favored method of pain management for labor and birth. It is suitable for all stages of labor and types of birth and for repair of episiotomy and lacerations.

ADVERSE EFFECTS

- Maternal hypotension
- Fetal bradycardia
- Fever
- Itching
- Inability to feel the urge to void
- Urinary retention
- Loss of the bearing-down reflex

NURSING ACTIONS

- Assist with administration of a bolus of IV fluids to help offset maternal hypotension. QEBP
- Help position and steady the client into a sitting or side-lying modified lateral semi-prone recumbent position with the back curved to widen the intervertebral space for insertion of the catheter.
- Encourage the client to remain in the side-lying position after insertion of the epidural catheter to avoid supine hypotension syndrome with compression of the vena cava.
- Coach the client in pushing efforts, and request an evaluation of epidural pain management by anesthesia personnel if pushing efforts are ineffective.
- Monitor maternal blood pressure and pulse, and observe for hypotension, respiratory depression, and decreased oxygen saturation.
- Assist with monitoring the FHR patterns continuously.
- Monitor the IV line, and have oxygen and suction available.
- Monitor for orthostatic hypotension. Be prepared to assist with positioning the client laterally and initiating oxygen. The RN may administer IV vasopressor (such as ephedrine) or increase the rate of IV fluid administration. Qs
- Provide for client safety, such as by raising the side rails of the bed.
  - Sequential compression device (SCD) may be used as a prophylactic treatment for deep vein thrombosis and hypotension following epidural placement.
- Check the bladder for distention at frequent intervals, and catheterize if necessary to prevent discomfort and interference with uterine contractions.
- Monitor for the return of sensation and motor control in the client's legs after delivery but prior to standing.
- Assist the client with standing and walking for the first time after a birth that included epidural anesthesia.

CLIENT EDUCATION: Use patient-controlled analgesia, if provided.

Spinal anesthesia (block): Consists of a local anesthetic that is injected into the subarachnoid space into the spinal fluid at the third, fourth, or fifth lumbar interspace. This can be done alone or in combination with an analgesic such as fentanyl. The spinal block eliminates all sensations from the level of the nipples to the feet. It is commonly used for cesarean births. A low spinal block can be used for a vaginal birth, but it is not used for labor. A spinal block is administered in the late second stage or before cesarean birth.

ADVERSE EFFECTS

- Maternal hypotension
- Fetal bradycardia
- Loss of the bearing-down reflex in the client with a higher incidence of operative births
- Potential headache from leakage of cerebrospinal fluid at the puncture site
- Higher incidence of maternal bladder and uterine atony following birth

NURSING ACTIONS

- Monitor maternal vital signs every 10 min.
- Manage maternal hypotension by assisting with the administration of an IV fluid bolus as prescribed, positioning the client laterally, increasing the rate of IV fluid administration, and initiating oxygen. Qs
- Monitor FHR patterns.
- Provide client safety to prevent injury by raising the side rails of the bed and assisting the client with repositioning.
- Monitor for manifestations of impending birth, including sitting on one buttock, making grunting sounds, and bulging of the perineum.
- Potential headache from leakage of cerebrospinal fluid at the puncture site. Encourage interventions to relieve a postpartum headache resulting from a cerebrospinal fluid leak. Interventions include placing the client in a supine position, promoting bed rest in a dark room, and administering oral analgesics, caffeine, and fluids. An autologous blood patch is the most beneficial and reliable relief measure for cerebrospinal fluid leaks.

CLIENT EDUCATION: Bear down for expulsion of the fetus because during a vaginal birth; contractions will not be felt.

General anesthesia

Rarely used for vaginal or cesarean births when there are no complications present. It is used only in the event of a birth complication or emergency when there is a contraindication to nerve block analgesia or anesthesia. General anesthesia produces unconsciousness.

NURSING ACTIONS

- Monitor maternal vital signs.
- Monitor FHR patterns.
- Ensure that the client has had nothing by mouth.
- Ensure that the IV infusion is in place.
- Apply antiembolic stockings or sequential compression devices.
- Premedicate the client with oral antacid to neutralize acidic stomach contents.

- Administer a histamine2-receptor antagonist, such as cimetidine, to decrease gastric acid production.
- Administer metoclopramide to increase gastric emptying as prescribed.
- Place a wedge under one of the client's hips to displace the uterus.
- Maintain an open airway and cardiopulmonary function.
- Monitor the client postpartum for decreased uterine tone, which can lead to hemorrhage and be produced by pharmacological agents used in general anesthesia. Qs

CLIENT EDUCATION: Facilitate parent-newborn attachment as soon as possible.

Therapeutic procedures to assist with labor and birth

Induction of labor is the deliberate initiation of uterine contractions to stimulate labor before spontaneous onset to bring about the birth by chemical or mechanical means.

METHODS

- Mechanical or chemical approaches
- Administration of IV oxytocin
- Nipple stimulation to trigger the release of endogenous oxytocin

INDICATIONS

Any condition in which augmentation or induction of labor is indicated. Elective induction for nonmedical indications must meet the criteria of at least 39 weeks of gestation. Elective inductions that do not meet recommended criteria can result in increased risk for infection, premature delivery, longer labor, and need for cesarean birth.

CLIENT PRESENTATION

- Postterm pregnancy (greater than 42 weeks of gestation)
- Dystocia (prolonged, difficult labor) due to inadequate uterine contractions
- Prolonged rupture of membranes, which predisposes the client and fetus to risk of infection
- Intrauterine growth restriction
- Maternal medical complications
  - Rh-isoimmunization
  - Diabetes mellitus
  - Pulmonary disease
  - Gestational hypertension
- Fetal demise
- Chorioamnionitis

CONSIDERATIONS

CLIENT PREPARATION

- Prepare the client for cervical ripening.
  - Ensure that the client gives informed consent.
  - If cervical-ripening agents are used, ensure that baseline data on fetal and maternal well-being is obtained.
  - Monitor FHR and uterine activity after administration of cervical-ripening agents.
  - Monitor for uterine tachysystole or fetal distress.
- Assist with preparing the client for misoprostol administration.
  - Misoprostol is a tablet inserted vaginally to ripen the cervix.
  - Encourage the client to void prior to the procedure.
- Assist with preparing the client for oxytocin administration.
  - Prior to the administration of oxytocin, it is essential that the nurse confirm that the fetus is engaged in the birth canal at a minimum of station 0.
  - Initiate oxytocin no sooner than 4 hr after the administration of misoprostol, and 6 to 12 hr after dinoprostone gel instillation or removal of a dinoprostone insert.
  - When oxytocin is administered, check maternal blood pressure, pulse, and respirations every 30 to 60 min and with every change in dose.
  - Monitor the FHR and contraction pattern every 15 min in the first stage of labor, every 5 min in the second stage of labor, and with every change in dose.
  - Monitor fluid intake and urinary output.
- Discontinue oxytocin if uterine tachysystole occurs. Clinical findings of uterine tachysystole include the following. Qs
  - Contraction frequency more often than every 2 min
  - Single contraction lasting greater than 2 minutes
  - No relaxation of uterus between contractions

COMPLICATIONS

Nonreassuring FHR

- Abnormal baseline less than 110 or greater than 160/min
- Loss of variability
- Late or prolonged decelerations

NURSING ACTIONS
- Notify the RN or provider.
- Position the client in a side-lying position to increase uteroplacental perfusion.
- Keep the IV line open and assist the nurse with administering an IV fluid bolus unless contraindicated.
- Administer O2 by a face mask at 8 to 10 L/min.
- Administer the tocolytic terbutaline 0.25 mg subcutaneously to diminish uterine activity.
- Monitor FHR and patterns in conjunction with uterine activity.
- Monitor responses to interventions.
- If unable to restore reassuring FHR, assist with preparing for an emergency cesarean birth.

Augmentation of labor

Augmentation of labor is the stimulation of hypotonic contractions once labor has spontaneously begun, but progress is inadequate.

Some providers favor active management of labor to establish effective labor with the aggressive use of oxytocin or rupture of membranes.

RISK FACTORS REQUIRING AUGMENTATION OF LABOR: Administration procedures, nursing data collection and interventions, and possible procedure complications are the same for labor induction.

Amniotomy

- An amniotomy is the artificial rupture of the amniotic membranes (AROM) by the provider using a hook, clamp, or other sharp instrument.
- Labor typically begins within 12 hr after the membranes rupture and can decrease the duration of labor by up to 2 hr.
- The client is at an increased risk for cord prolapse or infection.

INDICATIONS

- Labor progression is too slow, and augmentation or induction of labor is indicated.
- An amnioinfusion is indicated for cord compression.

CONSIDERATIONS

ONGOING CARE
- Ensure that the presenting part of the fetus is engaged prior to an amniotomy to prevent cord prolapse.
- Monitor FHR prior to and immediately following AROM to check for cord prolapse as evidenced by variable or late decelerations.
- Monitor and document characteristics of amniotic fluid including color, odor, and consistency.

INTERVENTIONS
- Note the time of rupture.
- Obtain a maternal temperature every 2 hr.
- Provide comfort measures (frequently changing pads, perineal cleansing).

Amnioinfusion

An amnioinfusion of normal saline or lactated Ringer's is instilled into the amniotic cavity through a transcervical catheter introduced into the uterus to supplement the amount of amniotic fluid. The instillation reduces the severity of variable decelerations caused by cord compression.

INDICATIONS

POTENTIAL DIAGNOSES
- Oligohydramnios (scant amount or absence of amniotic fluid) caused by any of the following
  - Uteroplacental insufficiency
  - Premature rupture of membranes
  - Postmaturity of the fetus
- Fetal cord compression secondary to postmaturity of fetus (macrosomic, large body), which places the fetus at risk for variable deceleration from cord compression

Vacuum-assisted birth

A vacuum-assisted birth involves the use of a cuplike suction device that is attached to the fetal head. Traction is applied during contractions to assist in the descent and birth of the head, after which the vacuum cup is released and removed preceding birth of the fetal body.

Follow recommendations by the manufacturer for product use to ensure safety.

CONDITIONS FOR USE
- Vertex presentation
- Cervical dilation of 10 cm
- Absence of cephalopelvic disproportion
- Ruptured membranes

ASSOCIATED RISKS
- Scalp lacerations
- Subdural hematoma of the neonate
- Cephalohematoma
- Maternal lacerations to the cervix, vagina, or perineum

INDICATIONS

- Maternal exhaustion and ineffective pushing efforts
- Fetal distress during second stage of labor
- Generally not used to assist birth before 34 weeks of gestation

CONSIDERATIONS

PREPARATION OF THE CLIENT

- Assist with providing the client and their partner with support and education regarding the procedure.
- Assist the client into the lithotomy position to allow for sufficient traction of the vacuum cup when it is applied to the fetal head.
- Check FHR before and during vacuum assistance.
- Check for bladder distention, and catheterize if necessary.

ONGOING CARE: Assist with preparing for a forceps-assisted birth if a vacuum-assisted birth is not successful.

INTERVENTIONS

- Reinforce with the postpartum care providers that vacuum assistance was used.
- Monitor the neonate for lacerations, cephalohematomas, or subdural hematomas after birth.
- Monitor the newborn for caput succedaneum. Caput succedaneum is swelling of the scalp in a newborn that usually disappears within 3 to 5 days.

Forceps-assisted birth

A forceps-assisted birth consists of using an instrument with two curved spoon-like blades to assist in the delivery of the fetal head. Traction is applied during contractions.

INDICATIONS

CLIENT PRESENTATION
- Prolonged second stage of labor and need to shorten duration (maternal exhaustion)
- Fetal distress during labor
- Abnormal presentation or a breech position requiring delivery of the head
- Arrest of rotation

CONSIDERATIONS

PREPARATION OF THE CLIENT

- Reinforce the procedure to the client and their partner.
- Assist the client into the lithotomy position.
- Check to ensure that the client's bladder is empty, and catheterize if necessary.
- Check to ensure that the fetus is engaged and that membranes have ruptured.

ONGOING CARE: Assist with the procedure as necessary.

INTERVENTIONS

- Monitor FHR before, during, and after forceps assistance.
- Compression of the cord between the fetal head and forceps will cause a decrease in the FHR.
  - If a FHR decrease occurs, the forceps are removed and reapplied.
- Monitor the neonate for bruising and abrasions at the site of forceps application after birth. Monitor for facial palsy.
- Check the client for any possible injuries after birth.
  - Vaginal or cervical lacerations indicated by bleeding in spite of contracted uterus
  - Urine retention resulting from bladder or urethral injuries
  - Hematoma formation in the pelvic soft tissues resulting from blood vessel damage
- Reinforce to the postpartum nursing caregivers that forceps or vacuum-assisted delivery methods were used.

COMPLICATIONS

- Lacerations of the cervix
- Lacerations of the vagina and perineum
- Injury to the bladder
- Facial nerve palsy of the neonate
- Facial bruising on the neonate
- Subdural hematoma in the neonate

Lacerations

Check for perineal lacerations, which usually occur as the fetal head is expulsed. Perineal lacerations (tears) are defined in terms of depth.

First degree: Laceration extends through the skin of the perineum and does not involve the muscles.

Second degree: Laceration extends through the skin and muscles into the perineum but not the anal sphincter.

Third degree: Laceration extends through the skin, muscles, perineum, and external anal sphincter muscle.

Fourth degree: Laceration extends through skin, muscles, anal sphincter, and the anterior rectal wall.

Episiotomy

An episiotomy is an incision made into the perineum to enlarge the vaginal opening to facilitate birth and minimize soft tissue damage.

INDICATIONS

- Shortens the second stage of labor
- Facilitates forceps-assisted or vacuum-assisted birth
- Prevents cerebral hemorrhage in a fragile preterm fetus
- Facilitates birth of a macrosomic (large) infant

CONSIDERATIONS

The site and direction of the incision designates the type of episiotomy.

- A median (midline) episiotomy extends from the vaginal outlet toward the rectum, and is the most commonly used.
  - Effective
  - Easily repaired
  - Generally least painful
  - Associated with a higher incidence of third- and fourth-degree lacerations
- A **mediolateral episiotomy** extends from the vaginal outlet posterolateral, either to the left or right of the midline, and is used when posterior extension is likely.
  - Third-degree laceration can occur.
  - Blood loss is greater, and the repair is more difficult and painful.

ONGOING CARE: Encourage alternate labor positions to reduce pressure on the perineum and promote perineal stretching to reduce the necessity for an episiotomy.

Cesarean birth

- A cesarean birth is the delivery of the fetus through a transabdominal incision of the uterus to preserve the life or health of the client and fetus when there is evidence of complications.
- Incisions are made vertically and horizontally into the lower segment of the uterus. Horizontal is the optimal incision.

INDICATIONS

POTENTIAL DIAGNOSES

- Malpresentation, particularly breech presentation
- Cephalopelvic disproportion
- Nonreassuring fetal status
- Placental abnormalities
- Placenta previa
- Abruptio placentae
- High-risk pregnancy
  - Positive HIV status
  - Hypertensive disorders (preeclampsia, eclampsia)
  - Diabetes mellitus
  - Active genital herpes lesions
- Previous cesarean birth
- Dystocia
- Multiple gestations
- Umbilical cord prolapse
- Congenital malformations
- Maternal cardiac or respiratory disease

CONSIDERATIONS

PREPROCEDURE

NURSING ACTIONS
- Monitor and record FHR and vital signs.
- Insert an indwelling urinary catheter.
- Ensure the client has signed the informed consent form.
- Apply a sequential compression device.
- Assist with the administration of preoperative medications.
- Assist with preparing the surgical site.
- Insert an IV catheter, and assist with the initiation of the administration of IV fluids.
- Determine whether the client has had nothing by mouth since midnight before the procedure. If the client has, notify the anesthesiologist.
- Reinforce the procedure to the client and their partner and provide emotional support.

POSTPROCEDURE

- Monitor for evidence of infection and excessive bleeding at the incision site.
- Check the uterine fundus for firmness or tenderness.
- Check the lochia for amount and characteristics.

> A tender uterus and foul-smelling lochia can indicate endometritis.

- Monitor for productive cough or chills, which could be a manifestation of pneumonia.
- Check for indications of thrombophlebitis, which include tenderness, pain, and heat on palpation.
- Monitor I&O.
- Monitor vital signs per protocol.
- Provide pain relief and antiemetics as prescribed.
- Encourage the client to turn, cough, and deeply breathe to prevent pulmonary complications.
- Encourage splinting of the incision with pillows.
- Encourage ambulation to prevent thrombus formation.
- Monitor the client for burning and pain on urination, which could be suggestive of a urinary tract infection.

COMPLICATIONS

MATERNAL
- Aspiration
- Amniotic fluid pulmonary embolism
- Wound infection
- Wound dehiscence
- Severe abdominal pain
- Thrombophlebitis
- Hemorrhage
- Urinary tract infection
- Injuries to the bladder or bowel
- Anesthesia-associated complications

FETAL
- Premature birth of fetus if gestational age is inaccurate
- Fetal injuries during surgery

Vaginal birth after cesarean (VBAC)

A vaginal birth after cesarean birth is when the client delivers vaginally after having had a previous cesarean birth.

INDICATIONS

CLIENT PRESENTATION: Selection criteria for VBAC
- No other uterine scars or history of previous rupture
- One or two previous low transverse cesarean births
- Clinically adequate pelvis
- Clients who have had a prior cesarean for dysfunctional labor, breech presentation, or abnormal FHR pattern, which are considered nonrecurring events
- Providers immediately available throughout active labor capable of monitoring labor and performing an emergency cesarean birth if necessary
- No current contraindications
  - Large-for-gestational-age newborn
  - Malpresentation
  - Cephalopelvic disproportion
  - Previous classical vertical uterine incision

CONSIDERATIONS

PREPROCEDURE

NURSING ACTIONS
- Review medical records for evidence of a previous low-segment transverse cesarean incision.
- Reinforce the procedure to the client and their partner.

POSTPROCEDURE

Nursing interventions for a vaginal delivery after a cesarean birth are the same as for a vaginal birth.

Complications related to the labor process

Complications occurring during the labor process are emergent and require immediate intervention in order to improve maternal fetal outcomes.

Prolapsed umbilical cord

A prolapsed umbilical cord occurs when the umbilical cord is displaced, preceding the presenting part of the fetus, or protruding through the cervix. This results in cord compression and compromised fetal circulation.

DATA COLLECTION

RISK FACTORS

- Rupture of amniotic membranes
- Abnormal fetal presentation (any presentation other than vertex [occiput as presenting part])
- Transverse lie: Presenting part is not engaged, which leaves room for the cord to descend.
- Small-for-gestational-age fetus
- Unusually long umbilical cord
- Multifetal pregnancy
- Unengaged presenting part
- Polyhydramnios

EXPECTED FINDINGS

Client reports the feeling of something coming through the vagina.

PHYSICAL FINDINGS

- Visualization or palpation of the umbilical cord protruding from the introitus
- FHR monitoring shows variable or prolonged deceleration
- Excessive fetal activity followed by cessation of movement; suggestive of severe fetal hypoxia

PATIENT-CENTERED CARE

NURSING CARE

- Call for assistance immediately.
- Notify the provider.
- The provider or RN will use a sterile-gloved hand, insert two fingers into the vagina, and apply finger pressure on either side of the cord to the fetal presenting part to elevate it off of the cord.
- Reposition the client in a knee-chest, Trendelenburg, or a modified lateral semi-prone recumbent position with a rolled towel under the client's right or left hip to relieve pressure on the cord.
- Apply a warm, sterile, saline-soaked towel to the visible cord to prevent drying and to maintain blood flow.
- Provide continuous electronic monitoring of FHR for variable decelerations, which indicate fetal asphyxia and hypoxia.
- Administer oxygen at 10 L/min via nonrebreather mask to improve fetal oxygenation.
- Assist in initiating IV access and administering IV fluid bolus.
- Prepare for an immediate vaginal birth if cervix is fully dilated or cesarean section if it is not.
- Reinforce to the client and support person about the interventions.

Meconium-stained amniotic fluid

- Meconium passage in the amniotic fluid during the antepartum period prior to the start of labor is typically not associated with an unfavorable fetal outcome.
- The fetus has had an episode of loss of sphincter control, allowing meconium to pass into amniotic fluid.

DATA COLLECTION

RISK FACTORS

- There is an increased incidence for meconium in the amniotic fluid after 38 weeks of gestation due to fetal maturity of normal physiological functions.
- Umbilical cord compression results in fetal hypoxia that stimulates the vagal nerve.
- Hypoxia stimulates the vagal nerve, which induces peristalsis of the fetal gastrointestinal tract and relaxation of the anal sphincter.

EXPECTED FINDINGS

PHYSICAL FINDINGS

- Amniotic fluid can vary in color (black to greenish, yellow, or brown), though meconium-stained amniotic fluid is often green. Consistency can be thin or thick.
- Criteria for evaluation of meconium-stained amniotic fluid
  - Often present in breech presentation and might not indicate fetal hypoxia
  - Present with no changes in FHR
  - Stained fluid accompanied by variable or late decelerations in FHR (ominous sign)

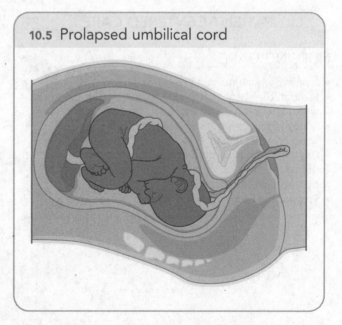

10.5 Prolapsed umbilical cord

DIAGNOSTIC PROCEDURES

Electronic fetal monitoring

PATIENT-CENTERED CARE

NURSING CARE

- Note and report color and consistency of stained amniotic fluid.
- Notify neonatal resuscitation team to be present at birth.
- Nonreassuring fetal status
- Fetal distress is present when:
  - FHR is below 110/min or above 160/min.
  - FHR shows decreased or no variability.
  - There is fetal hyperactivity or no fetal activity.

DATA COLLECTION

RISK FACTORS

- Fetal anomalies
- Uterine anomalies
- Complications of labor and birth

EXPECTED FINDINGS

Nonreassuring FHR pattern with decreased or no variability

DIAGNOSTIC PROCEDURES

- Monitor uterine contractions.
- Monitor FHR.
- Monitor findings of ultrasound and other diagnostics.

PATIENT-CENTERED CARE

NURSING CARE

- Monitor vital signs and FHR.
- Position the client in a left side–lying reclining position with legs elevated.
- Administer 8 to 10 L/min of oxygen via nonrebreather mask.
- Oxytocin should be discontinued.
- Prepare to assist with increasing IV fluid rate to treat hypotension if indicated.
- Prepare the client for an emergency cesarean birth.

Active Learning Scenario Key

Using the ATI Active Learning Template: Therapeutic Procedure

DESCRIPTION OF PROCEDURE: Delivery of the fetus through a transabdominal incision of the uterus to preserve the life or health of the client and fetus when there is evidence of complications; incisions are made vertically and horizontally into the lower segment of the uterus, with horizontally being the optimal incision

INDICATIONS
- Malpresentation, breech
- Cephalopelvic disproportion
- Nonreassuring fetal status
- Placenta previa
- Abruptio placentae
- HIV-positive status
- Dystocia
- Multiple gestations
- Umbilical cord prolapse
- Preeclampsia
- Eclampsia
- Active herpes lesions
- Previous cesarean birth

NURSING INTERVENTIONS
- Monitor FHR, vital signs.
- Position client in a supine position with a wedge under one hip.
- Insert an indwelling urinary catheter.
- Assist with administering preoperative medications.
- Insert an IV catheter, and assist with administering IV fluids.
- Ensure that the informed consent form is signed.
- Determine client's NPO status.
- Review preoperative testing results.
- Provide emotional support.

POTENTIAL COMPLICATIONS

Maternal
- Aspiration
- Amniotic fluid pulmonary embolism
- Wound infection
- Wound dehiscence
- Severe abdominal pain
- Thrombophlebitis
- Hemorrhage
- Urinary tract infection
- Injury to bladder or bowel
- Anesthesia-associated complications

Fetal
- Premature birth
- Fetal injury during surgery

Ⓝ *NCLEX® Connection: Reduction of Risk Potential, Therapeutic Procedures*

Active Learning Scenario

A nurse is planning care for a client who experienced a cesarean birth. What should the nurse include in the plan of care? Use the ATI Active Learning Template: Therapeutic Procedure to complete this item.

DESCRIPTION OF PROCEDURE: Describe the procedure.

INDICATIONS: Describe at least four.

NURSING INTERVENTIONS: Describe four that are preprocedure.

POTENTIAL COMPLICATIONS: Describe two that are maternal and two that are fetal.

Application Exercises

1. A nurse is assisting with the care of a client who is at 40 weeks of gestation and reports having a large gush of fluid from the vagina while walking from the bathroom. Which of the following actions should the nurse take first?

   A. Examine the amniotic fluid for meconium.

   B. Check the FHR.

   C. Dry the client and make them comfortable.

   D. Apply a tocotransducer.

2. A client calls a provider's office and reports having contractions for 2 hr that increased with activity and did not decrease with rest and hydration. The client denies leaking of vaginal fluid but did notice blood when wiping after voiding. Which of the following manifestations is the client experiencing?

   A. Braxton Hicks contractions

   B. Rupture of membranes

   C. Fetal descent

   D. True contractions

3. A nurse is teaching a client about the difference between true and false labor. Sort the following characteristics into true labor or false labor.

   A. Walking can increase the contraction intensity.

   B. Bloody show

   C. Contractions felt in the low back

   D. Cervix remains in the posterior position.

4. A nurse is assisting with the care for a client who is at 40 weeks of gestation and experiencing contractions every 3 to 5 min and becoming stronger. A vaginal exam by the registered nurse reveals that the client's cervix is 3 cm dilated, 80% effaced, and -1 station. The client asks for pain medication. Which of the following actions should the nurse prepare to take?

   A. Encourage use of patterned breathing techniques.

   B. Insert an indwelling urinary catheter.

   C. Administer opioid analgesic medication.

   D. Suggest application of cold.

   E. Provide ice chips.

5. A nurse is assisting with the care for a client who is at 42 weeks of gestation and is having an ultrasound. For which of the following conditions should the nurse prepare for an amnioinfusion?

   A. Oligohydramnios

   B. Hydramnios

   C. Fetal cord compression

   D. Hydration

   E. Fetal immaturity

6. A nurse is reinforcing teaching about an episiotomy with a client who is in labor. Which of the following information should the nurse include?

   A. An episiotomy is a perineal tear that is created while pushing during labor.

   B. A fourth-degree episiotomy extends into the rectal area.

   C. An episiotomy is an incision that is made by the provider to facilitate birth of the fetus.

   D. A mediolateral episiotomy is easier to repair than a median episiotomy.

7. A nurse is assisting with the care of a client in active labor. The nurse observes clear fluid and a loop of pulsating umbilical cord outside the client's vagina. Which of the following actions should the nurse perform first?

   A. Place the client in the Trendelenburg position.

   B. Apply finger pressure to the presenting part.

   C. Administer oxygen at 10 L/min via a nonrebreather.

   D. Call for assistance.

Application Exercises Key

1. B. **CORRECT:** The greatest risk to the client and fetus is umbilical cord prolapse, leading to fetal distress following rupture of membranes. The first action to take is to check the FHR for clinical findings of distress. Check the color, clarity, odor, and amount of amniotic fluid, but this is not the first action to take. Provide comfort by drying the client following rupture of the membranes, but this is not the first action to take. Apply a tocotransducer to the client's uterine contraction pattern after rupture of the membranes, but this is not the first action to take.

   Ⓝ *NCLEX® Connection: Health Promotion and Maintenance, Ante-/Intra-/Postpartum and Newborn*

2. D. **CORRECT:** The nurse should recognize the client is reporting true contractions, which do not go away with hydration or walking. They are regular in frequency, duration, and intensity and become stronger with walking. Braxton Hicks contractions decrease with hydration and walking. Rupture of membranes would be indicated by the presence of a gush of fluid that is unrelated to the client's activity. Fetal descent is the downward movement of the fetus in the birth canal and cannot be evaluated based on the client's report.

   Ⓝ *NCLEX® Connection: Health Promotion and Maintenance, Ante-/Intra-/Postpartum and Newborn*

3. **TRUE LABOR:** A, B; **FALSE LABOR:** C, D

   The nurse should include manifestations of true labor, which includes walking, which can increase the intensity of the contractions, and bloody show can occur. Also, contractions felt in the low back and a cervix that remains in the posterior position are findings of false labor.

   Ⓝ *NCLEX® Connection: Health Promotion and Maintenance, Ante-/Intra-/Postpartum and Newborn*

4. A, C, D. **CORRECT:** The nurse should take the following actions when the client is requesting pain medication during labor. The use of patterned breathing techniques can assist with pain management at this time. Administer an opioid analgesic. Also, the use of a nonpharmacological approach, such as the application of cold, is an appropriate intervention at this time. However, there is no indication for the insertion of an indwelling urinary catheter at this time. Also, providing ice chips does not address the client's request for assistance with pain management.

   Ⓝ *NCLEX® Connection: Basic Care and Comfort, Nonpharmacological Comfort Interventions*

5. A, C. **CORRECT:** The nurse recognizes that an amnioinfusion should be prepared for clients who have the following. Oligohydramnios is an indication for an amnioinfusion because inadequate amniotic fluid can contribute to intrauterine growth restriction of the fetus, restrict fetal movement, and cause fetal distress during labor. Oligohydramnios results in fetal cord compression, which decreases fetal oxygenation. Amnioinfusion prevents cord compression. Hydramnios is excessive amniotic fluid. Amnioinfusion does not increase hydration. IV fluids or oral intake would provide hydration. Fetal immaturity is not a reason for performing an amnioinfusion.

   Ⓝ *NCLEX® Connection: Physiological Adaptation, Unexpected Response to Therapies*

6. C. **CORRECT:** A laceration is a perineal tear that can occur during labor while pushing. A fourth-degree laceration extends into the rectal area. An episiotomy is an incision that is made by the provider during labor to facilitate the delivery of the fetus. A median episiotomy is easier to repair than a mediolateral episiotomy because it is most commonly used and less invasive.

   Ⓝ *NCLEX® Connection: Physiological Adaption, Alterations in Body Systems*

7. D. **CORRECT:** The nurse should place the client in the Trendelenburg position. However, another action is the priority. The nurse should apply pressure to the presenting part with their fingers. However, another action is the priority. The nurse should administer oxygen at 10 L/min via a face mask. However, another action is the priority. According to evidence-based practice, the nurse should first call for assistance

   Ⓝ *NCLEX® Connection: Physiological Adaptation, Unexpected Response to Therapies*

UNIT 2 **INTRAPARTUM NURSING CARE**
SECTION: LABOR AND DELIVERY

CHAPTER 11 ## *Fetal Monitoring During Labor*

The diagnostic procedures mentioned in this chapter include Leopold maneuvers and fetal heart rate (FHR) pattern and uterine contraction monitoring.

Leopold maneuvers

Leopold maneuvers consist of performing external palpations of the maternal uterus through the abdominal wall to determine the following.
- Presenting part, fetal lie, and fetal attitude
- Degree of descent of the presenting part into the pelvis
- Location of the fetus's back to monitor for fetal heart tones
  - **Vertex presentation:** Fetal heart tones should be monitored below the client's umbilicus in either the right- or left-lower quadrant of the abdomen.
  - **Breech presentation:** Fetal heart tones should be monitored above the client's umbilicus in either the right- or left-upper quadrant of the abdomen.

CONSIDERATIONS

PREPARATION OF THE CLIENT
- Ask the client to empty the bladder prior to collecting data.
- Place the client in the supine position with a pillow under the head, and have both knees slightly flexed.
- Place a small, rolled towel under the client's right or left hip to displace the uterus off the major blood vessels to prevent supine hypotensive syndrome.

ONGOING CARE
- Identify the fetal part occupying the fundus. The head should feel round, firm, and move freely. The breech should feel irregular and soft. This maneuver identifies the fetal lie (longitudinal or transverse) and presenting part (cephalic or breech).
- Locate and palpate the smooth contour of the fetal back using the palm of one hand and the irregular small parts of the hands, feet, and elbows using the palm of the other hand. This maneuver validates the presenting part.

- Determine the part that is presenting over the true pelvic inlet by gently grasping the lower segment of the uterus between the thumb and fingers. If the head is presenting and not engaged, determine whether the head is flexed or extended. This maneuver assists in identifying the descent of the presenting part into the pelvis.
- Face the client's feet, and outline the fetal head using the palmar surface of the fingertips on both hands to palpate the cephalic prominence. If the cephalic prominence is on the same side as the small parts, the head is flexed with vertex presentation. If the cephalic prominence is on the same side as the back, the head is extended with a face presentation. This maneuver identifies the fetal attitude.

INTERVENTIONS
- Auscultate the FHR post-maneuvers to determine fetal tolerance to the procedure.
- Document the findings from the maneuvers.

Intermittent auscultation and uterine contraction palpation

Intermittent auscultation of the FHR is a low-technology method that can be performed during labor using a handheld Doppler ultrasound device, ultrasound stethoscope, or fetoscope to monitor FHR. In conjunction, palpation of contractions at the fundus for frequency, intensity, duration, and resting tone is used to evaluate fetal well-being. During labor, uterine contractions compress the uteroplacental arteries, temporarily stopping maternal blood flow into the uterus and intervillous spaces of the placenta, decreasing fetal circulation and oxygenation. Circulation to the uterus and placenta resumes during uterine relaxation between contractions. For low-risk labor and delivery, this procedure allows the client freedom of movement and can be done at home or a birthing center.

Guidelines for intermittent auscultation or continuous electronic fetal monitoring
- During latent phase: < 4 cm at least hourly, (4 to 5 cm) every 15 to 30 min
- During active phase: every 15 to 30 min
- During second stage: every 5 to 15 min

INDICATIONS

- Determine active labor
- Rupture of membranes, spontaneously or artificially
- Preceding and subsequent to ambulation
- Prior to and following administration of or a change in medication analgesia
- At peak action of anesthesia
- Following vaginal examination
- Following expulsion of an enema
- After urinary catheterization
- Abnormal or excessive uterine contractions

CONSIDERATIONS

PREPARATION OF THE CLIENT

- Based on findings obtained using Leopold maneuvers, auscultate the FHR using a listening device.
- Palpate the uterine fundus to monitor uterine activity.
- Count FHR for 30 to 60 seconds between contractions to determine baseline rate.
- Auscultate FHR before, during, and after a contraction to determine FHR in response to the contractions.

ONGOING CARE: Identify FHR patterns and characteristics of uterine contractions.

INTERVENTIONS

- Monitor FHR patterns and characteristics of uterine contractions, assist with performing nursing interventions, and report nonreassuring patterns or abnormal uterine contractions to the registered nurse or provider.
- Cultural considerations, as well as the emotional, educational, and comfort needs of the client and the family must be considered for the plan of care while continuing to monitor the FHR pattern's response to uterine contractions during the labor process. **Q**PCC

> The method and frequency of fetal surveillance during labor will vary and depend on maternal/fetal risk factors, as well as the preference of the facility, provider, and client.

INTERPRETATION OF FINDINGS

- A normal, reassuring FHR is 110 to 160/min with increases and decreases from baseline.
- Tachycardia is a FHR greater than 160/min for 10 min or longer.
- Bradycardia is a FHR less than 110/min for 10 min or longer.

Continuous electronic fetal monitoring

Continuous external fetal monitoring is accomplished by securing an ultrasound transducer over the client's abdomen, which records the FHR pattern, and a tocotransducer on the fundus that records the uterine contractions.

ADVANTAGES

- Monitoring is noninvasive and reduces risk for infection.
- Membranes do not have to be ruptured.
- Cervix does not have to be dilated.
- Placement of transducers can be performed by the nurse.
- Provides permanent record of FHR and uterine contraction tracing

DISADVANTAGES

- Contraction intensity is not measurable.
- Movement of the client requires frequent repositioning of transducers.
- Quality of recording is affected by client obesity and fetal position.

INDICATIONS

- Multiple gestations
- Oxytocin infusion (augmentation or induction of labor)
- Placenta previa
- Fetal bradycardia
- Maternal complications (gestational diabetes mellitus, gestational hypertension, kidney disease)
- Intrauterine growth restriction
- Post-date gestation
- Active labor
- Meconium-stained amniotic fluid
- Abruptio placentae: suspected or actual
- Abnormal nonstress test or contraction stress test
- Abnormal uterine contractions

NONREASSURING FETAL STATUS

PREPARATION OF THE CLIENT

- Based on findings obtained using Leopold maneuvers, auscultate FHR using a listening device.
- Palpate the fundus to identify uterine activity for proper placement of the tocotransducer to monitor uterine contractions.

ONGOING CARE

- Reinforce education regarding the procedure to the client and the client's partner during placement and adjustments of the fetal monitor equipment. Client and family reinforcement of teaching is important when an electronic fetal monitor is used. Reinforce the purpose and reassure that use of monitoring does not necessarily imply fetal jeopardy.
- Encourage frequent maternal position changes, which can require adjustments of the transducers with position changes.
- If the client needs to void and can ambulate, and if it is not contraindicated, the nurse can disconnect the external monitor for the client to use the bathroom.
- If disconnecting the FHR monitor is contraindicated or an internal FHR monitor is being used, the nurse can bring the client a bedpan.

INTERPRETATION OF FINDINGS

- A normal fetal heart rate baseline at term is 110 to 160/min, excluding accelerations, decelerations, and periods of marked variability within a 10-min window. At least 2 min of baseline segments in a 10-min window should be present. A single number should be documented instead of a baseline range.
- Fetal heart rate baseline variability is described as fluctuations in the FHR baseline that are irregular in frequency and amplitude. Expected variability should be moderate variability. Classification of variability is as follows.
  - Absent or undetectable variability (considered nonreassuring)
  - Minimal variability (detectable but equal to or less than 5/min)
  - Moderate variability (6 to 25/min)
  - Marked variability (greater than 25/min)
- Changes in fetal heart rate patterns are categorized as episodic or periodic changes. Episodic changes are not associated with uterine contractions, and periodic changes occur with uterine contractions. These changes include accelerations and decelerations.

THREE-TIER SYSTEM

Current recommendations for fetal monitoring include a three-tier fetal heart rate interpretation system.

Category I

All of the following are included in the fetal heart rate tracing.
- Baseline fetal heart rate of 110 to 160/min
- Baseline fetal heart rate variability: moderate
- Accelerations: present or absent
- Early decelerations: present or absent
- Variable or late decelerations: absent

Category II

Category II tracings include all fetal heart rate tracings not categorized as Category I or Category III. Examples of Category II fetal heart rate tracings contain any of the following.

Baseline rate
- Tachycardia
- Bradycardia not accompanied by absent baseline variability

Baseline FHR variability
- Minimal baseline variability
- Absent baseline variability not accompanied by recurrent decelerations
- Marked baseline variability

Episodic or periodic decelerations
- Prolonged fetal heart rate deceleration equal or greater than 2 min but less than 10 min
- Recurrent late decelerations with moderate baseline variability
- Recurrent variable decelerations with minimal or moderate baseline variability
- Variable decelerations with additional characteristics, including "overshoots," "shoulders," or slow return to baseline fetal heart rate

Accelerations: Absence of induced accelerations after fetal stimulation

Category III

Category III fetal heart rate tracings include either:
- Sinusoidal pattern
- Absent baseline fetal heart rate variability and any of the following
  - Recurrent variable decelerations
  - Recurrent late decelerations
  - Bradycardia

Each uterine contraction is comprised of the following.
- **Increment:** the beginning of the contraction as intensity is increasing
- **Acme:** the peak intensity of the contraction
- **Decrement:** the decline of the contraction intensity as the contraction is ending

Nonreassuring FHR patterns are associated with fetal hypoxia and include the following.
- Fetal bradycardia
- Fetal tachycardia
- Absence of FHR variability
- Late decelerations
- Variable decelerations

FHR PATTERNS

Accelerations

Variable transitory increase in the FHR above baseline

CAUSES/COMPLICATIONS
- Healthy fetal/placental exchange
- Spontaneous fetal movement
- Vaginal exam
- Uterine contractions
- Fetal scalp stimulation
- Vibroacoustic stimulation
- Fundal pressure

NURSING INTERVENTIONS
- Be reassuring.
- No interventions required
- Indicate reactive nonstress test.

Fetal bradycardia

FHR less than 110/min for 10 min or more

CAUSES/COMPLICATIONS
- Uteroplacental insufficiency
- Umbilical cord prolapse
- Maternal hypotension
- Prolonged umbilical cord compression
- Fetal congenital heart block
- Anesthetic medications
- Viral infection
- Maternal hypoglycemia
- Fetal heart failure
- Maternal hypothermia

NURSING INTERVENTIONS
- Correct the underlying cause.
- Discontinue oxytocin if being administered.
- Assist the client to a side-lying position.
- Administer oxygen by mask at 10 L/min via nonrebreather face mask.
- Insert an IV catheter if one is not in place and assist with administering maintenance IV fluids.
- Assist with administering a tocolytic medication.
- Notify the provider.

Fetal tachycardia

FHR greater than 160/min for 10 min or more

CAUSES/COMPLICATIONS
- Maternal infection, chorioamnionitis
- Fetal anemia
- Fetal cardiac dysrhythmias
- Maternal use of caffeine or methamphetamines
- Maternal dehydration
- Maternal or fetal infection
- Maternal fever
- Maternal hyperthyroidism

11.1 Early decelerations

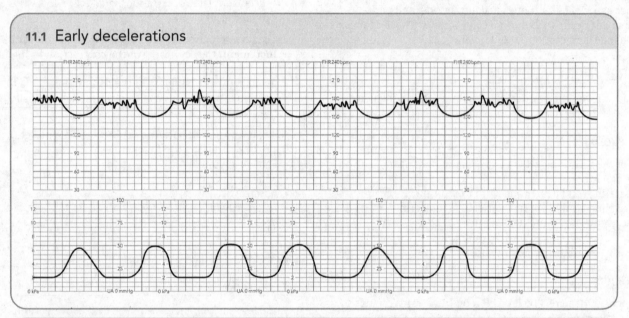

11.2 Late decelerations

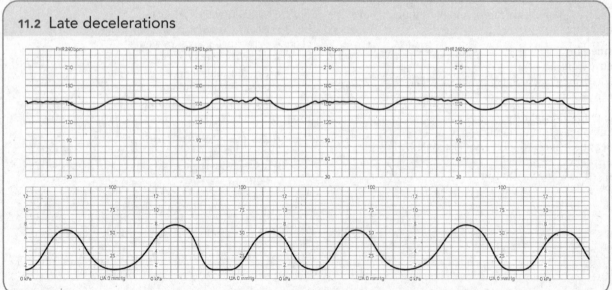

NURSING INTERVENTIONS

- Administer prescribed antipyretics for maternal fever, if present.
- Administer oxygen by mask at 10 L/min via nonrebreather face mask.
- Assist with administering IV fluid bolus.

Decrease or loss of FHR variability

Decrease or loss of irregular fluctuations in the baseline of the FHR

CAUSES/COMPLICATIONS

- Medications that depress the CNS (barbiturates, tranquilizers, general anesthetics)
- Fetal hypoxemia and metabolic acidemia
- Fetal sleep cycle (Minimal variability sleep cycles usually do not last longer than 30 min.)
- Congenital abnormalities

NURSING INTERVENTIONS

- Stimulation of the fetal scalp by the RN or provider
- Application of scalp electrode by provider
- Place client in left–lateral position.

Early deceleration of FHR

Slowing of FHR at the start of contraction with return of FHR to baseline at end of contraction

CAUSES/COMPLICATIONS

- Compression of the fetal head resulting from:
- Uterine contractions
- Vaginal exam
- Fundal pressure
- Placement of internal monitoring

NURSING INTERVENTIONS: No intervention required

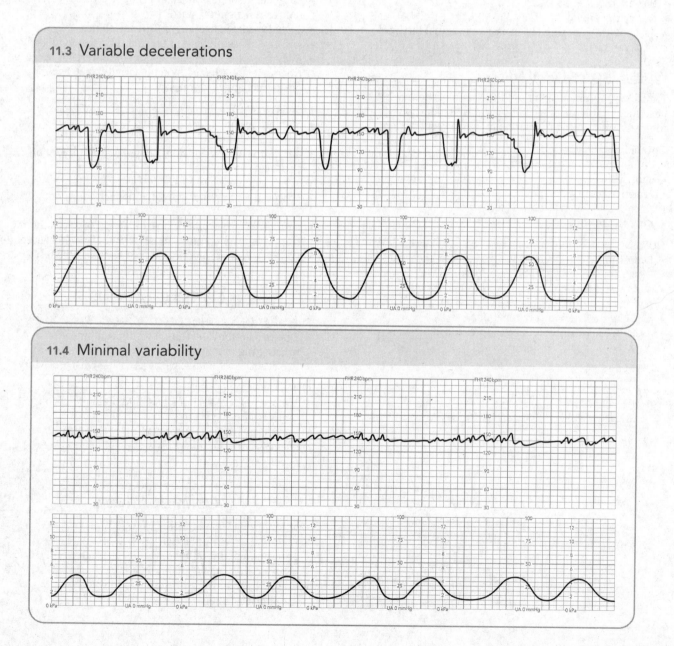

11.3 Variable decelerations

11.4 Minimal variability

Late deceleration of FHR

Slowing of FHR after contraction has started with return of FHR to baseline well after contraction has ended

CAUSES/COMPLICATIONS
- Uteroplacental insufficiency, causing inadequate fetal oxygenation
- Maternal hypotension, placenta previa, abruptio placentae, uterine tachysystole with oxytocin
- Preeclampsia
- Late- or post-term pregnancy
- Maternal diabetes mellitus

NURSING INTERVENTIONS
- Place client in side-lying position.
- Insert an IV catheter, if not in place, and increase rate of IV fluid administration.
- Discontinue oxytocin if being infused.
- Administer oxygen by mask at 10 L/min via nonrebreather face mask.
- Elevate the client's legs.
- Notify the provider.
- Assist with preparing for an assisted vaginal birth or cesarean birth.

Variable deceleration of FHR

Transitory, abrupt slowing of FHR 15/min or more below baseline for at least 15 seconds, variable in duration, intensity, and timing in relation to uterine contraction

CAUSES/COMPLICATIONS
- Umbilical cord compression
- Short cord
- Prolapsed cord
- Nuchal cord (such as around fetal neck)
- Knot in the cord

NURSING INTERVENTIONS
- Reposition client from side to side or into knee-chest.
- Discontinue oxytocin if being infused.
- Administer oxygen by mask at 10 to 15 L/min via nonrebreather face mask.
- Assist with a vaginal examination.
- Assist with an amnioinfusion if prescribed.

Continuous internal fetal monitoring

Continuous internal fetal monitoring with a scalp electrode is performed by attaching a small spiral electrode to the presenting part of the fetus to monitor the FHR. The electrode wires are then attached to a leg plate that is placed on the client's thigh and then attached to the fetal monitor.

INDICATIONS

Continuous internal fetal monitoring can be used in conjunction with an intrauterine pressure catheter (IUPC), which is a solid or fluid-filled transducer placed inside the client's uterine cavity to monitor the frequency, duration, and intensity of contractions.

ADVANTAGES
- Early detection of abnormal FHR patterns suggestive of nonreassuring fetal status
- Accurate data collection of FHR variability
- Accurate measurement of uterine contraction intensity
- Allows greater maternal freedom of movement because tracing is not affected by fetal activity, maternal position changes, or obesity

DISADVANTAGES
- Membranes must have ruptured to use internal monitoring.
- Cervix must be adequately dilated to a minimum of 2 to 3 cm.
- Presenting part must have descended to place electrode.
- Potential risk of injury to fetus if electrode is not properly applied
- A provider, nurse practitioner/midwife, or specially trained registered nurse must perform this procedure.
- Potential risk of infection to the client and the fetus

CONSIDERATIONS

PREPARATION OF THE CLIENT
- Ensure electronic fetal monitoring equipment is functioning properly.
- Use aseptic techniques when assisting with procedures.

ONGOING CARE
- Monitor maternal vital signs, and obtain maternal temperature every 1 to 2 hr.
- Encourage frequent repositioning of the client. If the client is lying supine, place a wedge under one of the client's hips to tilt the uterus.

COMPLICATIONS

- Misinterpretation of FHR patterns
- Maternal or fetal infection
- Fetal trauma if fetal monitoring electrode or IUPC are inserted into the vagina improperly
- Supine hypotension secondary to internal monitor placement

Application Exercises

1. A nurse is assisting with performing Leopold maneuvers on a client who is in labor. Which of the following techniques should the nurse use to identify the fetal lie?

   A. Apply palms of both hands to sides of uterus.

   B. Palpate the fundus of the uterus.

   C. Grasp lower uterine segment between thumb and fingers.

   D. Stand facing client's feet with fingertips outlining cephalic prominence.

2. A nurse is discussing intermittent fetal heart monitoring with a newly licensed nurse. Which of the following statements should the nurse include?

   A. "Count the fetal heart rate for 15 seconds to determine the baseline."

   B. "Auscultate the fetal heart rate every 5 minutes during the active phase of the first stage of labor."

   C. "Count the fetal heart rate after a contraction to determine baseline changes."

   D. "Auscultate the fetal heart rate every 30 minutes during the second stage of labor."

3. A nurse is assisting in the care of a client who is in active labor. The nurse notes tachycardia on the external fetal monitor tracing. Which of the following conditions should the nurse identify as a potential cause of the heart rate?

   A. Maternal fever

   B. Fetal heart failure

   C. Maternal hypoglycemia

   D. Fetal head compression

4. A nurse is assisting with caring for a client who is in labor and observes late decelerations on the electronic fetal monitor. Which of the following is the first action the nurse should identify that the registered nurse should take?

   A. Assist the client into the left-lateral position.

   B. Apply a fetal scalp electrode.

   C. Insert an IV catheter.

   D. Perform a vaginal exam.

5. A nurse is reinforcing teaching with a client about the benefits of internal fetal heart monitoring. Which of the following statements should the nurse include?

   A. "It is considered a noninvasive procedure."

   B. "It can detect abnormal fetal heart tones early."

   C. "It can determine the amount of amniotic fluid you have."

   D. "It allows for accurate readings with maternal movement."

   E. "It can measure uterine contraction intensity."

Active Learning Scenario

A nurse is assisting a nurse in labor and delivery with an in-service about intermittent fetal auscultation and uterine contraction palpation. What information should the nurse plan to include? Use the ATI Active Learning Template: Therapeutic Procedure to complete this item.

INDICATIONS: Describe four situations when this procedure should be performed.

OUTCOMES/EVALUATION: Describe normal, expected FHR findings.

NURSING INTERVENTIONS

• Preprocedure: Describe the three types of devices that are used to auscultate FHR.

• Intraprocedure: Identify the time frame for counting FHR to determine the baseline rate and when auscultation should take place.

Active Learning Scenario Key

Using the ATI Active Learning Template: Therapeutic Procedure

INDICATIONS
- Determine active labor
- Rupture of membranes, spontaneously or artificially
- Preceding and subsequent to ambulation
- Prior to and following administration of or a change in medication analgesia
- At the peak action of anesthesia
- Following vaginal examination
- Following expulsion of an enema
- After urinary catheterization
- Abnormal or excessive uterine contractions

OUTCOMES/EVALUATION: A normal, reassuring FHR is 110 to 160/min with increases and decreases from baseline.

NURSING INTERVENTIONS

Preprocedure
- Handheld Doppler ultrasound
- Ultrasound stethoscope
- Fetoscope

Intraprocedure
- Count FHR for 30 to 60 seconds between contractions to determine baseline rate.
- Auscultate FHR before, during, and after a contraction to determine FHR in response to the contractions.

Ⓝ *NCLEX® Connection: Health Promotion and Maintenance, Ante-/ Intra-/Postpartum and Newborn Care*

Application Exercises Key

1. B. **CORRECT:** Palpating the fundus of the uterus identifies the fetal part that is present, indicating the fetal lie (longitudinal or transverse).

   Ⓝ *NCLEX® Connection: Health Promotion and Maintenance, Data Collection Techniques*

2. C. **CORRECT:** Count the FHR for 30 to 60 seconds to determine the baseline. Auscultate the FHR every 15 min during the active phase of the first stage of labor. Count the FHR after contractions to identify any changes from baseline. Auscultate the FHR every 5 to 15 min during the second stage of labor.

   Ⓝ *NCLEX® Connection: Health Promotion and Maintenance, Ante-/Intra-/Postpartum and Newborn Care*

3. A. **CORRECT:** Tachycardia can be caused by maternal fever, infection, and chorioamnionitis. Fetal heart failure can cause bradycardia in the FHR. Maternal hypoglycemia can cause bradycardia in the FHR. Fetal head compression can cause early decelerations in the FHR.

   Ⓝ *NCLEX® Connection: Physiological Adaptation, Alterations in Body Systems*

4. A. **CORRECT:** The greatest risk to the fetus during late decelerations is uteroplacental insufficiency. The initial nursing action should be to place the client into the left-lateral position to increase uteroplacental perfusion. The application of a fetal scalp electrode will assist in the assessment of fetal well-being, but this is not the first action to take. Inserting an IV catheter is an intervention for late decelerations, but this is not the first action to take. The nurse may perform a vaginal exam to assess dilation, but this is not the first action to take.

   Ⓝ *NCLEX® Connection: Health Promotion and Maintenance, Ante-/Intra-/Postpartum and Newborn Care*

5. B, D, E. **CORRECT:** A disadvantage of internal fetal monitoring is that it is an invasive procedure. A benefit of internal fetal monitoring is that it can detect abnormal fetal heart tones early. Internal fetal monitoring cannot determine the amount of amniotic fluid. A benefit of internal fetal monitoring is that it allows for accurate readings with maternal movement, which external monitoring needs adjusting when the client moves. A benefit of internal fetal monitoring is that it can measure uterine contraction intensity, which external monitoring cannot.

   Ⓝ *NCLEX® Connection: Reduction of Risk Potential, Diagnostic Tests*

When reviewing the following chapters, keep in mind the relevant topics and tasks of the NCLEX outline.

Health Promotion and Maintenance

ANTE-/INTRA-/POSTPARTUM AND NEWBORN CARE
Perform care of postpartum client.

Monitor recovery of stable postpartum client.

DATA COLLECTION TECHNIQUES: Collect baseline physical data.

DEVELOPMENTAL STAGES AND TRANSITIONS: Assist client with expected life transition.

Pharmacological Therapies

EXPECTED ACTIONS/OUTCOMES
Apply knowledge of pathophysiology when addressing client pharmacological agents.

Evaluate client response to medication.

REDUCTION OF RISK POTENTIAL: Check and monitor client vital signs.

Physiological Adaptation

ALTERATIONS IN BODY SYSTEMS
Identify signs and symptoms of an infection.

Provide care for a client experiencing complications of pregnancy/labor or delivery.

UNIT 3 POSTPARTUM NURSING CARE
SECTION: ROUTINE POSTPARTUM CARE

CHAPTER 12 *Nursing Care of the Client During the Postpartum Period*

It is important to provide comfort measures for the client during the fourth stage of labor. This recovery period starts with delivery of the placenta and includes at least the first 2 hr after birth. Also during this stage, parent-newborn bonding should begin to occur.

The main goal during the immediate postpartum period is to monitor for postpartum hemorrhage. Other goals include assisting in a client's recovery, recognizing and reporting deviations in the expected recovery process, providing comfort measures and pharmacological pain relief, reinforcing client education about newborn and self-care, and providing baby-friendly activities to promote infant/family bonding.

The reinforcement of discharge teaching is also an important aspect of postpartum care. A client should be able to perform self-care and recognize effects that suggest complications prior to discharge.

A nurse should use a variety of strategies to reinforce learning. Return demonstrations are important to ensure that adequate learning has taken place.

PHYSICAL CHANGES

The postpartum period, also known as the puerperium, includes physiological and psychological adjustments. This period is the interval between birth and the return of the reproductive organs to their nonpregnant state. Although traditionally this has been considered to last 6 weeks, this time frame varies among postpartum clients.

- Physiological changes consist of uterine involution; lochia flow; cervical involution; decrease in vaginal distention; alteration in ovarian function and menstruation; and cardiovascular, urinary tract, breast, and gastrointestinal tract changes.
- The greatest risks during the postpartum period are hemorrhage, shock, and infection.
- Oxytocin, a hormone released from the pituitary gland, coordinates and strengthens uterine contractions.
  - Breastfeeding stimulates the release of endogenous oxytocin from the pituitary gland.
  - Exogenous oxytocin can be administered postpartum to improve the quality of the uterine contractions. A firm and contracted uterus prevents excessive bleeding and hemorrhage.
  - Uncomfortable uterine cramping is referred to as afterpains.
- After delivery of the placenta, hormones (estrogen, progesterone, and placental enzyme insulinase) decrease, thus resulting in decreased blood glucose, estrogen, and progesterone levels.
  - Decreased estrogen is associated with breast engorgement, diaphoresis (profuse perspiration), and diuresis (increased formation and excretion of urine) of excess extracellular fluid accumulated during pregnancy.
  - Decreased estrogen diminishes vaginal lubrication. Local dryness and intercourse discomfort can persist until ovarian function returns and menstruation resumes.
  - Decreased progesterone results in an increase in muscle tone throughout the body.
  - Decreased placental enzyme insulinase results in reversal of the diabetogenic effects of pregnancy, which lowers blood glucose levels immediately in the puerperium.
  - Human chorionic gonadotropin (hCG) disappears from the blood quickly, but some can be detected for up to 4 weeks postpartum.
- Lactating and nonlactating clients differ in the timing of the first ovulation and the resumption of menstruation.
  - In lactating clients, the blood prolactin levels remain elevated and suppress ovulation.
    - The return of ovulation is influenced by breastfeeding frequency, the length of each feeding, and the use of supplementation.
    - The newborn's suck is also believed to affect prolactin levels.
    - Length of time to the first postpartum ovulation is approximately 6 months.
- In nonlactating clients, prolactin declines and reaches the prepregnant level by the third week postpartum.
  - Ovulation occurs 7 to 9 weeks after birth.
  - Menses resume by 12 weeks postpartum.

DATA COLLECTION

Data collection in the immediate postpartum period includes monitoring vital signs, uterine firmness and its location in relation to the umbilicus, uterine position in relation to the midline of the abdomen, and amount of vaginal bleeding.

American Academy of Pediatrics and American College of Obstetricians and Gynecologists recommends that blood pressure and pulse be checked at least every 15 min for the first 2 hr after birth. Temperature should be checked every 4 hr for the first 8 hr after birth and then at least every 8 hr.

Data collection for the postpartum client include checking the client's:
- **B: Breasts**
- **U: Uterus** (fundal height, uterine placement, and consistency)
- **B: Bowel** and GI function
- **B: Bladder** function
- **L: Lochia** (color, odor, consistency, and amount [COCA])
- **E: Episiotomy** (edema, ecchymosis, approximation)
- Vital signs, to include collecting data for pain
- Reinforcement of teaching needs

LABORATORY TESTS

- Can include urinalysis and CBC with monitoring of Hgb, Hct, and WBC and platelet counts.
- If the rubella and Rh status are unknown, tests should be performed to determine their status.

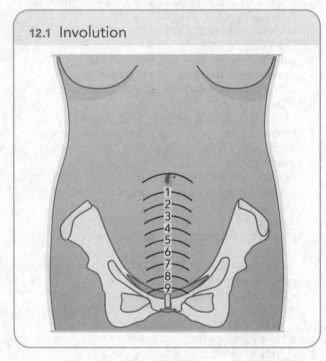

12.1 Involution

Uterus

Physical changes of the uterus include involution of the uterus. Involution occurs with contractions of the uterine smooth muscle, whereby the uterus returns to its prepregnant state. The uterus also rapidly decreases in size from approximately 1 kg (2.2 lb) at the end of the third stage of labor to 60 to 80 g at 6 weeks postpartum with the fundal height steadily descending into the pelvis approximately one fingerbreadth (1 cm) per day.
- Immediately after delivery, the fundus (top portion of the uterus) should be palpable firm at the midline and 2 cm below the umbilicus.
- 1 hour after delivery, the fundus will rise to the umbilicus; at 12 hr after delivery, the fundus can be palpated at 1 cm above the umbilicus.
- Every 24 hr, the fundus should descend approximately 1 to 2 cm. It should be halfway between the symphysis pubis and the umbilicus by the sixth postpartum day.
- After about 2 weeks, the uterus should lie within the true pelvis and should not be palpable.

DATA COLLECTION

The nurse should assist with determining the fundal height, uterine placement, and uterine consistency at least every 8 hr after the recovery period has ended.
- Explain the procedure to the client.
- Position the client supine with their knees slightly flexed so that the fundal height is not influenced by positioning.
- Apply clean gloves and a lower perineal pad, and observe lochia flow as the fundus is palpated.
- Cup one hand just above the symphysis pubis to support the lower segment of the uterus, and with the other hand, palpate the abdomen to locate the fundus. Never palpate the fundus without cupping the uterus.
- Document the fundal height, location, and uterine consistency.
  - Determine the fundal height by placing fingers on the abdomen and measuring how many fingerbreadths (centimeters) fit between the fundus and the umbilicus above, below, or at the umbilical level.
  - Determine whether the fundus is midline in the pelvis or displaced laterally (caused by a full bladder).
  - Determine whether the fundus is firm or boggy. If the fundus is boggy (not firm), lightly massage the fundus in a circular motion. ⓆEBP
  - If the uterus does not firm after massaging, keep massaging and notify the provider.
- Document the position and location of the uterus by the number of fingerbreadths and according to facility policy.
  - If above the umbilicus, document as +1, U+1, 1/U.
  - If below the umbilicus, document as −1, U−1, U/1.

PATIENT-CENTERED CARE

- Monitor for adverse effects of oxytocic medications.
  - Oxytocin and misoprostol can cause hypotension.
  - Methylergonovine, ergonovine, and carboprost can cause hypertension.
- Encourage early breastfeeding for a client who is lactating. This will stimulate the production of natural oxytocin and prevent hemorrhage.
- Encourage emptying of the bladder to prevent possible uterine displacement and loss of uterine muscle tone (atony).

Lochia

Lochia is post-birth uterine discharge that contains blood, mucus, and uterine tissue. The amount of lochia is similar to a heavy menstrual period about 2 hr after birth then decreases gradually at a consistent rate.

Three stages of lochia

Lochia rubra: Dark red color, menstrual-period-like discharge that contains debris from the sloughing of the uterine lining. It has a bloody consistency, fleshy odor and can contain small clots, and transient flow increases during breastfeeding and upon rising. Lasts 1 to 3 days after birth. Remind the client that they can experience a surge of discharge upon arising after lying in bed for an extended period of time. This should not be mistaken for hemorrhage.

Lochia serosa: Pinkish-brown color and serosanguineous consistency. Can contain small clots and leukocytes. Lasts from approximately day 4 to day 10 after birth.

Lochia alba: Yellowish-white creamy color, fleshy odor. Can consist of mucus and leukocytes. Lasts from approximately day 10 up to 6 weeks postpartum.

DATA COLLECTION

- Lochia amount is determined by the quantity of saturation on the perineal pad as follows.
  - Scant: less than 2.5 cm
  - Light: 2.5 to 10 cm
  - Moderate: more than 10 cm
  - Heavy: one pad saturated within 2 hr
  - Excessive blood loss: one pad saturated in 15 min or less, or pooling of blood under buttocks Qs
    - This is an indication of postpartum hemorrhage and should be reported to the charge nurse or provider immediately.

- Check the lochia for normal color, amount, odor, and consistency.
  - Monitor lochia frequently to determine the amount of bleeding. Check at least every 15 min for the first hour after delivery, then every 1 hr for the next 4 hr, and then every 4 to 8 hr depending on facility policy.
  - Lochia typically trickles from the vaginal opening but flows more steadily during uterine contractions.
  - Check for pooled lochia on the pad under the client, which they might not feel. This can identify heavy bleeding, which can be unnoticed.
  - Massaging the uterus or ambulation can result in a gush of lochia with the expression of clots and dark blood that has pooled in the vagina but should soon decrease back to a trickle of bright red lochia when in the early puerperium.
  - Soiled pads can be weighed to give a better estimation as to the extent of bleeding.
  - If a cesarean section was performed, the amount of bleeding will be decreased because the provider cleans out the uterus after surgery.

PATIENT-CENTERED CARE

Nursing interventions for abnormal lochia include notifying the charge nurse or provider and assisting with prescribed interventions based on the cause of the abnormality.

MANIFESTATIONS OF ABNORMAL LOCHIA

- Excessive spurting of bright red blood from the vagina, possibly indicating a cervical or vaginal tear
- Numerous large clots and excessive blood loss (saturation of one pad in 15 min or less), which can indicate hemorrhage
- Foul odor, which is suggestive of infection
- Persistent heavy lochia rubra in the early postpartum period beyond day 3, which can indicate retained placental fragments
- Continued flow of lochia serosa or alba beyond the normal length of time can indicate endometritis, especially if it is accompanied by fever, pain, or abdominal tenderness.

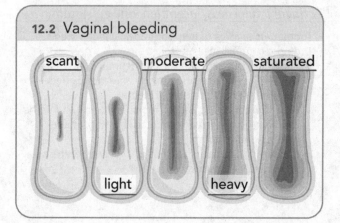

12.2 Vaginal bleeding

scant   moderate   saturated
light   heavy

CLIENT EDUCATION

- Change pads frequently.
- Perform hand hygiene after perineal care and changing of soiled pads.
- Do not use tampons due to the increased risk for infection.

Cervix, vagina, and perineum

PHYSICAL CHANGES

- The cervix is soft directly after birth and can be edematous, bruised, and have small lacerations.
  - Within 2 to 3 days postpartum, it shortens, regains its form, and becomes firm, with the os gradually closing.
  - Lacerations to the cervix can decrease the amount of cervical mucus.
  - External os will no longer have a round-dimple shape and will have a slit-like appearance.
- The vagina, which has distended, gradually returns to its prepregnancy size with the reappearance of rugae and a thickening of the vaginal mucosa.
  - Muscle tone is never restored completely.
  - Breastfeeding increases the incidence of vaginal dryness and atrophy.
- The soft tissues of the perineum can be erythematous and edematous, especially in areas of an episiotomy or lacerations.
  - Hematomas or hemorrhoids can be present.
  - Pelvic floor muscles can be overstretched and weak.

DATA COLLECTION

- Check the perineum for erythema, edema, hematoma, and signs of healing.
- Inspect episiotomy and lacerations for approximation, drainage, quantity, and quality. A bright red trickle of blood from the episiotomy site in the early postpartum period is a normal finding.
- Initial healing occurs in 2 to 3 weeks, and complete healing occurs within 4 to 6 months.

PATIENT-CENTERED CARE

Perineal tenderness, laceration, and episiotomy

- Promote measures to help soften the client's stools.
- Promote comfort measures.
  - Apply ice/cold packs to the perineum for the first 24 hr to reduce edema and provide anesthetic effect. Do not apply directly to the perineum.
  - Heat therapies (hot packs), moist heat, and sitz baths can be used to increase circulation and promote healing and comfort.
  - Encourage sitz baths at a hot or cool temperature for 20 min at least twice a day. Q̇EBP

- Administer analgesics, such as non-opioids (acetaminophen), nonsteroidal anti-inflammatories (ibuprofen), and opioids (codeine, hydrocodone) for pain and discomfort.
  - Opioid analgesia can be administered via a patient-controlled analgesia (PCA) pump after cesarean birth. Continuous epidural infusions can also be used for pain control after cesarean birth.
  - Apply topical anesthetic cream or spray, or witch hazel compresses to the perineum after cleansing. Witch hazel compresses or hemorrhoidal creams can be applied to the rectal area for hemorrhoid discomfort.
- Reinforce with the client about proper cleansing to prevent infection.
- Encourage the use of distraction, imagery, and other relaxation methods.

CLIENT EDUCATION

- Wash both hands thoroughly before and after voiding.
- Use a squeeze bottle filled with warm water or antiseptic solution after each voiding to cleanse the perineal area.
- Blot the perineal area to clean it after toileting, starting from front to back (urethra to anus).
- Use topical antiseptic cream or spray sparingly.
- Change the perineal pad by removing the front part first, peeling it toward the back after voiding or defecating.

SEXUAL ACTIVITY

- Clients can safely resume sexual intercourse by the second to forth week after birth, when bleeding has stopped and the perineum has healed. Over-the-counter lubricants might be needed during the first 6 weeks to 6 months.
- Physiological reactions to sexual activity can be slower and less intense for the first 3 months following birth.

CONTRACEPTION

Discuss the use of contraception upon the resumption of sexual activity and reinforce to the client that pregnancy can occur while breastfeeding even though menses has not returned.

CLIENT EDUCATION

- If breastfeeding, do not take oral contraceptives until milk production is well-established (usually 6 weeks).
- Menses for nonlactating clients might not resume until around 4 to 10 weeks. However, ovulation can occur as early as 1 month after delivery.
- Menses for lactating clients might not resume for 6 months or until cessation of breastfeeding.

Breasts

Physical changes of the breasts include the secretion of clear yellow fluid called colostrum, which occurs during pregnancy and 2 to 3 days immediately after birth. Milk is produced 72 to 96 hr after the birth of the newborn.

DATA COLLECTION

The nurse should inspect the client's breasts, and determine the client's choice regarding breastfeeding.

- Colostrum (early milk) transitions to mature milk by about 72 to 96 hr after birth; this transition is referred to as the milk coming in.
- Engorgement (fullness) of the breast tissue is a result of lymphatic circulation, milk production, and temporary vein congestion. The breast will appear tight, tender, warm, and full.
  - Inform clients who do not plan to breastfeed that this will resolve on its own, but breast binders or support bras can be used, or an ice pack or cabbage leaves can be applied.
  - Inform clients who plan to breastfeed that breast care and frequent feedings will prevent or manage engorgement.
- Observe for erythema, breast tenderness, cracked nipples, and indications of mastitis (infection in a milk duct of the breast with concurrent flu-like manifestations).
- Determine the client's ability to assist the newborn with latching on, and ensure the newborn has latched on correctly to prevent sore nipples.
- Ineffective newborn feeding patterns are related to maternal dehydration, maternal discomfort, newborn positioning, or difficulty with the newborn latching onto the breast. Deviations from expected findings and complications with breastfeeding should be reported to the charge nurse.

PATIENT-CENTERED CARE

- Reinforce early breastfeeding within the first 1 to 2 hr after birth.
- Encourage early demand feeding for the client who chooses to breastfeed. This will also stimulate the production of natural oxytocin and help prevent uterine hemorrhage.
- Assist the client into a comfortable position and have them try various positions during breastfeeding. The four traditional positions for breastfeeding are football hold (under the arm), cradle, across the lap (modified cradle), and side-lying. Explain how varying positions can prevent nipple soreness.
- Reinforce with the client the importance of proper latch techniques (the newborn takes in part of the areola and nipple, not just the tip of the nipple) to prevent nipple soreness.
- Inform the client that breastfeeding causes the release of oxytocin, which stimulates uterine contractions. This is a normal occurrence and beneficial to uterine tone.
- Advise clients who do not plan to breastfeed to not stimulate the breast or express breast milk.

12.3 Breastfeeding positions

Football hold

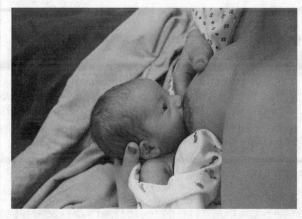

Cradle

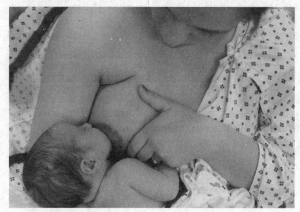

Modified cradle

The mother positions the baby as in the cradle position shown above but reverses the function of each arm.

Side-lying

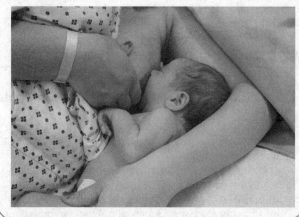

Cardiovascular system and fluid and hematologic status

PHYSICAL CHANGES

In the cardiovascular system during the postpartum period

- The cardiovascular system undergoes a decrease in blood volume during the postpartum period related to:
  - Blood loss during childbirth (Average blood loss is 300 to 500 mL [10% of blood volume] in an uncomplicated vaginal birth and 500 to 1,000 mL [15% to 30% of blood volume] for a cesarean birth.)
  - Diaphoresis and diuresis occur within the first 2 to 5 days after birth, and rid the body of the excess fluid accumulated during the last part of pregnancy.
  - Weight loss (due to lochia, delivery, and diuresis of about 19 lb [8.6 kg]) during the first 5 days after birth
- Hypovolemic shock does not usually occur in response to the normal blood loss of labor and birth because of the expanded blood volume of pregnancy and the readjustment in the maternal vasculature, which occurs in response to the following.
  - Elimination of the placenta
  - Rapid reduction in the size of the uterus, putting more blood into the maternal systemic circulation

In blood values, coagulation factors, and fibrinogen levels during the puerperium

- Hematocrit levels drop moderately for 3 to 4 days then begin to increase and reach nonpregnant levels by 8 weeks postpartum.
- During the first 4 to 7 days after birth, WBC values between 20,000 and 25,000mm^3 are common and can rise as high as 30,000/mm^3. This is called postpartum leukocytosis, and it is how the body prevents infection and aids in healing.
- Coagulation factors and fibrinogen levels increase during pregnancy and remain elevated in the immediate postpartum period. Hypercoagulability predisposes the postpartum client to thrombus formation and thromboembolism.

VITAL SIGN CHANGES

- Blood pressure is usually unchanged with an uncomplicated pregnancy but can have an insignificant, slight transient increase. Significant decrease from baseline could indicate bleeding. Significant increase could indicate gestational hypertension or preeclampsia and requires evaluation.
- Possible orthostatic hypotension within the first 48 hr postpartum can occur immediately after standing up with manifestations of faintness or dizziness resulting from splanchnic (viscera/internal organs) engorgement that can occur after birth. Encourage the client to sit on the side of the bed prior to standing up.

- Elevation of pulse, stroke volume, and cardiac output for the first hour postpartum occurs and then gradually decreases to a prepregnant state baseline by 6 to 8 weeks. Due to elevations in stroke volume during the first 2 days after birth, the heart rate can be as low as 40/min. This is called puerperal bradycardia, and this is common finding. Tachycardia in the postpartum period should be evaluated.
- Elevation of temperature to 38° C (100.4° F) resulting from dehydration after labor during the first 24 hr can occur but should return to normal after 24 hr postpartum. Elevation after 24 hr or that persists after 2 days could indicate infection.

DATA COLLECTION

Monitor for cardiovascular and vital sign changes and blood component changes. Compare with baseline pregnancy vital signs.

- Check pedal pulses, skin turgor, and the legs and feet for edema.
- Inspect the legs for redness, swelling, and warmth, which are additional indications of venous thrombosis.

PATIENT-CENTERED CARE

Nursing actions for alterations in findings include notifying the charge nurse and provider and assisting with performing prescribed interventions based on the cause of the alteration.

- Encourage adequate fluid intake.
- Encourage early ambulation to prevent venous stasis and thrombosis.
- Encourage the use of distraction, imagery, and other relaxation methods.
- Administer medications as prescribed.

Gastrointestinal system and bowel function

Operative vaginal birth (forceps- and vacuum-assisted) and anal sphincter lacerations increase the risk of temporary postpartum anal incontinence that usually resolves within 6 months.

PHYSICAL CHANGES IN THE GASTROINTESTINAL SYSTEM

- Increased appetite following birth
- Constipation
- Hemorrhoids

DATA COLLECTION

The nurse should check the gastrointestinal system including bowel function.
- Check for reports of hunger. Expect the client to have a good appetite.
- Check for bowel sounds and the return of normal bowel function. Spontaneous bowel movement might not occur for 2 to 3 days after birth secondary to decreased intestinal muscle tone during labor and puerperium, prelabor diarrhea, dehydration, or medication adverse effects.
- Check for discomfort with defecation due to perineal tenderness, episiotomy, lacerations, or hemorrhoids.
- Check the rectal area for varicosities (hemorrhoids).

PATIENT-CENTERED CARE

- Encourage interventions to promote bowel function (early ambulation, increased fluids, and intake of high-fiber foods).
- Administer stool softeners (docusate sodium) to prevent constipation.
- Enemas and suppositories are contraindicated for clients who have third- or fourth-degree perineal lacerations. Qs
- Flatus is common after a cesarean birth. Encourage the client to ambulate or rock in a chair to promote passage of flatus, and to avoid gas-forming foods. Anti-flatulence medications can be required.

Urinary system and bladder function

The urinary system can show evidence of the following.
- Urinary retention secondary to loss of bladder elasticity and tone and/or loss of bladder sensation resulting from trauma, medications, or anesthesia. A distended bladder as a result of urinary retention can cause infection, uterine atony, and displacement to one side. The ability of the uterus to contract is also lessened.
- Postpartal diuresis with increased urinary output begins within 12 hr of birth.

DATA COLLECTION

Check the urinary system and bladder function.
- Check the client's ability to void (perineal/urethral edema can cause pain and difficulty in voiding during the first 24 to 48 hr).
- Check bladder elimination pattern. Excessive urine diuresis (more than 3,000 mL/day) is normal within the first 2 to 3 days after birth.
- Check for evidence of a distended bladder.
  - Fundal height above the umbilicus or baseline level
  - Fundus displaced from the midline over to the side
  - Bladder bulges above the symphysis pubis
  - Excessive lochia
  - Tenderness over the bladder area
- Frequent voiding of less than 150 mL of urine is indicative of urinary retention with overflow.

PATIENT-CENTERED CARE

- Assist the client to void within 6 to 8 hr after birth. If unable to void, catheterization can be required.
- Encourage the client to empty their bladder frequently to prevent possible displacement of the uterus and atony.
- Measure the client's first few voidings after birth to monitor for bladder emptying.
- Encourage the client to increase their oral fluid intake to replace fluids lost at delivery and to prevent or correct dehydration.
- Catheterize if necessary for bladder distention if the client is unable to void to ensure complete emptying of the bladder and allow uterine involution.

Musculoskeletal system

Physical changes of the musculoskeletal system involve a reversal of the musculoskeletal adaptations that occurred during pregnancy. By 6 to 8 weeks after birth:
- The joints return to their prepregnant state and are completely restabilized. The feet, however, can remain permanently increased in size.
- Muscle tone begins to be restored throughout the body with the removal of progesterone's effect following delivery of the placenta. The rectus abdominis muscles of the abdomen and the pubococcygeus muscle tone are restored following placental expulsion and return to the prepregnant state about 6 weeks postpartum.

DATA COLLECTION

- Check the musculoskeletal system for changes.
- Check the abdominal wall for diastasis recti (separation of the rectus muscle). It usually resolves within 6 weeks.

PATIENT-CENTERED CARE

Prevent falls by encouraging the client to wear nonskid slippers or socks, assisting the client with getting out of bed, and instructing the client to call for assistance initially when getting out of bed.

CLIENT EDUCATION

- Perform postpartum strengthening exercises, starting with simple exercises and then gradually progressing to more strenuous ones.
- Following cesarean birth, postpone abdominal exercises until about 4 to 6 weeks after birth, or follow recommendations of the provider.
- Use good body mechanics and proper posture.
- Ambulate soon after delivery.
- Perform Kegel exercises to strengthen pelvic muscles.

Immune system

Review the status of the following.

Rubella: A client who is nonimmune to rubella or has a negative or low titer is administered a subcutaneous injection of rubella vaccine or a measles, mumps, and rubella (MMR) vaccine during the postpartum period to protect a subsequent fetus from malformations. The client should not get pregnant for 28 days following the immunization. Qs

Rh: All Rh-negative clients who have newborns who are Rh-positive must be given Rho(D) immune globulin administered IM within 72 hr of the newborn being born to suppress antibody formation in the mother. The nurse should check to see if the client has not been sensitized prior to administering Rho(D) immune globulin. Observe the client for at least 20 minutes post administration for an allergic reaction.

Test the client who receives both a live virus vaccine, such as the rubella vaccine, and Rho(D) immune globulin after 3 months to determine whether immunity to rubella has been developed. QEBP

Varicella: If the client has no immunity, varicella vaccine is administered before discharge. The client should not get pregnant for 1 month following the immunization. A second dose of vaccine is given at 4 to 8 weeks.

Tetanus-diphtheria-acellular pertussis vaccine: The vaccine is recommended for clients who have not previously received it. It is also recommended for people who are going to be around the baby frequently if they have not received the vaccine previously. Administer prior to discharge or as soon as possible in the postpartum period. Breastfeeding is not contraindicated.

Comfort level

DATA COLLECTION AND INTERVENTIONS
- Check pain related to episiotomy, lacerations, incisions, afterpains, and sore nipples.
- Determine location, type, and quality of the pain to guide nursing interventions and client education.
- Administer pain medications as prescribed.
- Reinforce nonpharmacological measures (distraction, imagery, heating pads, position changes, cold packs).

Nutrition

- Encourage nonlactating clients to consume 1,800 to 2,200 kcal/day.
- Reinforce to the lactating client to increase their caloric intake and to include calcium-enriched foods in the diet.
  - The American Academy of Pediatrics recommends that clients who are lactating add an additional 450 to 500 calories/day to their prepregnancy diet.
  - Iron supplements can be prescribed for clients who have low hemoglobin and hematocrit levels.

CLIENT EDUCATION
- Consume a nutritious diet including all food groups and high in protein, which will aid in tissue repair.
- Continue taking prenatal vitamins until 6 weeks following birth.

Psychosocial

During the postpartum period, a client can experience many different emotions due to hormonal changes. Monitor for conditions such as postpartum blues and depression during the postpartum period.

DATA COLLECTION AND INTERVENTIONS
- Allow verbalization of feelings.
- Check emotional status.
- Observe for bonding with newborn.
- Monitor for manifestations of postpartum blues or depression.
  - Decreased appetite
  - Difficulty sleeping
  - Decreased interactions with others
  - Lack of communication

PATIENT-CENTERED CARE

- Encourage skin-to-skin contact with their baby after birth.
- Document interactions and bonding concerns.
- Encourage rooming in with the baby in the client's room at all times.
- Provide support, and initiate referrals as needed for counseling.

Discharge education

The client should be discharged with an appointment date and time for a postpartum follow-up visit or a number to call and schedule an appointment.
- Following a vaginal delivery, the follow-up visit should take place in 4 to 6 weeks. However, current recommendations by the American College of Obstetricians and Gynecologists suggest follow-up visits as early as 3 weeks postpartum. Following a cesarean birth, the visit should take place in 2 to 4 weeks.
- The date and time of the follow-up appointment should be written on the client's discharge paperwork and discussed in the discharge instructions.

CLIENT EDUCATION: Report indications of potential complications to the provider, such as the following.
- Chills or fever greater than 38° C (100.4° F) after 24 hr
- Change in vaginal discharge with increased amount, large clots, change to a previous lochia color (bright red bleeding), and a foul odor
- Normal lochial flow patterns
  - Rubra: Dark red vaginal drainage for 1 to 3 days
  - Serosa: Brownish-red or pink vaginal drainage from days 3 to 10
  - Alba: Yellowish-white vaginal discharge after day 10 to 8 weeks

- Episiotomy, laceration, or incisional pain that does not resolve with analgesics, foul-smelling drainage, redness, or edema
- Pain or tenderness in the abdominal or pelvic areas that does not resolve with analgesics
- Breast(s) with localized areas of pain and tenderness with firmness, heat, and swelling, and/or nipples with cracks, redness, bruising, blisters, or fissures
- Calves with localized pain, tenderness, redness, and swelling. A lower extremity with either areas of redness and warmth or tenderness
- Urination with burning, pain, frequency, urgency
- Indications of possible depression, including apathy toward the infant, inability to provide self- or infant-care, or feelings that they might hurt themselves or the infant

Active Learning Scenario

A nurse on the postpartum unit is assisting with providing education with a group of clients about perineal care after delivery. What information should the nurse prepare to include? Use the ATI Active Learning Template: Basic Concept to complete this item.

UNDERLYING PRINCIPLES: Describe three concepts that are the basis for perineal hygiene.

NURSING INTERVENTIONS

- Describe four actions the client should take to prevent infection.
- Describe four actions the nurse can take to promote client comfort.

Application Exercises

1. As a nurse, what information should you discuss with the client regarding the three stages of lochia?

2. During ambulation to the bathroom, a postpartum client experiences a gush of dark red blood that soon stops. On data collection, a nurse finds the uterus to be firm, midline, and at the level of the umbilicus. Which of the following findings should the nurse interpret this data as being?

   A. Evidence of a possible vaginal hematoma
   B. An indication of a cervical or perineal laceration
   C. A normal postural discharge of lochia
   D. Abnormally excessive lochia rubra flow

3. A nurse is checking the fundus of a client who is 2 days postpartum and observes the perineal pad for lochia. The pad is saturated approximately 12 cm with lochia that is bright red and contains small clots. Which of the following findings should the nurse document in the client's medical record?

   A. Moderate lochia rubra
   B. Excessive lochia serosa
   C. Light lochia rubra
   D. Scant lochia serosa

4. A nurse is preparing to reinforce education to a client who is 2 hr postpartum and has perineal laceration. Which of the following information should the nurse include? (Select all that apply.)

   A. Use a perineal squeeze bottle to cleanse the perineum.
   B. Sit on the perineum while resting in bed.
   C. Apply a topical anesthetic cream or spray to the perineum.
   D. Wipe the perineum thoroughly with a back-and-forth motion.
   E. Apply cold or ice packs to the perineum.

5. A nurse is reinforcing discharge instructions for a client. At 4 weeks postpartum, the client should contact the provider for which of the following client findings?

   A. Scant, nonodorous, white vaginal discharge
   B. Uterine cramping during breastfeeding
   C. Sore nipple with cracks and fissures
   D. Decreased response with sexual activity

6. A nurse is reinforcing postpartum discharge teaching to a client who had no immunity to varicella and was given the varicella vaccine. Which of the following statements by the client indicates understanding?

   A. "I will need to use contraception for 3 months before considering pregnancy."
   B. "I need a second vaccination at my postpartum visit."
   C. "I was given the vaccine because my baby is O-positive."
   D. "I will be tested in 3 months to see if I have developed immunity."

1. The nurse should include the following information about the three stages of lochia with the client. Lochia rubra: dark red color; bloody consistency; fleshy odor; can contain small clots; transient flow increases during breastfeeding and upon rising; lasts 1 to 3 days after birth. Lochia serosa: pinkish-brown color; serosanguineous consistency; can contain small clots and leukocytes; lasts from approximately day 4 to day 10 after birth. Lochia alba: yellowish-white creamy color; fleshy odor; can consist of mucus and leukocytes; lasts from approximately day 10 up to 6 weeks postpartum

   Ⓝ *NCLEX® Connection: Health Promotion and Maintenance, Ante-/Intra-/Postpartum and Newborn Care*

2. C. **CORRECT:** A client who has a vaginal hematoma is expected to report excessive pain or vaginal pressure. Excessive spurting of bright red blood from the vagina indicates a possible cervical or perineal laceration. Lochia typically trickles from the vaginal opening but flows more steadily during uterine contractions. Massaging the uterus or ambulation can result in a gush of lochia with the expression of clots and dark blood that has been pooled in the vagina, but it should soon decrease back to a trickle of bright red lochia in the early puerperium. Excessive blood loss consists of one pad saturated in 15 min or less or the pooling of blood under the buttocks, which is not affected by the client's postural changes.

   Ⓝ *NCLEX® Connection: Health Promotion and Maintenance, Ante-/Intra-/Postpartum and Newborn Care*

3. A. **CORRECT:** The client has moderate lochia rubra containing small clots, which is an expected finding for the second day postpartum. Excessive lochia serosa is indicated by saturation of a perineal pad in 15 min or less or pooling of blood under the buttocks. Light lochia rubra is a perineal pad that is saturated less than 10 cm with lochia. Scant lochia serosa (less than 2.5 cm on perineal pad) is pinkish brown in color and serosanguineous in consistency. It occurs on day 4 to 12 following delivery.

   Ⓝ *NCLEX® Connection: Health Promotion and Maintenance, Ante-/Intra-/Postpartum and Newborn Care*

4. A, C, E. **CORRECT:** Use a perineal squeeze bottle filled with warm water to cleanse the perineum and promote healing. Sitting supine on the perineum while resting in bed will apply more pressure to the area. Instead, the client should lay on one side when possible. The application of a topical anesthetic cream or spray to the perineum will promote comfort. The client should blot the perineum to dry it from front to back using toilet paper or wipes. The application of cold or ice packs to the perineum will promote comfort and decrease swelling

   Ⓝ *NCLEX® Connection: Health Promotion and Maintenance, Ante-/Intra-/Postpartum and Newborn Care*

5. C. **CORRECT:** Lochia alba, a white vaginal discharge, is normal from the 11th day postpartum to approximately 6 weeks following birth. Oxytocin, which is released with breastfeeding, causes the uterus to contract and can cause discomfort. A sore nipple that has cracks and fissures is an indication of mastitis. Physiological reactions to sexual activity can be slower and less intense for the first 3 months following birth.

   Ⓝ *NCLEX® Connection: Health Promotion and Maintenance, Ante-/Intra-/Postpartum and Newborn Care*

6. B. **CORRECT:** A client is instructed to not get pregnant for 1 month following administration of varicella vaccine. A second varicella immunization is needed at 4 to 8 weeks following delivery by clients who had no history of immunity. Rho(D) immune globulin is administered to an Rh-negative client who has an Rh-positive newborn. A client requires testing for immunity at 3 months following administration of rubella vaccine and Rho(D) immune globulin.

   Ⓝ *NCLEX® Connection: Health Promotion and Maintenance, Ante-/Intra-/Postpartum and Newborn Care*

Active Learning Scenario Key

Using the ATI Active Learning Template: Basic Concept

UNDERLYING PRINCIPLES
- Increase tissue perfusion.
- Prevent infection.
- Promote comfort.

NURSING INTERVENTIONS
- Prevent infection.
  - Wash hands thoroughly before and after voiding.
  - Use a squeeze bottle with warm water or antiseptic solution after each voiding.
  - Clean the perineal area from front to back.
  - Blot dry; do not wipe.
  - Use topical application of antiseptic cream or spray sparingly.
  - Change perineal pad from front to back after voiding and defecating.
- Promote comfort.
  - Apply ice or cold packs to the perineum.
  - Encourage sitz baths at least twice a day.
  - Administer analgesics.
  - Apply topical anesthetics to perineal area or witch hazel compresses to the rectal area.

Ⓝ *NCLEX® Connection: Health Promotion and Maintenance, Ante-/Intra-/Postpartum and Newborn Care*

CHAPTER 13 *Baby-Friendly Care*

Bonding and integration of a newborn into the family structure should start during pregnancy and continue into the fourth stage of labor and throughout hospitalization.

Observation of bonding and integration of a newborn into the family structure requires that a nurse understand the normal postpartum psychological changes the client undergoes in the attainment of the maternal role and the recognition of deviations. Baby-friendly care can be promoted by delaying nursing procedures during the first hour after birth and through the first attempt of the client to breastfeed to allow for immediate parent-newborn contact.

A client's emotional and physical condition (unwanted pregnancy, adolescent pregnancy, history of depression, difficult pregnancy and birth) and the newborn's physical condition (prematurity, congenital anomalies) after birth can affect the family's bonding process. Culture, age, and socioeconomic status are factors that can influence the bonding process. Bonding can be delayed secondary to maternal or neonatal factors.

PSYCHOSOCIAL AND MATERNAL ADAPTION

Psychosocial adaptation and maternal adjustment begin during pregnancy as the client goes through commitment, attachment, and preparation for the birth of the newborn.

- During the first 2 to 6 weeks after birth, the client goes through a period of acquaintance with the newborn, as well as physical restoration. During this time the client also focuses on competently caring for the newborn.
- Finally, the act of achieving maternal identity is accomplished around 4 months following birth.
- These stages can overlap and are variable based on maternal, newborn, and environmental factors.

PHASES OF MATERNAL ROLE ATTAINMENT

Dependent: taking-in phase
- First 24 to 48 hr
- Focus on meeting personal needs
- Rely on others for assistance
- Excited, talkative
- Need to review birth experience with others

Dependent-independent: taking-hold phase
- Begins on day 2 or 3
- Lasts 10 days to several weeks
- Focus on baby care and improving caregiving competency
- Want to take charge but need acceptance from others
- Want to learn and practice
- Dealing with physical and emotional discomforts, can experience "baby blues"

Interdependent: letting-go phase
- Focus on family as a unit
- Resumption of role (intimate partner, individual)

DATA COLLECTION

Data collection by the nurse includes noting the client's condition after birth, observing the maternal adaptation process, monitoring maternal emotional readiness to care for the newborn, and monitoring how comfortable the client appears in providing newborn care.
- Monitor for behaviors that facilitate and indicate parent-newborn bonding.
  - Considers the newborn a family member
  - Holds the newborn face-to-face (en face position), maintaining eye contact
  - Assigns meaning to the newborn's behavior and views this positively
  - Identifies the newborn's unique characteristics and relates them to those of other family members
  - Names the newborn, indicating bonding is occurring
  - Touches the newborn and maintains close physical proximity and contact
  - Provides physical care for the newborn (feeding, diapering)
  - Responds to the newborn's cries
  - Smiles at, talks to, and sings to the newborn
- Monitor for behaviors that impair and indicate a lack of parent-newborn bonding.
  - Apathy when the newborn cries
  - Disgust when the newborn voids, stools, or spits up
  - Expresses disappointment in the newborn
  - Turns away from the newborn
  - Does not seek close physical proximity to the newborn
  - Does not talk about the newborn's unique features
  - Handles the newborn roughly
  - Ignores the newborn entirely
  - Does not include the newborn in the family context
  - Perceives newborn behavior as uncooperative

- Monitor for manifestations of mood swings, conflict about maternal role, or personal insecurity.
  - Feelings of being "down"
  - Feelings of inadequacy
  - Feelings of anxiety
  - Emotional lability with frequent crying
  - Flat affect and being withdrawn
- Feeling unable to care for the newborn

NURSING ACTIONS
- Facilitate the bonding process by placing the newborn skin-to-skin or in the en face position with the client immediately after birth.
- Promote rooming-in as a quiet and private environment that enhances the family bonding process.
- Promote early initiation of breastfeeding and encourage the client to recognize newborn readiness cues. Offer assistance as needed.
- Reinforce newborn care to facilitate bonding as the client's confidence improves.
- Encourage parents to bond with the newborn through cuddling, bathing, feeding, diapering, and watching the newborn.
- Provide frequent praise, support, and reassurance to the client as they move toward independence in caring for the newborn and adjusting to their parental role.
- Encourage parents to express feelings, fears, and anxieties about caring for the newborn.

CO-PARENT ADAPTATION

Co-parent adaptation occurs through bonding with the newborn through the following behaviors.
- Using skin-to-skin contact, holding the newborn, and engaging in eye-to-eye contact with the newborn.
- Observing the newborn for similarities to the parent's own features
- Talking, singing, and reading to the newborn

TRANSITION

Research on the transition to co-parenthood has revealed the following phases.

Expectations and intentions: Desires to be deeply and emotionally connected with the newborn

Confronting reality: Understands that reality does not always meet expectations. Commonly expressed emotions include feeling sad, frustrated, and jealous. Can feel like they are unable to talk with the other parent, who is consumed with newborn caregiving and their own transition to parenthood

Creating the role of the involved co-parent: Decides to become actively involved in the care of the newborn

Reaping rewards: Rewards include newborn smiles and a sense of completeness and meaning.

DATA COLLECTION

Data collection of paternal adaptation includes observing for the characteristics of newborn bonding.

NURSING ACTIONS
- Provide reinforcement about newborn care with each parent or caregiver and encourage a hands-on approach.
- Assist the co-parent to transition to the parental role by providing guidance and encouraging equal participation in newborn care.
- Encourage the parents to verbalize concerns and expectations related to newborn care.

SIBLING ADAPTATION

The addition of a newborn into the family unit affects everyone in the family, including siblings who can experience a temporary separation from parents. Siblings become aware of changes in the parents' behavior because the newborn requires much more of parents' time.

DATA COLLECTION

Data collection of sibling adaptation to the newborn includes the following.
- Observe for positive responses from the sibling.
  - Interest and concern for the newborn
  - Increased independence
- Monitor for adverse responses from the sibling.
  - Indications of sibling rivalry and jealousy
  - Regression in toileting and sleep habits
  - Aggression toward the newborn
  - Increased attention-seeking behaviors and whining

NURSING ACTIONS
- Take the sibling on a tour of the obstetric unit.
- Encourage the parents to do the following.
  - Let the sibling be one of the first to see the newborn.
  - Provide a gift from the newborn to give the sibling.
  - Arrange for one parent to spend time with the sibling while the other parent is caring for the newborn.
  - Allow older siblings to help in providing care for the newborn.
  - Provide preschool-aged siblings with a doll to care for.

COMPLICATIONS

NURSING ACTIONS
- Emphasize verbal and nonverbal communication skills between the client, caregivers, and the newborn.
- Collect continuous data of the client's parenting abilities, as well as any other caregivers for the newborn.
- Encourage continued support of grandparents and other family members.
- Provide home visits and group sessions for discussion regarding newborn care and parenting problems.
- Give the client and caregivers information about social networks that provide a support system where they can seek assistance.
- Notify programs that provide prompt and effective community interventions to prevent more serious problems from occurring.

Application Exercises

1. A client in the early postpartum period is very excited and talkative. They repeatedly tell the nurse every detail of the labor and birth. Because the client will not stop talking, the nurse is having difficulty completing their nursing care. Discuss the action the nurse should take.

2. A nurse is assisting with the care of a client who is 1 day postpartum. The nurse is assessing for maternal adaptation and parent-newborn bonding. Which of the following behaviors by the client indicates a need for the nurse to intervene?

   A. Demonstrates apathy when the newborn cries

   B. Touches the newborn and maintains close, physical proximity

   C. Views the newborn's behavior as uncooperative during diaper changing

   D. Identifies and relates newborn's characteristics to those of family members

   E. Interprets the newborn's behavior as meaningful and a way of expressing needs

3. A nurse concludes that the parent of a newborn is not showing positive indications of parent-newborn bonding. The parent appears very anxious and nervous when the nurse brings the newborn to the room. Which of the following actions should the nurse use to promote parent-newborn bonding?

   A. Hand the parent the newborn and suggest that they change the diaper.

   B. Ask the parent why they are so anxious and nervous.

   C. Tell the parent that they will grow accustomed to the newborn.

   D. Provide education about newborn care when the parent is present.

4. A nurse is assisting in the care of a client who is 2 days postpartum. The client states, "My 4-year-old son was toilet trained, and now they are frequently wetting themselves." Which of the following responses should the nurse provide to the client?

   A. "Your child was probably not ready for toilet training and should wear training pants."

   B. "Your child is displaying a common negative response to the birth of a sibling."

   C. "Your child may need counseling."

   D. "You should try sending your child to preschool to resolve the behavior."

Active Learning Scenario

A nurse is assisting with preparing a parenting class on paternal adaptation for expectant clients and their partners. What concepts on paternal adaptation should the nurse include in the presentation? Use the ATI Active Learning Template: Basic Concept to complete this item.

RELATED CONTENT: Describe three ways the co-parent develops a parent-newborn bond.

UNDERLYING PRINCIPLES

• Describe three stages of co-parent transition to parenthood.

• Describe three stages of the development of the co-parent-newborn bond.

NURSING INTERVENTIONS: Describe three actions to assist in the co-parent-newborn bonding process.

Active Learning Scenario Key

Using the ATI Active Learning Template: Basic Concept

RELATED CONTENT

- Development of parent-newborn bond
- Touching, holding, skin-to-skin contact, and maintaining eye-to-eye contact
- Recognizing personal features in the newborn, and validating their claim to the newborn
- Talking, reading, singing, and verbally interacting with the newborn

UNDERLYING PRINCIPLES

Stages of co-parent transition to parenthood
- Expectations: Having preconceived ideas about parenthood
- Reality: Recognizing expectations might not be met, facing these feelings, and then embracing the need to become actively involved in parenting
- Transition to mastery: Taking an active role in parenting

Development of the co-parent-newborn bond
- Making a commitment and assuming responsibility for parenting
- Becoming connected and having feelings of attachment to the newborn
- Modifying lifestyle to make room to care for the newborn

NURSING INTERVENTIONS

- Provide reinforcement about newborn care when the co-parent is present.
- Encourage the co-parent to take a hands-on role in care when present.
- Provide guidance.
- Involve the co-parent as a full partner, not a helper, in the parenting process.
- Encourage the couple to verbalize concerns and expectations about newborn care.

(N) *NCLEX® Connection: Psychosocial Integrity, Coping Mechanisms*

Application Exercises Key

1. The nurse should give the client time to express their feelings and recognize that the client is excited about the birth of their baby by giving them the opportunity to discuss the birth. This also helps to develop rapport with the client and allows for therapeutic communication.

(N) *NCLEX® Connection: Health Promotion, Ante-/Intra-/Postpartum and Newborn Care*

2. A, C. **CORRECT:** Demonstrating apathy when the newborn cries demonstrates a lack of interest in the newborn and impaired parent-newborn bonding. Touching the newborn and maintaining close proximity are indications of effective parent-newborn bonding. A client's view of their newborn as being uncooperative during diaper changing is a sign of impaired parent-newborn bonding. Endowing the newborn with family characteristics indicates effective parent-newborn bonding. Recognizing the newborn's behavior as meaningful and a way to express needs is an indication of effective parent-newborn bonding.

(N) *NCLEX® Connection: Psychosocial Integrity, Coping Mechanisms*

3. D. **CORRECT:** It is not helpful to push the parent into newborn care activities without first providing education. Asking the parent why they are anxious and nervous is a nontherapeutic statement and presumes the nurse knows what the parent is feeling. Telling the parent that they will grow accustomed to the newborn is a nontherapeutic statement and offers the nurse's opinion. Nursing interventions to promote paternal bonding include providing education about newborn care and encouraging the parent to take a hands-on approach.

(N) *NCLEX® Connection: Psychosocial Integrity, Coping Mechanisms*

4. B. **CORRECT:** Recommending that the child wear training pants because they were not ready for toilet training is not an appropriate intervention because it overlooks the child's emotional response to a new family member. Adverse responses by a sibling to a newborn can include regression in toileting habits. Recommending that the child receive counseling is not an appropriate nursing intervention for a child who is demonstrating an adverse sibling response. Recommending that the child be sent to preschool is not an appropriate nursing intervention for a child who is demonstrating an adverse sibling response.

(N) *NCLEX® Connection: Psychosocial Integrity, Therapeutic Communication*

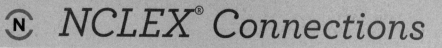
When reviewing the following chapters, keep in mind the relevant topics and tasks of the NCLEX outline.

Health Promotion and Maintenance

ANTE-/INTRA-/POSTPARTUM AND NEWBORN CARE
Perform care of postpartum client.

Monitor recovery of stable postpartum client.

DATA COLLECTION TECHNIQUES: Collect baseline physical data.

DEVELOPMENTAL STAGES AND TRANSITIONS: Assist client with expected life transition.

Pharmacological Therapies

EXPECTED ACTIONS/OUTCOMES
Apply knowledge of pathophysiology when addressing client pharmacological agents.

Evaluate client response to medication.

REDUCTION OF RISK POTENTIAL: Check and monitor client vital signs.

Physiological Adaptation

ALTERATIONS IN BODY SYSTEMS
Identify signs and symptoms of an infection.

Provide care for a client experiencing complications of pregnancy/labor or delivery.

CHAPTER 14 # *Complications of the Postpartum Period*

Postpartum disorders are unexpected events or occurrences that can happen during the postpartum period. It is imperative for a nurse to have a thorough understanding of each disorder and initiate appropriate nursing interventions to achieve positive outcomes.

Postpartum disorders reviewed in this chapter include superficial and deep-vein thrombosis, pulmonary embolus, postpartum hemorrhage, uterine atony, subinvolution of the uterus, inversion of the uterus, retained placenta, lacerations, and hematomas.

Deep-vein thrombosis

- Thrombophlebitis refers to a thrombus that is associated with inflammation.
- Thrombophlebitis of the lower extremities can be of superficial or deep veins, which are most often of the femoral, saphenous, or popliteal veins. The postpartum client is at greatest risk for a deep-vein thrombosis (DVT) that can lead to a pulmonary embolism.

DATA COLLECTION

RISK FACTORS

- Pregnancy
- Cesarean birth (doubles the risk)
- Operative vaginal birth
- Pulmonary embolism or varicosities
- Immobility
- Obesity
- Smoking
- Multiparity
- Age greater than 35 years
- History of thromboembolism

EXPECTED FINDINGS

Leg pain and tenderness

PHYSICAL FINDINGS

- Unilateral area of swelling, warmth, and redness
- Hardened vein over the thrombosis
- Calf tenderness

DIAGNOSTIC PROCEDURES

Noninvasive

- Doppler ultrasound scanning
- Computed tomography
- Magnetic resonance imaging

PATIENT-CENTERED CARE

NURSING CARE

Prevention of thrombophlebitis

- Maintain sequential compression device until ambulation is established.
- If bed rest is prolonged longer than 8 hr, use active and passive range of motion to promote circulation in the legs if warranted.
- Initiate early and frequent ambulation postpartum.
- Measure the lower extremities for fitted elastic thromboembolic hose to lower extremities.

CLIENT EDUCATION

- Avoid prolonged periods of standing, sitting, or immobility.
- Elevate both legs when sitting.
- Avoid crossing the legs, which will reduce the circulation and exacerbate venous stasis.
- Maintain fluid intake of 2 to 3 L each day from food and beverage sources to prevent dehydration, which causes circulation to be sluggish.
- Discontinue smoking.

Management of thrombophlebitis

- Facilitate bed rest and elevation of the client's extremity above the level of the heart. (Avoid using a knee gatch or pillow under knees.) Encourage the client to change positions frequently.
- Administer intermittent or continuous warm, moist compresses.
- Do **NOT** massage the affected limb to prevent thrombus from dislodging and becoming an embolus.
- Measure and monitor the client's leg circumferences.
- Provide thigh-high antiembolism stockings for the client at high risk for venous insufficiency.
- Administer analgesics (nonsteroidal anti-inflammatory agents).
- Administer anticoagulants for DVT.

MEDICATIONS

Heparin

CLASSIFICATION: Anticoagulant

THERAPEUTIC INTENT: Given IV to prevent formation of other clots and to prevent enlargement of the existing clot

NURSING ACTIONS

- Initially, IV heparin is administered by the RN via continuous infusion for 3 to 5 days with doses adjusted according to coagulation studies. Protamine sulfate, the heparin antidote, should be readily available to counteract the development of heparin-induced antiplatelet antibodies.
- Monitor aPTT (1.5 to 2.5 times the control level of 30 to 40 seconds).

CLIENT EDUCATION: Report bleeding from the gums or nose, increased vaginal bleeding, blood in the urine, and frequent bruising.

Warfarin

CLASSIFICATION: Anticoagulant

THERAPEUTIC INTENT: Used for treatment of clots

NURSING ACTIONS

- Phytonadione, the warfarin antidote, should be readily available for prolonged clotting times.
- Monitor PT.

CLIENT EDUCATION

- Watch for bleeding from the gums or nose, increased vaginal bleeding, blood in the urine, and frequent bruising. Qs
- Use birth control to avoid pregnancy due to the teratogenic effects of warfarin. Oral contraceptives are contraindicated because of the increased risk for thrombosis.

CLIENT EDUCATION

PRECAUTIONS WHILE RECEIVING ANTICOAGULANTS QEBP

- Avoid taking aspirin or ibuprofen (increases bleeding tendencies).
- Use an electric razor for shaving.
- Avoid alcohol use (inhibits warfarin).
- Brush teeth gently using a soft toothbrush.
- Avoid rubbing or massaging legs.
- Avoid periods of prolonged sitting or crossing legs.

Pulmonary embolus

- An embolus occurs when fragments or an entire clot dislodges and moves into circulation.
- A pulmonary embolism is a complication of DVT that occurs if the embolus moves into the pulmonary artery or one of its branches and lodges in a lung, occluding the vessel and obstructing blood flow to the lungs.
- Acute pulmonary embolus is an emergent situation.

DATA COLLECTION

RISK FACTORS

Risk factors are the same as those for DVT.

EXPECTED FINDINGS

- Apprehension
- Pleuritic chest pain
- Dyspnea
- Tachypnea
- Hemoptysis
- Tachycardia
- Cough
- Syncope
- Crackles with breath sounds
- Elevated temperature
- Hypoxia

DIAGNOSTIC AND THERAPEUTIC PROCEDURES

- Ventilation/perfusion lung scan
- Magnetic resonance angiography
- Spiral computed tomography
- Pulmonary angiogram
- Embolectomy to surgically remove the embolus

PATIENT-CENTERED CARE

NURSING CARE

- Place the client in a semi-Fowler's position with the head of the bed elevated to facilitate breathing.
- Administer oxygen by mask.

MEDICATIONS

- Medications prescribed include the medications listed under DVT.
- Thrombolytic therapy to break up blood clots can be prescribed.
  - **Alteplase, streptokinase:** Similar adverse effects and contraindications as anticoagulants

Postpartum hemorrhage

Postpartum hemorrhage is considered to occur if the client loses more than 500 mL blood after a vaginal birth or more than 1,000 mL blood after a cesarean birth. Two complications that can occur following postpartum hemorrhage include hypovolemic shock and anemia. Current evidence-based guidelines recommend early identification of risk factors, which could cause postpartum hemorrhage. The nurse should collaborate with the interprofessional team to ensure prompt identification and inventions are implemented. AWHONN recommends that quantification of blood loss (QBL) be measured with every birth.

DATA COLLECTION

RISK FACTORS

- Uterine atony or history of uterine atony
- Overdistended uterus
- Prolonged labor, oxytocin-induced labor
- High parity
- Ruptured uterus
- Complications during pregnancy (placenta previa, abruptio placentae)
- Precipitous delivery
- Administration of magnesium sulfate therapy during labor
- Lacerations and hematomas
- Inversion of uterus
- Subinvolution of the uterus
- Retained placental fragments
- Coagulopathies (DIC)

EXPECTED FINDINGS

Increase or change in lochial pattern (return to previous stage, large clots)

PHYSICAL FINDINGS

- Uterine atony (hypotonic or boggy)
- Blood clots larger than a quarter
- Perineal pad saturation in 15 min or less
- Constant oozing, trickling, or frank flow of bright red blood from the vagina
- Tachycardia and hypotension
- Pallor of skin and mucous membranes; cool, and clammy with loss of turgor
- Oliguria

LABORATORY TESTS

- Hgb and Hct
- Coagulation profile (PT)
- Blood type and crossmatch

PATIENT-CENTERED CARE

NURSING CARE

- Determine QBL immediately following birth.
- Weigh all blood-saturated items and clots, measure fluids in suction cannisters, and subtract any irrigation fluids.
- Firmly massage the uterine fundus.
- Monitor vital signs.
- Monitor for source of bleeding.
  - Palpate fundus for height, firmness, and position. If uterus is boggy, massage fundus to increase muscle contraction.
  - Monitor lochia for color, quantity, and clots.
  - Observe for clinical findings of bleeding from lacerations, episiotomy site, or hematomas.
- Palpate bladder for distention. Insert an indwelling urinary catheter to check kidney function and obtain an accurate measurement of urinary output.

- Maintain or assist initiating IV fluids to replace fluid volume loss with IV isotonic solutions, such as lactated Ringer's or 0.9% sodium chloride; colloid volume expanders, such as albumin; and blood products (packed RBCs and fresh frozen plasma).
- Provide oxygen at 10 to 12 L/min per nonrebreather face mask, and monitor oxygen saturation.
- Elevate the client's legs to increase circulation to essential organs.

MEDICATIONS

Oxytocin

CLASSIFICATION: Uterine stimulant

THERAPEUTIC INTENT: Promotes uterine contractions

NURSING ACTIONS
- Monitor uterine tone and vaginal bleeding.
- Monitor vital signs.

Methylergonovine

CLASSIFICATION: Uterine stimulant

THERAPEUTIC INTENT: Controls postpartum hemorrhage

NURSING ACTIONS
- Monitor uterine tone and vaginal bleeding. Do not administer to clients who have hypertension or cardiovascular disease.
- Monitor for adverse reactions, including hypertension, nausea, vomiting, and headache.

Misoprostol

CLASSIFICATION: Uterine stimulant

THERAPEUTIC INTENT: Controls postpartum hemorrhage

NURSING ACTIONS: Monitor uterine tone and vaginal bleeding.

Carboprost tromethamine

CLASSIFICATION: Uterine stimulant

THERAPEUTIC INTENT: Controls postpartum hemorrhage

NURSING ACTIONS
- Monitor uterine tone and vaginal bleeding.
- Monitor for adverse reactions, including fever, chills, headache, nausea, vomiting, diarrhea, and hypertension.

Tranexamic acid

CLASSIFICATION: Antifibrinolytics

THERAPEUTIC INTENT: Works to improve blood clotting

NURSING ACTIONS: Monitor vaginal bleeding. It is recommended to administer to clients who experience postpartum hemorrhage within 3 hr of birth.

CLIENT EDUCATION

Limit physical activity to conserve strength, to increase iron and protein intake to promote the rebuilding of RBC volume, and to take iron with vitamin C to enhance absorption.

Uterine atony

Uterine atony results from the inability of the uterine muscle to contract adequately after birth. This can lead to postpartum hemorrhage.

DATA COLLECTION

RISK FACTORS

- Retained placental fragments
- Prolonged or precipitous labor
- Oxytocin induction or augmentation of labor
- Overdistention of the uterine muscle (multiparity, multiple gestations, polyhydramnios [hydramnios], macrosomic fetus)
- Magnesium sulfate administration as a tocolytic
- Anesthesia and analgesia administration
- Trauma during labor and birth from operative delivery (forceps- or vacuum-assisted birth, cesarean birth)

EXPECTED FINDINGS

Increased vaginal bleeding

PHYSICAL FINDINGS
- Uterus that is larger than normal and boggy with possible lateral displacement on palpation
- Prolonged lochial discharge
- Irregular or excessive bleeding
- Tachycardia and hypotension
- Pallor of skin and mucous membranes; cool, and clammy with loss of turgor

DIAGNOSTIC PROCEDURES

- Bimanual compression or manual exploration of the uterine cavity for retained placental fragments by the provider
- Surgical intervention may be necessary if all other methods fail to decrease the bleeding and promote a firm uterus.
- Uterine tamponage is an intrauterine balloon that is placed inside the uterus to treat the postpartum hemorrhage.
- Surgical management, such as a hysterectomy

PATIENT-CENTERED CARE

NURSING CARE

- Ensure that the urinary bladder is empty.
- Monitor the following.
  ○ Fundal height, consistency, and location
  ○ Lochia for quantity, color, and consistency
- Perform fundal massage if indicated.
  ○ If the uterus becomes firm, continue monitoring.
  ○ If uterine atony persists, anticipate surgical intervention, such as a hysterectomy.
- Express clots that can have accumulated in the uterus, but only after the uterus is firmly contracted. It is critical not to express clots prior to the uterus becoming firmly contracted, because pushing on an uncontracted uterus can invert the uterus and result in extensive hemorrhage. Q EBP
- Monitor vital signs.
- Maintain IV fluids.
- Provide supplemental oxygen if needed.

MEDICATIONS

As noted for postpartum hemorrhage

CLIENT EDUCATION

- Rapid intervention is required. The health care team will explain the purpose of the interventions as they are performed.
- After becoming stable, limit physical activity to conserve strength. Increase iron and protein intake to promote the rebuilding of RBC volume.

Subinvolution of the uterus

Subinvolution is when the uterus remains enlarged with continued lochial discharge and can result in postpartum hemorrhage.

DATA COLLECTION

RISK FACTORS

- Pelvic infection and endometritis
- Retained placental fragments not completely expelled from the uterus

EXPECTED FINDINGS

- Prolonged vaginal bleeding
- Irregular or excessive vaginal bleeding

PHYSICAL FINDINGS
- Uterus that is enlarged and higher than normal in the abdomen relative to the umbilicus
- Boggy uterus
- Prolonged lochia discharge with irregular or excessive bleeding

LABORATORY TESTS

Blood, intracervical, and intrauterine bacterial cultures to check for evidence of infection and endometritis

THERAPEUTIC PROCEDURES

Dilation and curettage (D&C) is performed by the provider to remove retained placental fragments or to debride placenta insertion site, if indicated.

PATIENT-CENTERED CARE

NURSING CARE

- Monitor fundal position and consistency.
- Monitor lochia for color, amount, consistency, and odor.
- Monitor vital signs.
- Encourage the client to use activities that can enhance uterine involution.
  - Breastfeeding
  - Early and frequent ambulation
  - Frequent voiding

MEDICATIONS

Oxytocin, methylergonovine, ergonovine

CLASSIFICATION: Uterine stimulant

THERAPEUTIC INTENT: To promote uterine contractions and expel the retained fragments of placenta

NURSING ACTIONS: Monitor uterine tone and vaginal bleeding.

Antibiotic therapy

Can be prescribed to prevent or treat infection.

Inversion of the uterus

Inversion of the uterus is the turning inside out of the uterus and can be partial or complete. Uterine inversion is an emergency situation that can result in postpartum hemorrhage and requires immediate intervention.

DATA COLLECTION

RISK FACTORS

- Retained placenta
- Tocolysis
- Fetal macrosomia
- Nulliparity
- Uterine atony
- Vigorous fundal pressure
- Abnormally adherent placental tissue

- Fundal implantation of the placenta
- Excessive traction applied to the umbilical cord
- Short umbilical cord
- Prolonged labor

EXPECTED FINDINGS

Sudden pain in lower abdomen

PHYSICAL FINDINGS
- Vaginal bleeding: hemorrhage
  - Prolapsed inversion as evidenced by a large, red, rounded mass that protrudes 20 to 30 cm outside the introitus
  - Complete inversion as evidenced by the palpation of a smooth mass through the dilated cervix
- Dizziness
- Low blood pressure, increased pulse (shock)
- Pallor

THERAPEUTIC PROCEDURES

Manual replacement of the uterus into the uterine cavity and repositioning of the uterus by the provider

PATIENT-CENTERED CARE

NURSING CARE

- Monitor for an inverted uterus.
  - Visualize the introitus.
- Maintain IV fluids.
- Administer oxygen.
- Stop oxytocin if it is being administered at the time uterine inversion occurred.
- Anticipate surgery if nonsurgical interventions and management are unsuccessful.

MEDICATIONS

Terbutaline

CLASSIFICATION: Tocolytic

THERAPEUTIC INTENT: To relax the uterus prior to the provider's attempt at replacement of the uterus into the uterine cavity and uterus repositioning

NURSING ACTIONS: Following replacement of the uterus into the uterine cavity:
- Closely observe the client's response to treatment and monitor for stabilization of hemodynamic status.
- Avoid aggressive fundal massage.
- Administer oxytocics as prescribed.
- Administer broad-spectrum antibiotics for infection prophylaxis.

Retained placenta

The placenta or fragments of the placenta remain in the uterus and prevent the uterus from contracting, which can lead to uterine atony or subinvolution. A placenta that has not been delivered within 30 min of the birth is a retained placenta.

DATA COLLECTION

RISK FACTORS

- Partial separation of a normal placenta
- Entrapment of a partially or completely separated placenta by a constricting ring of the uterus
- Excessive traction on the umbilical cord prior to complete separation of the placenta
- Placental tissue that is abnormally adherent to the uterine wall
- Preterm births between 20 and 24 weeks of gestation

EXPECTED FINDINGS

PHYSICAL FINDINGS
- Uterine atony, subinvolution, or inversion
- Excessive bleeding or blood clots larger than a quarter
- Return of lochia rubra once lochia has progressed to serosa alba
- Malodorous lochia or vaginal discharge
- Elevated temperature

LABORATORY TESTS

Hgb and Hct

DIAGNOSTIC PROCEDURES

- Manual separation and removal of the placenta is done by the provider.
- D&C if oxytocics are ineffective in expelling the placental fragments.

PATIENT-CENTERED CARE

NURSING CARE

- Monitor the uterus for fundal height, consistency, and position.
- Monitor lochia for color, amount, consistency, and odor.
- Monitor vital signs.
- Maintain or initiate IV fluids.
- Provide supplemental oxygen.
- Anticipate surgical interventions (D&C, hysterectomy) if postpartum bleeding is present and continues.

MEDICATIONS

Oxytocin

To expel retained fragments of the placenta

CLASSIFICATION: Uterine stimulant

THERAPEUTIC INTENT: Promotes uterine contractions and expels the retained fragments of placenta

NURSING ACTIONS: Monitor uterine tone and vaginal bleeding.

CLIENT EDUCATION

After becoming stable, limit physical activity to conserve strength. Increase iron and protein intake to promote the rebuilding of RBC volume.

Lacerations and hematomas

- Lacerations that occur during labor and birth consist of the tearing of soft tissues in the birth canal and adjacent structures including the cervical, vaginal, vulvar, perineal, and/or rectal areas.
- An episiotomy can extend and become a third- or fourth-degree laceration.
- A hematoma is a collection of clotted blood within tissues that can appear as a bulging, bluish mass. Hematomas can occur in the pelvic region or higher in the vagina or broad ligament.
- Pain, rather than noticeable bleeding, is the distinguishable clinical finding of hematomas.
- The client is at risk for hemorrhage or infection due to a laceration or hematoma.

DATA COLLECTION

RISK FACTORS

- Operative vaginal birth (forceps-assisted, vacuum-assisted birth)
- Precipitous birth
- Cephalopelvic disproportion
- Size (macrosomic infant) and abnormal presentation or position of the fetus
- Prolonged pressure of the fetal head on the vaginal mucosa
- Previous scarring of the birth canal from infection, injury, or operation

EXPECTED FINDINGS

LACERATION
- Sensation of oozing or trickling of blood
- Excessive bleeding (with or without clots)

HEMATOMA
- Pain
- Pressure sensation in rectum (urge to defecate) or vagina
- Difficulty voiding

PHYSICAL FINDINGS
- **Laceration**
  - Vaginal bleeding even though the uterus is firm and contracted
  - Continuous slow trickle of bright red blood from vagina, laceration, episiotomy
- **Hematoma:** Bulging, bluish mass or area of red-purple discoloration on vulva, perineum, or rectum

PATIENT-CENTERED CARE

NURSING CARE

- Monitor for pain.
- Visually or manually inspect the vulva, perineum, and rectum for lacerations and/or hematomas.
- Evaluate lochia.
- Continue to monitor vital signs and hemodynamic status.
- Attempt to identify the source of the bleeding.
- Assist the provider with repair procedures.
- Use ice packs to treat small hematomas.
- Administer pain medication.
- Encourage sitz baths and frequent perineal hygiene.

THERAPEUTIC PROCEDURES

- Repair and suturing of the episiotomy or lacerations is done by the provider.
- Ligation of the bleeding vessel or surgical incision for evacuation of the clotted blood from the hematoma is done by the provider.

Postpartum infections

Postpartum infections are complications that can occur up to 28 days following childbirth or a spontaneous or induced abortion. Fever of 38° C (100.4° F) or higher after the first 24 hr or for 2 days during the first 10 days of the postpartum period is indicative of a postpartum infection and requires further investigation.

Uterine infection, wound infection, mastitis, and a urinary tract infection are examples of postpartum infections. Early identification and prompt treatment are necessary to promote positive outcomes.

Infections (endometritis, mastitis, and wound infections)

The immediate postpartum period following birth is a time of increased risk for all clients for micro-organisms entering the reproductive tract and migrating into the blood and other parts of the body, which can result in life-threatening septicemia.

Uterine infection is also referred to as **endometritis**.
- Endometritis is an infection of the uterine lining or endometrium. It is the most frequently occurring puerperal infection.
- Endometritis usually begins on the third to fourth postpartum day, generally starting as a localized infection at the placental attachment site and spreading to include the entire uterine endometrium.

Sites of **wound infections** include cesarean incisions, episiotomies, lacerations, and any trauma wounds present in the birth canal following labor and birth.

Mastitis is an infection of the breast involving the interlobular connective tissue and is usually unilateral. Mastitis can progress to an abscess if untreated.
- It usually occurs during the first 6 weeks of breastfeeding but can occur at any time during breastfeeding.
- *Staphylococcus aureus* is usually the infecting organism.

DATA COLLECTION

RISK FACTORS

- Urinary tract infection, mastitis, pneumonia, or history of previous venous thrombus
- History of diabetes mellitus, immunosuppression, anemia, or malnutrition
- History of alcohol or substance use disorder
- Cesarean birth
- Premature rupture of membranes
- Retained placental fragments and manual extraction of the placenta
- Bladder catheterization
- Chorioamnionitis
- Internal fetal/uterine pressure monitoring
- Multiple vaginal examinations after rupture of membranes
- Prolonged labor
- Postpartum hemorrhage
- Operative vaginal birth
- Epidural analgesia/anesthesia
- Hematomas
- Episiotomy or lacerations

Mastitis

- Milk stasis, which can be caused by a blocked duct, engorgement, or a bra with an underwire
- Nipple trauma and cracked or fissured nipples
- Poor breastfeeding technique with improper latching of the infant onto the breast, which can lead to sore and cracked nipples
- Decrease in breastfeeding frequency due to supplementation with bottle feeding
- Contamination of breasts due to poor hygiene

EXPECTED FINDINGS

PUERPERAL INFECTIONS

- Flu-like manifestations (body aches, chills, fever, malaise)
- Anorexia and nausea

ENDOMETRITIS

- Pelvic pain
- Chills
- Fatigue
- Loss of appetite

MASTITIS

- Painful or tender localized hard mass and reddened area, usually on one breast
- Influenza-like manifestations (chills, fever, headache, body ache)
- Fatigue

PHYSICAL FINDINGS

- **Puerperal infections**
- Elevated temperature of at least 38° C (100.4°F) for 2 or more consecutive days after the first 24 hr
- Tachycardia
- **Endometritis**
- Uterine tenderness
- Profuse lochia
- Lochia that is either malodorous or purulent
- Temperature greater than 38° C (100.4° F), typically on the third or fourth postpartum day
- Tachycardia
- **Wound infection**
- Wound warmth, erythema, tenderness, pain, edema, seropurulent drainage, and wound dehiscence (separation of wound or incision edges) or evisceration (protrusion of internal contents through the separated wound edges)
- Temperature greater than 38° C (100.4° F) for 2 or more consecutive days
- **Mastitis:** Axillary adenopathy in the affected side (enlarged tender axillary lymph nodes) with an area of inflammation that can be red, swollen, warm, and tender

LABORATORY TESTS

- Blood, intracervical, or intrauterine bacterial cultures to reveal the offending organism
- WBC count: leukocytosis
- RBC sedimentation rate: distinctly increased
- RBC count: anemia

PATIENT-CENTERED CARE

NURSING CARE

- Obtain frequent vital signs.
- Monitor for pain.
- Check fundal height, position, and consistency.
- Observe lochia for color, quantity, and consistency.
- Inspect incisions, episiotomy, and lacerations.
- Inspect breasts.

Puerperal infections

- Use aseptic technique for appropriate procedures; perform proper hand hygiene; and don gloves for labor, birth, and postpartum care.
- Maintain IV access.
- Administer IV broad-spectrum antibiotic therapy (penicillins, cephalosporins, clindamycin, gentamicin).
- Provide comfort measures (warm blankets, cool compresses), depending on findings.

CLIENT EDUCATION

- Report manifestations of worsening conditions.
- Adhere to the treatment plan with the completion of a full course of antibiotics.
- Preventative measures include thorough handwashing and good perineal hygiene.
- A diet high in protein promotes tissue healing.

Endometritis

- Assist with collecting vaginal and blood cultures.
- Administer IV antibiotics.
- Administer analgesics.

CLIENT EDUCATION

- Perform effective hand hygiene techniques.
- Maintain interaction with the infant to facilitate bonding.

Wound infection

- Perform wound care.
- Administer IV antibiotics.
- Provide or encourage comfort measures (sitz baths, perineal care, warm or cold compresses).

CLIENT EDUCATION: Good hygiene techniques include changing perineal pads from front to back and performing thorough hand hygiene prior to and after perineal care.

Mastitis

Administer antibiotics.

CLIENT EDUCATION: Breast hygiene can prevent and manage mastitis.

- Thoroughly wash hands prior to breastfeeding.
- Maintain cleanliness of breasts with frequent changes of breast pads.
- Allow nipples to air-dry.
- Proper infant positioning and latching-on techniques include both the nipple and the areola. Release the infant's grasp on the nipple prior to removing the infant from the breast.

- Completely empty the breasts with each feeding to prevent milk stasis, which provides a medium for bacterial growth.
- Use ice packs or warm packs on affected breasts for discomfort.
- Continue breastfeeding frequently (at least every 2 to 4 hr), especially on the affected side.
- Manually express breast milk or use a breast pump if breastfeeding is too painful.
- Breastfeed or pump frequently, emptying the affected side.
- Rest, take analgesics, and maintain fluid intake of at least 3,000 mL per day.
- Wear a well-fitting bra for support. The bra should not have an underwire because that increases the risk for infection.
- Report redness and fever.
- Complete the entire course of antibiotics as prescribed.

MEDICATIONS

For endometritis

Clindamycin

Cephalosporins, penicillins, and gentamicin

CLASSIFICATION: Antibiotic

THERAPEUTIC INTENT: Treatment of bacterial infections

CLIENT EDUCATION
- Take all the medication as prescribed.
- Notify the provider of the development of watery, bloody diarrhea.
- Notify the provider if breastfeeding.

THERAPEUTIC PROCEDURES

The provider might need to open and drain the wound or perform wound debridement if indicated.

Urinary tract infection

- Urinary tract infections (UTIs) are a common postpartum infection secondary to bladder trauma incurred during the delivery or a break in aseptic technique during bladder catheterization.
- A potential complication of a UTI is the progression to pyelonephritis with permanent kidney damage, leading to kidney failure.

DATA COLLECTION

RISK FACTORS

- Postpartal hypotonic bladder or urethra (urinary stasis and retention)
- Epidural anesthesia
- Urinary bladder catheterization
- Frequent pelvic examinations

- Genital tract injuries
- History of UTIs
- Cesarean birth

EXPECTED FINDINGS

- Reports of urgency, frequency, dysuria, and pelvic area discomfort
- Fever
- Chills
- Malaise

PHYSICAL FINDINGS
- Change in vital signs, elevated temperature
- Urine (cloudy, blood-tinged, malodorous, sediment visible)
- Urinary retention
- Pain in the suprapubic area
- Pain at the costovertebral angle (pyelonephritis)

DIAGNOSTIC PROCEDURES

Urinalysis for WBCs, RBCs, protein, bacteria

PATIENT-CENTERED CARE

NURSING CARE

- Obtain a random or clean-catch urine sample.
- Administer antibiotics, and reinforce with the client about the importance of completing the entire course of antibiotics as prescribed.
- Acetaminophen is taken to reduce discomfort and pain associated with a urinary tract infection.
- Reinforce with the client proper perineal hygiene, such as wiping from front to back.
- Encourage the client to increase their fluid intake to 3,000 mL/day to dilute the bacteria and flush the bladder.

Postpartum mental health disorders

Postpartum blues can occur in up to 85% of clients during the first few days after birth and generally continues for up to 10 days. It is characterized by mood swings, anxiety, tearfulness, insomnia, and lack of appetite. A parent can experience an intense fear, anxiety, anger, and inability to cope with the slightest problems and become despondent. Postpartum blues typically resolves in 10 days without intervention.

Postpartum depression occurs within 12 months of birth and is characterized by persistent feelings of sadness and intense mood swings. Depression and anxiety occurs in 10% to 15% of new parents and usually does not resolve without intervention. It is similar to nonpostpartum mood disorders. According to ACOG, perinatal depression has been identified as one of the most common medical conditions during pregnancy and the postpartum period. It affects one in seven clients.

According to AWHONN, perinatal mood disorders (PMSs) can occur any time during pregnancy and during the first year postpartum. This includes depression, bipolar disorder, anxiety, and postpartum psychosis.

Postpartum psychosis develops within the first 2 to 3 weeks of the postpartum period. Clients who have a history of bipolar disorder are at a higher risk. Clinical findings are severe and can include confusion, disorientation, hallucinations, delusions, obsessive behaviors, and paranoia. The client might attempt to harm themselves or their newborn.

A nurse should monitor clients for suicidal or delusional thoughts. The nurse should monitor newborns for failure to thrive secondary to an inability of the parent to provide care.

DATA COLLECTION

RISK FACTORS

- Hormonal changes with a rapid decline in estrogen and progesterone levels
- Individual socioeconomic factors
- Decreased social support system
- Anxiety about assuming new role as a parent
- Unintended pregnancy
- History of previous depressive disorder
- Low self-esteem
- History of partner violence
- Medical conditions (thyroid imbalance, diabetes, infertility)
- Complications with breastfeeding
- Parent of multiples

EXPECTED FINDINGS

Postpartum blues

- Feelings of sadness
- Lack of appetite
- Sleep pattern disturbances
- Feeling of inadequacies
- Crying easily for no apparent reason
- Restlessness, insomnia, fatigue
- Headache
- Anxiety, anger, sadness

PHYSICAL FINDINGS: Crying

Postpartum depression

- Feelings of guilt and inadequacies
- Irritability
- Anxiety
- Fatigue persisting beyond a reasonable amount of time
- Feelings of loss
- Lack of appetite
- Persistent feelings of sadness
- Intense mood swings
- Sleep pattern disturbances
- Thoughts of harming self or newborn

PHYSICAL FINDINGS
- Crying
- Weight loss
- Flat affect
- Irritability
- Rejection of the newborn
- Severe anxiety and panic attack

Postpartum psychosis

- Pronounced sadness
- Disorientation
- Confusion
- Paranoia
- Impulsive behaviors
- Obsessive concerns
- Suspicious
- Irrational statements
- Initially: fatigue, insomnia, restless, and tearful
- Rapid mood swings

PHYSICAL FINDINGS: Behaviors indicating hallucinations or delusional thoughts of self-harm or harming the newborn

PATIENT-CENTERED CARE

NURSING CARE

- All clients should receive an assessment throughout pregnancy and during the postpartum period for perinatal mood disorders (PMDs). This assessment should include questions that address the client's mood and anxiety. This screening is recommended by ACOG. Postpartum depression should be assessed during the postpartum period before discharge and then reassessed four weeks after birth.
- Monitor interactions between the client and their newborn. Encourage bonding activities.
- Monitor interactions between the client and their infant. Encourage bonding activities.
- Monitor the client's mood and affect.
- Reinforce that feeling down in the postpartum period is normal and self-limiting. Encourage the client to notify the provider if the condition persists.
- Encourage the client to communicate feelings, validate and address personal conflicts, and reinforce personal power and autonomy.
- Reinforce the importance of compliance with any prescribed medication regimen.
- Assist with contacting a community resource to schedule a follow-up visit after discharge for clients who are at high risk for postpartum depression.
- Ask the client if they have thoughts of self-harm, suicide, or harming their newborn. Provide for the safety of the infant and client as the priority of care.

MEDICATIONS

- **Antidepressants** can be prescribed by the provider if indicated.
- **Antipsychotics** and **mood stabilizers** can be prescribed for clients who have postpartum psychosis.

CLIENT EDUCATION

CARE AFTER DISCHARGE

- Get plenty of rest and nap when the newborn sleeps.
- Remember the importance of taking time out for self.
- Schedule a follow-up visit prior to the traditional postpartum visit if at risk for developing postpartum depression.
- Consider community resources (La Leche League, community mental health centers).
- Seek counseling, and consider social agencies as indicated.

Active Learning Scenario

A nurse is contributing to the plan of care for a client who has endometritis with a group of newly hired nurses. What information should the nurse reinforce in the teaching? Use the ATI Active Learning Template: System Disorder to complete this item.

ALTERATION IN HEALTH (DIAGNOSIS)

EXPECTED FINDINGS: Describe at least six.

NURSING CARE: Describe at least three nursing interventions.

Application Exercises

1. A nurse is caring for a client who is postpartum. The nurse should identify which of the following findings as an early indicator of hypovolemia caused by hemorrhage?

   A. Increasing pulse and decreasing blood pressure

   B. Dizziness and increasing respiratory rate

   C. Cool, clammy skin and pale mucous membranes

   D. Altered mental status and level of consciousness

2. A nurse is reinforcing teaching with a client who is breastfeeding and has mastitis. What response should the nurse make?

3. A nurse is caring for a client who has mastitis. What is a typical causative agent of mastitis?

4. A nurse is discussing risks factors for urinary tract infections and endometritis for clients with a newly licensed nurse. Which of the following conditions should the nurse include in the teaching? Sort the following options into risk factors based on the following conditions: Urinary Tract Infection or Endometritis

   A. Epidural

   B. Premature rupture of membranes

   C. History of UTIs

   D. Prolonged labor

   E. Chorioamnionitis

5. A nurse is assisting with the care of a client who has postpartum psychosis. Which of the following actions is the nurse's priority?

   A. Reinforce the need to take antipsychotics as prescribed.

   B. Ask the client if they have thoughts of harming themselves or their infant.

   C. Monitor the infant for indications of failure to thrive.

   D. Review the client's medical record for a history of bipolar disorder.

Active Learning Scenario Key

Using the ATI Active Learning Template: System Disorder

ALTERATION IN HEALTH (DIAGNOSIS): Endometritis is an infection of the uterine lining or endometrium. It usually begins as a localized infection at the placental attachment site and spreads to include the entire endometrium. It is the most frequently occurring puerperal infection.

EXPECTED FINDINGS
- Uterine tenderness
- Profuse lochia
- Malodorous or purulent lochia
- Temperature greater than 38° C (100.4° F) on the third or fourth postpartum day
- Tachycardia
- Pelvic pain
- Chills
- Fatigue, loss of appetite

NURSING CARE
- Assist with obtaining vaginal and blood cultures.
- Administer IV antibiotics.
- Administer analgesics.
- Reinforce with client hand hygiene techniques.
- Encourage client interaction with their infant to facilitate bonding.

Ⓝ *NCLEX® Connection: Physiological Adaptation, Alterations in Body Systems*

Application Exercises Key

1. A. **CORRECT:** The nurse should recognize a rising pulse rate and decreasing pressure are often the first indications of inadequate blood volume. Dizziness and increased respiratory rate are findings that occur in hypovolemia but are not the earliest indicators of hypovolemia. Skin that is cool, clammy, and pale, along with pale mucous membranes, are changes that occur in the physical status of a client who has decreased blood volume, but they are not the first indicators of inadequate blood volume. Altered mental status and changes in level of consciousness are late manifestations of decreased blood volume, which leads to hypoxia and low oxygen saturation.

   Ⓝ *NCLEX® Connection: Psychosocial Integrity, Alterations in Body Systems*

2. The nurse should instruct the client to completely empty each breast at each feeding to prevent milk stasis, which provides a medium for bacterial growth. Continue breastfeeding frequently (at least every 2 to 4 hr), especially on the affected side. Use ice packs or warms packs on the affected breasts for discomfort. Take analgesics, and antibiotics as prescribed. Also, rest and maintain fluid intake of at least 3,000 mL per day.

   Ⓝ *NCLEX® Connection: Psychosocial Integrity, Illness Management*

3. *Staphylococcus aureus, Escherichia coli,* and streptococcus are usually the infecting agents that enter the breast due to sore or cracked nipples, which result in mastitis

   Ⓝ *NCLEX® Connection: Psychosocial Integrity, Alterations in Body Systems*

4. **URINARY TRACT INFECTION:** A, C; **ENDOMETRITIS:** B, D, E

   The nurse is discussing risks factors for urinary tract infections and endometritis for clients with a newly licensed nurse. The nurse should include an epidural and history of UTIs as risks for the development of a urinary tract infection. Also, premature rupture of membranes, prolonged labor, and chorioamnionitis are risk factors for the development of endometritis.

   Ⓝ *NCLEX® Connection: Physiological Adaptation, Illness Management*

5. B. **CORRECT:** The priority action the nurse should take when using Maslow's hierarchy of needs is to meet the client's need for the client's safety. The nurse should ask the client if they are having any thoughts of harming themselves or their newborn. Reinforcing the need to take antipsychotics as prescribed is important because it will assist with symptom management; however, there is another intervention that is the priority. Monitoring the newborn for indications of failure to thrive is important because the nurse should intervene should manifestations of failure to thrive exist; however, there is another intervention that is the priority. Reviewing the client's medical record for a history of bipolar disorder is important because the nurse should identify any perinatal mood disorders in order to implement appropriate interventions and care; however, there is another intervention that is the priority.

   Ⓝ *NCLEX® Connection: Health Promotion and Maintenance, Health Screening*

When reviewing the following chapters, keep in mind the relevant topics and tasks of the NCLEX outline.

Safe and Effective Care Environment

HOME SAFETY: Reinforce client education on home safety precautions.

SECURITY PLAN: Initiate and participate in security alert.

Health Promotion and Maintenance

ANTE-/INTRA-/POSTPARTUM AND NEWBORN CARE
Contribute to newborn plan of care.

Reinforce client teaching on infant care skills.

DATA COLLECTION TECHNIQUES
Collect data for health history.

Collect baseline physical data.

DEVELOPMENTAL STAGES AND TRANSITIONS: Assist client with expected life transition.

Pharmacological Therapies

EXPECTED ACTIONS/OUTCOMES
Apply knowledge of pathophysiology when addressing client pharmacological agents.

Evaluate client response to medication.

Reduction of Risk Potential

POTENTIAL FOR COMPLICATIONS OF DIAGNOSTIC TESTS/ TREATMENTS/PROCEDURES: Use precautions to prevent injury or complications associated with a procedure or diagnosis.

LABORATORY VALUES: Monitor diagnostic or laboratory test results.

UNIT 4   NEWBORN NURSING CARE
SECTION: LOW-RISK NEWBORN

CHAPTER 15 ## Newborn Data Collection

Understanding physiologic responses of a newborn to birth and physical findings are imperative for providing newborn nursing care. Key responsibilities include assisting with the physical examination of the newborn, obtaining newborn vital signs and measurements, classifying a newborn by gestational age and weight, performing diagnostic and therapeutic procedures, and identifying complications of a newborn.

PHYSIOLOGIC RESPONSE OF NEWBORN TO BIRTH

- Adjustments to extrauterine life occur as a newborn's respiratory and circulatory systems are required to rapidly adjust to life outside of the uterus.
- The establishment of respiratory function with the cutting of the umbilical cord is the most critical extrauterine adjustment as air inflates the lungs with the first breath.
- Circulatory changes occur due to changes in pressures of the cardiovascular system related to cutting of the umbilical cord as a newborn begins breathing independently. The three shunts (ductus arteriosus, ductus venosus, foramen ovale) functionally close during a newborn's transition to extrauterine life with the flow of oxygenated blood in the lungs and readjustment of atrial blood pressure in the heart.

PHYSICAL DATA COLLECTION OF NEWBORN FOLLOWING BIRTH

Apgar scoring and a brief physical exam is done immediately following birth as newborns transition to extrauterine life to rule out abnormalities.

EQUIPMENT FOR NEWBORN DATA COLLECTION

Bulb syringe: Used for suctioning excess mucus from the mouth and nose

Stethoscope with a pediatric head: Used to evaluate heart rate, breath sounds, and bowel sounds

Axillary thermometer: Used to monitor temperature and prevent hypothermia. Rectal temperatures are avoided because they can injure the delicate rectal mucosa.

Blood pressure cuff: Electronic method. Blood pressure can be done in all four extremities if evaluating the newborn for cardiac problems.

Scale with protective cover in place: Scale should be at 0; weight should include pounds, ounces, and grams.

Tape measure in centimeters: Measure from crown to heel of foot for length. Measure head circumference at greatest diameter (occipital to frontal). Measure chest circumference beginning at the nipple line and abdominal circumference above the umbilicus.

Clean gloves: Worn for all physical data collection until discharge

INITIAL DATA COLLECTION

External data collection: Skin color, peeling, birthmarks, foot creases, breast tissue, nasal patency, and meconium staining (can indicate fetal hypoxia)

Chest: Point of maximal impulse location; ease of breathing; auscultation for heart rate and quality of tones; and respirations for crackles, wheezes, and equality of bilateral breath sounds

Abdomen: Rounded abdomen and umbilical cord with one vein and two arteries

Neurologic: Muscle tone and reflex reaction (Moro reflex); palpation for the presence and size of fontanels and sutures; data collection of fontanels for fullness or bulge

Other observations: Inspection for gross structural malformations

EXPECTED REFERENCE RANGES

Weight: 2,500 to 4,000 g (5.5 to 8.8 lb); normal variation 2,700–4,000 g (6 to 9 lb)

Length: 45 to 55 cm (18 to 22 in)

Head circumference: 32 to 36.8 cm (12.6 to 14.5 in)

Chest circumference: 30 to 33 cm (12 to 13 in)

CLASSIFICATION
Following data collection, classification of the newborn by gestational age and birth weight is determined.

Appropriate for gestational age (AGA): Weight is between the 10th and 90th percentile.

Small for gestational age (SGA): Weight is less than the 10th percentile.

Large for gestational age (LGA): Weight is greater than the 90th percentile.

Low birth weight (LBW): Weight is 2,500 g or less at birth.

Intrauterine growth restriction (IUGR): Growth rate does not meet expected norms.
- Early term is defined as occurring from 37 0/7 weeks through 38 6/7 weeks.
- Full term is defined as occurring from 39 0/7 through 40 6/7 weeks.
- Late term is defined as occurring from 41 0/7 weeks through 41 6/7 weeks.

Preterm or premature: Born prior to 37 0/7 weeks of gestation

Late preterm is defined as occurring from 34 0/7 through 36 6/7 weeks.

Postterm: Born after the completion of 42 0/7 weeks of gestation

Postmature: Born after the completion of 42 weeks of gestation with evidence of placental insufficiency

VITAL SIGNS

Vital signs are checked in the following sequence: respirations, heart rate, blood pressure, and temperature. The nurse observes the respiratory rate first before the newborn becomes active or agitated by use of the stethoscope, thermometer, and/or blood pressure cuff.

Respiratory rate varies from 30 to 60 breaths/min with short periods of apnea (less than 20 seconds) occurring most frequently during the rapid eye movement sleep cycle. Periods of apnea lasting longer than 20 seconds should be evaluated. Crackles and wheezing are manifestations of fluid or infection in the lungs. Grunting and nasal flaring are clinical findings of respiratory distress.

Expected heart rate ranges from 110 to 160/min with brief fluctuations above and below this range depending on activity level (crying, sleeping). Apical pulse rate is counted for 1 full minute, preferably when the newborn is sleeping. The pediatric stethoscope head is placed on the fourth or fifth intercostal space at the left midclavicular line over the apex of the newborn's heart. Heart murmurs are documented and reported.

Blood pressure should be 60 to 80 mm Hg systolic and 40 to 50 mm Hg diastolic.

Normal temperature range is 36.5° C to 37.5° C (97.7° F to 99.5° F), with 37° C (98.6° F) being average. The newborn is at risk for hypothermia and hyperthermia until thermoregulation (ability to produce heat and maintain normal body temperature) stabilizes. If the newborn becomes chilled (cold stress), oxygen demands can increase and acidosis can occur.

A more extensive physical exam is performed on the neonate within 24 hr of birth. Vital signs are obtained. A head-to-toe exam is performed. Neurologic and behavioral exams are completed by eliciting reflexes and observing responses. Laboratory data are monitored.

PHYSICAL EXAM FROM HEAD TO TOE

Posture

- Lying in a curled-up position with arms and legs in moderate flexion
- Resistant to extension of extremities

Skin

- Skin color should be initially deep red to purple, with acrocyanosis (bluish tint to hands and feet). Skin color should fade to a color congruent to the newborn genetic background. Secondary to increased bilirubin, jaundice can appear on the third day of life but then decrease spontaneously.
- Skin turgor should be quick, indicating that the newborn is well-hydrated. The skin should spring back immediately when pinched.
- Texture should be dry, soft, and smooth, showing good hydration. Cracks in hands and feet can be present. In full-term newborns, desquamation (peeling) occurs a few days after birth.
- Vernix caseosa (protective, thick, cheesy covering) amounts vary, with more present in creases and skin folds.
- Lanugo (fine, downy hair) varies regarding the amount present. It is usually found on the pinnae of ears, forehead, and shoulders.

NORMAL DEVIATIONS

- **Milia** (small, raised, pearly or white spots on the nose, chin, and forehead) can be present. These spots disappear spontaneously without treatment (parents should not squeeze the spots).
- **Mongolian spots** (spots of pigmentation that are blue, gray, brown, or black) are commonly noted on the back and buttocks. These spots are more commonly present on newborns who have dark skin and can be linked to genetics. Be sure the parents are aware of Mongolian spots, and document location and presence.

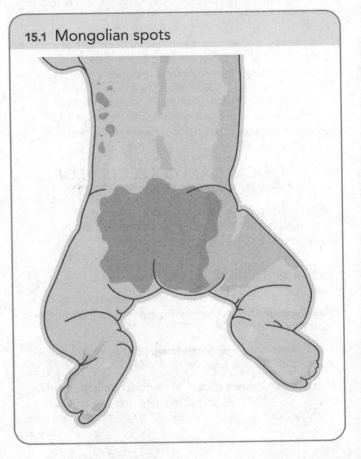

15.1 Mongolian spots

- **Telangiectatic nevi** (stork bites) are flat pink or red marks that easily blanch and are found on the back of the neck, nose, upper eyelids, and middle of the forehead. They usually fade by the second year of life.
- **Nevus flammeus** (port wine stain) is a capillary angioma below the surface of the skin that is purple or red, varies in size and shape, is commonly seen on the face, and does not blanch or disappear.
- **Erythema toxicum** (erythema neonatorum) is a pink rash that appears suddenly anywhere on the body of a term newborn during the first 3 weeks. This is frequently referred to as newborn rash. No treatment is required.

Head

- Head should be 2 to 3 cm larger than chest circumference. If the head circumference is greater than or equal to 4 cm larger than the chest circumference, this can be an indication of **hydrocephalus** (excessive cerebral fluid within the brain cavity surrounding the brain). If the head circumference is less than or equal to 32 cm, this can be an indication of **microcephaly** (abnormally small head).
- Anterior fontanel should be palpable and approximately 5 cm on average and diamond-shaped. Posterior fontanel is smaller and triangle-shaped. Fontanels should be soft and flat. Fontanels can bulge when the newborn cries, coughs, or vomits but should be flat when the newborn is quiet. Bulging fontanels at rest can indicate increased intracranial pressure, infection, or hemorrhage. Depressed fontanels can indicate dehydration.
- Sutures should be palpable, separated, and can be overlapping (molding), a normal occurrence resulting from head compression during labor.
- **Caput succedaneum** (localized swelling of the soft tissues of the scalp caused by pressure on the head during labor) is an expected finding that can be palpated as a soft edematous mass and can cross over the suture line. Caput succedaneum usually resolves in 3 to 4 days and does not require treatment.
- **Cephalohematoma** is a collection of blood between the periosteum and the skull bone that it covers. It does not cross the suture line. It results from trauma during birth such as pressure of the fetal head against the maternal pelvis in a prolonged difficult labor or forceps delivery. It appears in the first 1 to 2 days after birth and resolves in 2 to 8 weeks.

Eyes

- Check eyes for symmetry in size and shape.
- Each eye from the inner to outer canthus and the space between the eyes should equal one-third the distance across both eyes to rule out chromosomal abnormalities, such as Down syndrome.
- Lacrimal glands are immature, with minimal or no tears.
- Subconjunctival hemorrhages can result from pressure during birth.
- Pupillary and red reflex are present.
- Eyeball movement will demonstrate random, jerky movements.

Ears

- When examining the placement of ears, draw an imaginary line through the inner to the outer canthus of the newborn's eye. The line should be even with the top notch of the newborn's ear, where the ear meets the scalp. Ears that are low-set can indicate a chromosome abnormality, such as Down syndrome, or a kidney disorder.
- Cartilage should be firm and well-formed. Lack of cartilage indicates prematurity.
- The newborn should respond to voices and other sounds.
- Inspect ears for skin tags.

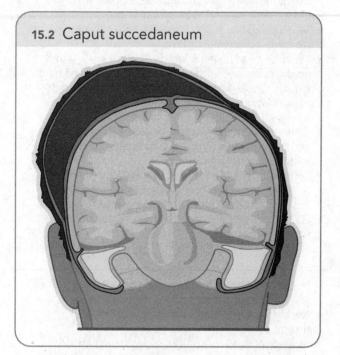

15.2 Caput succedaneum

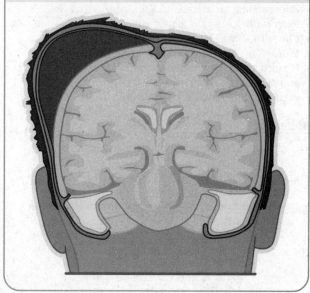

15.3 Cephalohematoma

Nose

- The nose should be midline, flat, and broad with lack of a bridge.
- Some mucus should be present, but with no drainage.
- Newborns are obligate nose breathers and do not develop the response of opening the mouth with a nasal obstruction until 3 weeks after birth. Therefore, a nasal blockage can result in flaring of the nares, cyanosis, or asphyxia.
- Newborns sneeze to clear nasal passages.

Mouth

- Check for palate closure and strength of sucking.
- Lip movements should be symmetrical.
- Saliva should be scant. Excessive saliva can indicate a tracheoesophageal fistula.
- Epstein's pearls (small, whitish-yellow cysts found on the gums and at the junction of the soft and hard palates) are expected findings. They result from the accumulation of epithelial cells and disappear a few weeks after birth.
- Tongue should move freely, be symmetrical in shape, and not protrude. (A protruding tongue can be an indication of Down syndrome.)
- Soft and hard palate should be intact.
- Gray-white patches on the tongue and gums can indicate thrush, a fungal infection caused by *Candida albicans*, sometimes acquired from the mother's vaginal secretions.

Neck

- Neck should be short, thick, surrounded by skin folds, and exhibit no webbing.
- Neck should move freely from side to side and up and down.
- Absence of head control can indicate prematurity or Down syndrome.

Chest

- Chest should be barrel-shaped.
- Respirations are primarily diaphragmatic.
- Clavicles should be intact.
- Retractions should be absent.
- Nipples should be prominent, well-formed, and symmetrical.
- Breast nodules can be 3 to 10 mm.

Abdomen

- Umbilical cord should be odorless and exhibit no intestinal structures.
- Abdomen should be round, dome-shaped, and nondistended.
- Bowel sounds should be present within a few minutes following birth.

Anogenital

- Anus should be present, patent, and not covered by a membrane.
- Meconium should be passed within 24 to 48 hr after birth.
- Genitalia of a male newborn should include rugae on the scrotum.
- Testes should be present in the scrotum.
- Male urinary meatus should be located at penile tip.
- Genitalia of a female should include labia majora covering the labia minora and clitoris and are usually edematous.
- Vaginal blood-tinged discharge can occur in female newborns, which is caused by maternal pregnancy hormones. This is an expected finding.
- A hymenal tag should be present.
- Urine should be passed within 24 hr after birth. Uric acid crystals will produce a rust color in the urine the first couple of days of life.

Extremities

- Check for full range, symmetry of motion, and spontaneous movements.
- Extremities should be flexed.
- Check for bowed legs and flat feet, which should be present because lateral muscles are more developed than the medial muscles.
- No click should be heard when abducting the hips.
- Gluteal folds should be symmetrical.
- Soles should be well-lined over two-thirds of the feet.
- Nail beds should be pink, and no extra digits are present.

Spine

Spine should be straight, flat, midline, and easily flexed.

Reflexes

Sucking and rooting reflex
- EXPECTED FINDING: Elicit by stroking the cheek or edge of mouth. Newborn turns the head toward the side that is touched and starts to suck.
- EXPECTED AGE: Usually disappears after 3 to 4 months but can persist up to 1 year

Palmar grasp
- EXPECTED FINDING: Elicit by placing examiner's finger in palm of newborn's hand. The newborn's fingers curl around examiner's fingers.
- EXPECTED AGE: Lessens by 3 to 4 months

Plantar grasp
- EXPECTED FINDING: Elicit by placing examiner's finger at base of newborn's toes. The newborn responds by curling toes downward.
- EXPECTED AGE: Birth to 8 months

Moro reflex
- EXPECTED FINDING: Elicit by allowing the head and trunk of the newborn in a semi-sitting position to fall backward to an angle of at least 30°. The newborn will symmetrically extend and then abduct the arms at the elbows and fingers spread to form a "C."
- EXPECTED AGE: Complete response can be seen until 8 weeks, body jerk only until 8 to 18 weeks, and then absent by 6 months.

Tonic neck reflex (fencing position)
- EXPECTED FINDING: With newborn in supine, neutral position, examiner turns newborn's head quickly to one side. The newborn's arm and leg on that side extend, and opposing arm and leg flex.
- EXPECTED AGE: Birth to 3 to 4 months

Babinski reflex
- EXPECTED FINDING: Elicit by stroking the outer edge of sole of the foot, moving up towards the toes on the lateral side and then across the ball of the foot.
- EXPECTED AGE: Birth to 1 year

Stepping
- EXPECTED FINDING: Elicit by holding the newborn upright with feet touching a flat surface. The newborn responds with stepping movements.
- EXPECTED AGE: Birth to 4 weeks

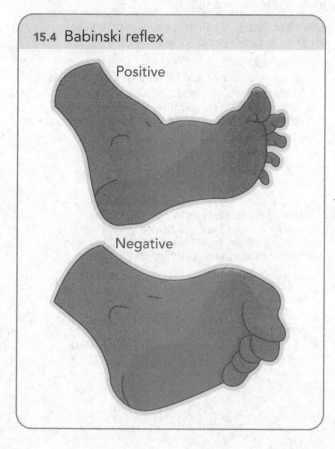

15.4 Babinski reflex

Positive

Negative

Senses

Vision: The newborn should be able to focus on objects 8 to 12 inches away from face. This is approximately the distance from the mother's face when the newborn is breastfeeding. The eyes are sensitive to light, so newborns prefer dim lighting. Pupils are reactive to light, and the blink reflex is easily stimulated. The newborn can track high-contrast objects and prefers black and white patterns. Term newborns can see objects as far away as 2.5 feet. Within 2 to 3 months, they can discriminate colors.

Hearing: Hearing is similar to that of an adult once the amniotic fluid drains from the ears. Newborns exhibit selective listening to familiar voices and rhythms of intrauterine life. The newborn turns toward the general direction of a sound.

Touch: Newborns should respond to tactile messages of pain and touch. The mouth, hands, and soles of the feet are the areas most sensitive to touch in the newborn.

Taste: Newborns can taste and prefer sweet to salty, sour, or bitter.

Smell: Newborns have a highly developed sense of smell, prefer sweet smells, and can recognize the mother's smell.

Habitation: This is a protective mechanism whereby the newborn becomes accustomed to environmental stimuli. Response to a constant or repetitive stimulus is decreased. This allows the newborn to select stimuli that promotes continued learning, avoiding overload.

> **!** Reinforce to the parent and family about the neonate's appearance, and give reassurance about expected findings that the family can be concerned about (milia, Epstein's pearls, caput succedaneum).

PAIN DATA COLLECTION

Measure newborn pain using a combination of behavioral observation and physiological findings. Several pain scales have been developed as a tool to measure newborn pain.
- CRIES scale
- Neonatal Infant Pain Scale (NIPS)

Behavioral responses to pain

- Alterations in sleep-wake cycles, feeding, or activity
- Fussiness or irritability
- Limb withdrawal; thrashing or fist-clenching; muscle rigidity or flaccidity
- Facial grimacing; chin quivering; furrowed brow; tightly closed eyes; open, square-shaped mouth
- Crying, groaning, or whimpering vocalizations

Physiologic responses to pain

Vital signs: Rapid or shallow respirations; decreased oxygen saturation; increased heart rate and blood pressure

Skin: Pallor or flushing; palmar or general diaphoresis

Laboratory findings: Hyperglycemia, decreased pH, increased blood corticosteroid levels

Other: Increased muscle tone, decreased vagal nerve tone, increased intracranial pressure, dilated pupils

DIAGNOSTIC AND THERAPEUTIC PROCEDURES FOLLOWING BIRTH

Cord blood is collected at birth. Laboratory tests are conducted to determine ABO blood type and Rh status if the parent's blood type is "O" or they are Rh-negative. A CBC can be done by a capillary stick to evaluate for anemia, polycythemia, infection, or clotting problems. Blood glucose levels are usually evaluated only in newborns who have risk factors for hypoglycemia.

EXPECTED LABORATORY VALUES

- **Hgb:** 14 to 24 g/dL
- **Platelets:** 150,000 to 300,000/mm³
- **Hct:** 44% to 64%
- **Glucose:** 40 to 45 mg/dL
- **RBC count:** 4.8×10^6 to 7.1×10^6
- **Bilirubin**
  - 24 hr: 2 to 6mg/dL
  - 48 hr: 6 to 7 mg/dL
  - 3 to 5 days: 4 to 6 mg/dL
- **WBC count:** 9,000 to 30,000/mm³

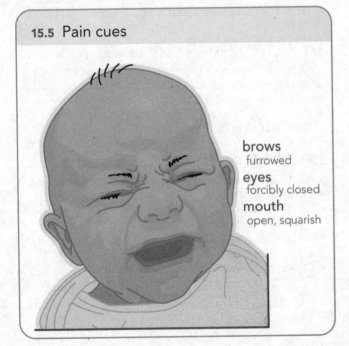

15.5 Pain cues

brows furrowed
eyes forcibly closed
mouth open, squarish

COMPLICATIONS

Airway obstruction related to mucus

NURSING ACTIONS: Suction mouth first and then nose with a bulb syringe to prevent aspiration.

Hypothermia

NURSING ACTIONS

- Monitor axillary temperature. Healthy newborn temperature averages 37° C (98.6° F), with a range of 36.5° C to 37.5° C (97.7° F to 99.5° F).
- If temperature is unstable, place the newborn in a radiant warmer, and maintain skin temperature at approximately 36.5° C (97.7° F). Ideal method for promoting warmth and maintaining neonate's body temperature for a stable newborn is early skin-to-skin contact with parent. If the newborn does not remain skin-to-skin with parent during the first 1 to 2 hr after birth, place the thoroughly dried newborn under the radiant warmer or in a warm incubator until body temperature stabilizes.
- Check axillary temperature every hour until stable.
- All exams and collection of data should be performed while the newborn is under a radiant warmer or during skin-to-skin contact with the parent.

Inadequate oxygen supply

Related to obstructed airway, poorly functioning cardiopulmonary system, or hypothermia

NURSING ACTIONS

- Monitor respirations and for indication of cyanosis (changes in skin, mucous membrane color).
- Stabilize the body temperature or clear airway as indicated, administer oxygen, and if needed, prepare for resuscitation.

Active Learning Scenario

A nurse in the nursery is assisting with admitting a newborn 2 hr following birth. What nursing actions should the nurse use to evaluate newborn physical development? Use the ATI Active Learning Template: Growth and Development to complete this item.

PHYSICAL DEVELOPMENT

- Describe at least three tools for data collection.
- Describe four reflex responses present at birth and how they are elicited.
- Describe newborn heart rate and how it is evaluated.

Application Exercises

1. A nurse is caring for a newborn who was born at 38 weeks of gestation, weighs 3,200 g, and is in the 60th percentile for weight. Based on the weight and gestational age, the nurse should assign the newborn which of the following classifications?

   A. Low birth weight

   B. Appropriate for gestational age

   C. Small for gestational age

   D. Large for gestational age

2. A nurse is checking the heart rate of a newborn immediately following birth. Auscultate the heart rate using your stethoscope on the apex of the newborn's heart.

   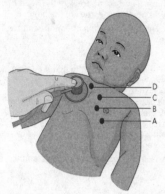

   A. Apex

   B. Tricuspid

   C. Pulmonic

   D. Aortic

3. A nurse is assisting with collecting data from a newborn following birth. Which of the following data indicate the newborn is adapting to extrauterine life? (Select all that apply.)

   A. Expiratory grunting

   B. Inspiratory nasal flaring

   C. Apnea for 10-second periods

   D. Obligatory nose breathing

   E. Crackles and wheezing

4. A nurse is teaching a newly licensed nurse how to bathe a newborn and observes a bluish-brown marking across the newborn's lower back. The nurse should include which of the following information in the teaching?

   A. "This is more commonly seen in newborns who have dark skin."

   B. "This is a finding indicating hyperbilirubinemia."

   C. "This is a forceps mark from an operative delivery."

   D. "This is related to prolonged birth or trauma during delivery."

5. A nurse is collecting data from a newborn and observes small, pearly white nodules on the roof of the newborn's mouth. This finding is a characteristic of which of the following conditions?

   A. Mongolian spots

   B. Milia spots

   C. Erythema toxicum

   D. Epstein's pearls

6. A nurse is checking the reflexes of a newborn. In checking for the Moro reflex, the nurse should perform which of the following?

   A. Hold the newborn vertically under the arms and allow one foot to touch table.

   B. Stimulate the pads of the newborn's hands with stroking or massage.

   C. Stimulate the soles of the newborn's feet on the outer lateral surface of each foot.

   D. Hold the newborn in a semi-sitting position, then allow the newborn's head and trunk to fall backward.

Active Learning Scenario Key

Using the ATI Active Learning Template:
Growth and Development

PHYSICAL DEVELOPMENT

Data collection tools
- Brief initial data collection of all systems
- Gestational age: Physical measurements
- Vital signs
- Head-to-toe data collection

Reflexes
- Sucking and rooting: Turns head to side that is touched and begins to suck when cheek or edge of mouth is stroked
- Palmar grasp: Grasps object when placed in palm
- Plantar grasp: Toes curl downward when sole of the foot is touched.
- Moro reflex: Arms and legs symmetrically extend and then abduct while fingers spread to form a "C" when newborn's head and trunk are allowed to fall backward to an angle of at least 30°.
- Tonic neck (fencer position): Extends arm and leg on same side when head is turned to that side and flexes arm and leg of opposite side
- Babinski: Toes fan upward and out when outer edge of sole of foot is stroked, moving up toward toes.
- Stepping: Makes stepping movements when held upright with feet touching flat surface

Heart rate
- 100 to 160/min with brief fluctuations above and below, depending on activity level
- When newborn is sleeping, place pediatric stethoscope head on fourth or fifth intercostal space at the left midclavicular line over apex of the heart. Listen for 1 full minute.
- Note any murmurs.

Ⓝ *NCLEX® Connection: Health Promotion and Maintenance, Data Collection Techniques*

Application Exercises Key

1. B. **CORRECT:** The nurse should identify that a newborn who was born at 38 weeks of gestation and weighs 3,200 g is in the 60th percentile for weight. This newborn is classified as appropriate for gestational age because the weight is between the 10th and 90th percentile. A newborn who has a low birth weight would weigh less than 2,500 g. A newborn who is small for gestational age would weigh less than the 10th percentile. A newborn who is large for gestational age would weigh greater than the 90th percentile.

   Ⓝ *NCLEX® Connection: Health Promotion and Maintenance, Data Collection Techniques*

2. A. **CORRECT:** The nurse should auscultate an apical pulse rate for 1 full minute, preferably when the newborn is sleeping. The pediatric stethoscope head is placed on the fourth or fifth intercostal space at the left midclavicular line over the apex of the newborn's heart. The nurse should auscultate at the tricuspid, pulmonic, and aortic areas of the heart but should obtain an apical pulse at the apex of the heart.

   Ⓝ *NCLEX® Connection: Health Promotion and Maintenance, Data Collection Techniques*

3. C, D. **CORRECT:** The nurse should identify that the following findings indicate the newborn is adapting to extrauterine life. Periods of apnea lasting less than 20 seconds are an expected finding. Newborns are obligatory nose breathers. Crackles and wheezing are manifestations of fluid or infection in the lungs. Nasal flaring and expiratory grunting are manifestations of respiratory distress and not indicators of the newborn adapting to extrauterine life.

   Ⓝ *NCLEX® Connection: Health Promotion and Maintenance, Data Collection Techniques*

4. A. **CORRECT:** The nurse should tell the newly licensed nurse that Mongolian spots are commonly found over the lumbosacral area of newborns who have dark skin and can be linked to genetics. Hyperbilirubinemia would present as jaundice. Forceps marks would most likely present as a cephalohematoma. Birth trauma would present as ecchymosis.

   Ⓝ *NCLEX® Connection: Health Promotion and Maintenance, Data Collection Techniques*

5. D. **CORRECT:** The nurse should identify that Epstein's pearls are small, yellow-white nodules that appear on the roof of a newborn's mouth. Mongolian spots are areas of darkened pigmentation that occur on the back or sacrum. Milia are small, pearly white bumps that occur on the nose due to clogged sebaceous glands. Erythema toxicum is a transient maculopapular rash seen in newborns.

   Ⓝ *NCLEX® Connection: Health Promotion and Maintenance, Data Collection Techniques*

6. D. **CORRECT:** The Moro reflex is elicited by the nurse holding the newborn in a semi-sitting position and then allowing the head and trunk to fall backward. Holding the newborn vertically under the arms and allowing one foot to touch the table elicits the stepping reflex. Stimulating the pads of the newborn's hands elicits the grasp reflex. Stimulating the outer lateral portion of the newborn's soles elicits the Babinski reflex.

   Ⓝ *NCLEX® Connection: Health Promotion and Maintenance, Data Collection Techniques*

CHAPTER 16 *Nursing Care of Newborns*

Nurses play an important role in the care of newborns after birth. Initial nursing care includes maintaining a patent airway, monitoring vital signs, ensuring proper identification, maintaining thermoregulation, monitoring elimination patterns, preventing infection, and reinforcing discharge teaching for parents.

LOW-RISK NEWBORN

DATA COLLECTION

- Vital signs should be checked frequently following birth according to facility protocol or as indicated by the status of the newborn.
- Weight should be checked daily at the same time, using the same scale.
- Inspect the umbilical cord. Observe for any bleeding from the cord and ensure that the cord is clamped securely to prevent hemorrhage.
- Using the facility's preferred pain data collection tool, conduct pain data collection on the newborn with routine data collection and following painful procedures. Q EBP

LABORATORY TESTS

Hgb and Hct, if prescribed

Cord blood for type and Rh immediately following birth per facility policy

Blood glucose for hypoglycemia, per facility policy or as prescribed

Metabolic screening
- Newborn genetic screening is mandated in all states. A capillary heel stick should be done 24 hr following birth. For results to be accurate, the newborn must have received formula or breast milk for at least 24 hr. If the newborn is discharged before 24 hr of age, the test should be repeated in 1 to 2 weeks.
- All states require testing for phenylketonuria (PKU). PKU is a defect in protein metabolism in which the accumulation of the amino acid phenylalanine can result in permanent damage to the brain, leaving the infant severely cognitively challenged.

Other genetic testing that can be done includes testing for galactosemia, cystic fibrosis, maple syrup urine disease, hypothyroidism, and sickle cell disease.

Serum bilirubin on all newborns prior to discharge

Collecting blood samples

- Heel stick blood samples are obtained by the nurse, who dons clean gloves.
- Administer oral sucrose and offer a pacifier for pain management.
- Warm the newborn's heel first to increase circulation.
- Cleanse the area with an appropriate antiseptic and allow for drying.
- A spring-activated lancet is used so that the skin incision is made quickly and painlessly.
- The outer aspect of the heel should be used, and the lancet should go no deeper than 2.4 mm to prevent necrotizing osteochondritis resulting from penetration of bone with the lancet.
- Follow facility protocol for specimen collection, equipment to be used, and labeling of specimens.
- Apply pressure with dry gauze (do not use alcohol because it will cause bleeding to continue) until bleeding stops, and cover with an adhesive bandage.
- Skin to skin, non-nutritive sucking with or without oral sucrose, or swaddling can be implemented to reduce procedural pain.
- Cuddle and comfort the newborn when the procedure is completed to reassure the newborn and promote feelings of safety.

DIAGNOSTIC PROCEDURES

A newborn hearing screening is recommended for all newborns prior to discharge. Newborns are screened so that hearing impairments can be detected and treated early. Q EBP

Screening for critical congenital heart disease (CCHD). Newborns are screened at 24 to 48 hours of age. Pulse oximetry testing can detect some congenital heart defects. The oxygen saturation is measured in the right foot and right hand. The nurse should recognize that a "passing" result is an oxygen saturation greater than 95% in either extremity, with a less than 3% difference between the lower and upper extremities.

THERAPEUTIC PROCEDURES

Circumcision is the surgical removal of the foreskin of the penis.
- The newborn's family makes the choice regarding whether to circumcise, depending on health, hygiene, religion (Judaism on eighth day after birth), tradition, culture, or social norms. Parents should make a well-informed decision in consultation with the provider.
- Circumcision should not be performed immediately following birth because the newborn's level of vitamin K is at a low point, and the newborn would be at risk for hemorrhage. The newborn is also at increased risk for cold stress.
- Circumcision is usually performed within the first few days of life but might be postponed due to cultural reasons or for preterm or medically unstable newborns.

HEALTH BENEFITS

- Easier hygiene
- Decreased risk of STIs (HIV, human papillomavirus [HPV])
- Decreased risk of penile cancer and cervical cancer in female partners Qpcc

POSSIBLE RISKS

- Hemorrhage
- Infection
- Inflammation or stenosis of the urinary meatus
- Urethral fistula
- Adhesions or dehiscence of the skin
- Concealed penis

CONTRAINDICATIONS

- Hypospadias (abnormal positioning of urethra on ventral under-surface of the penis) and epispadias (urethral canal terminates on dorsum of penis) because the prepuce skin can be needed for surgical repair of the defect
- Family history of bleeding disorders
- Newborns who do not receive vitamin K, making them more likely to experience bleeding at the circumcision site

Preprocedure

- A signed informed consent is needed.
- The newborn will not be able to be bottle fed for up to 2 to 3 hr prior to the procedure to prevent vomiting and aspiration. Newborns can breastfeed up until the procedure.

NURSING ACTIONS

- Check the newborn for the following.
  - Family history of bleeding tendencies (hemophilia, clotting disorders)
  - Hypospadias or epispadias
  - Ambiguous genitalia (can include both male and female characteristics)
  - Illness or infection
- Ensure that parents have signed informed consent.
- Gather and prepare supplies.
- Administer medication as prescribed.
- Assist with procedure.
  - Place the newborn on the restraining board, and provide a radiant heat source to prevent cold stress. Do not leave the newborn unattended. Have bulb syringe readily available.
  - Comfort the newborn as needed.
  - Document time and type of circumcision, amount of bleeding, and newborn voiding following procedure.

Intraprocedure

ANESTHESIA: Anesthesia is required for circumcision. Types of anesthesia include a ring block, dorsal-penile nerve block, topical anesthetic (eutectic mixture of local anesthetics), and concentrated oral sucrose. Nonpharmacological methods (swaddling, nonnutritive sucking) can be used to enhance pain management.

EQUIPMENT FOR PERFORMING CIRCUMCISION: Gomco (Yellen) or Mogen clamp, or Plastibell device

- The provider applies the Gomco (Yellen) or Mogen clamp to the penis, loosens the foreskin, and inserts the cone under the foreskin to provide a cutting surface for removal of the foreskin and to protect the penis. Using the clamp reduces the amount of blood lost. The wound is covered with sterile petroleum gauze to prevent infection and control bleeding.
- The provider slides the Plastibell device between the foreskin and the glans of the penis. The provider ties a suture tightly around the foreskin at the coronal edge of the glans. This applies pressure as the excess foreskin is removed from the penis. After 5 to 7 days, the Plastibell drops off, leaving a clean, healed excision. No petroleum is used for circumcision with the Plastibell.

Postprocedure

NURSING ACTIONS

- Remove the newborn from the restraining board, and swaddle to provide comfort.
- Monitor for bleeding and voiding per facility protocol. Apply gauze lightly to penis if bleeding or oozing is observed. Check bleeding every 15 to 30 min for the first hour and then hourly for the next 4 to 6 hr. Check for first void following circumcision.
- Fan-fold diapers to prevent pressure on the circumcised area.
- Liquid acetaminophen 10 to 15 mg/kg can be administered orally after the procedure and repeated every 4 to 6 hr as prescribed for a maximum of 30 to 45 mg/kg/day.

16.1 Circumcision plastibell

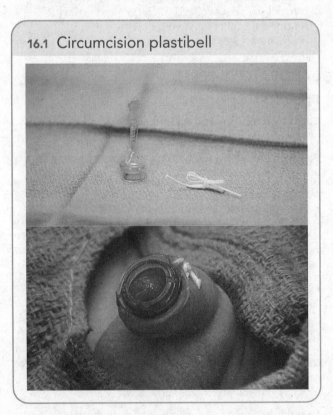

CLIENT EDUCATION

- Keep the area clean. Change the newborn's diaper at least every 4 hr and clean the penis with warm water with each diaper change. With clamp procedures, apply petroleum jelly with each diaper change for at least 24 hr after the circumcision to keep the diaper from adhering to the penis.
- Avoid wrapping the penis in tight gauze, which can impair circulation to the glans.
- Do not give a tub bath until the circumcision is healed. Until then, trickle warm water gently over the penis.
- Notify the provider if there is any redness, discharge, swelling, strong odor, tenderness, decrease in urination, or excessive crying from the newborn.
- A film of yellowish mucus can form over the glans by day two. Do not wash it off.
- Avoid using premoistened towelettes to clean the penis because they contain alcohol.
- The newborn can be fussy or can sleep for several hours after the circumcision. Provide comfort measures for 24 to 48 hr, to include acetaminophen as prescribed.
- The circumcision should heal completely within a couple of weeks.
- Reinforce discharge instructions to the parents about manifestations of infection, comfort measures, medications, and when to notify the provider.

Complications and nursing management

Hemorrhage
- Monitor for bleeding.
- Provide gentle pressure on the penis using a small gauze square. Gelfoam powder or sponge can be applied to stop bleeding. If bleeding persists, notify the provider that a blood vessel might need to be ligated. Have a nurse continue to hold pressure until the provider arrives while another nurse prepares the circumcision tray and suture material.

Cold stress/hypoglycemia
- Monitor for excessive loss of heat resulting in increased respirations and lowered body temperature.
- Swaddle and feed the newborn as soon as the procedure is over.

Other complications: Report any frank bleeding, foul-smelling drainage, or lack of voiding to the provider.

PATIENT-CENTERED CARE

NURSING CARE

Stabilize and/or give resuscitation to the newborn.

Respiratory complications

Monitor for clinical findings of respiratory complications.
- **Bradypnea:** respirations less than 25/min
- **Tachypnea:** respirations greater than or equal to 60/min
- **Abnormal breath sounds:** expiratory grunting, crackles, wheezes
- **Respiratory distress:** nasal flaring, retractions, grunting, gasping, labored breathing

---

16.2 Case study

Scenario introduction

A nurse is discussing with a newly licensed nurse how to reinforce teaching with the parents about circumcision care. Their newborn is postoperative following a circumcision and has been monitored per facility protocol. The newborn is ready to be transported to the parents' room via bassinet, and instructions are provided on how to care for the circumcision.

Scene 1

Nurse Quinn: "Demetria, now that you have monitored Baby Wen for bleeding every 15 minutes for the first hour, it is time to take the baby out to the parents. Be certain you teach them how to care for the circumcision."

Newly Licensed Nurse Demetria: "What should I tell them regarding checking the site for bleeding?"

Scene 2

Quinn: "Instruct them to check the circumcision site for bleeding with every diaper change. If bleeding should occur, they should apply gentle pressure with folded sterile gauze and notify the nurse."

Demetria: "Sounds good. I will tell them that and the other things they should know about how to provide circumcision care to their newborn."

Scene 3

Demetria: "Good morning to each of you. Your baby has been circumcised, per your request, and is doing well. I have a few things I need to go over with you to ensure you understand how to care for the circumcision."

Parents: "Good. Our first baby was a girl, so we know nothing about what to do when we change the diaper. Should the diaper be applied tightly after changing him?"

Demetria: "No, you should loosely apply the diaper over the penis to prevent pressure on the penis. Check the site for bleeding with diaper changes. Also, let us know when the baby voids following the circumcision. Cleanse the site with water and avoid using baby wipes. Your baby's provider used a Plastibell for the circumcision. It is a plastic ring and should fall off in about 1 week. Here is an information sheet with additional information about how to care for your baby's circumcision. Please let me know if you have any questions."

Scenario conclusion

The parents discuss with the newly licensed nurse how to provide comfort measures, such as holding the newborn skin to skin, swaddling, rocking, and breastfeeding the baby. Also, they are aware that a yellow exudate will appear around 24 to 48 hours and will last about 2 to 3 days and not to remove it. They discussed notifying the provider of swelling, discharge, redness, or odor, which are findings that indicate infection.

INTERVENTIONS FOR STABILIZATION AND RESUSCITATION OF AIRWAY

- The newborn is able to clear most secretions in their airway passages. However, if the newborn is unable to clear the secretions suctioning of the mouth, then the nasal passages with a bulb syringe can be done to remove excess mucus in the respiratory tract.
- Newborns delivered by cesarean birth are more susceptible to fluid remaining in the lungs than newborns who were delivered vaginally.
- If bulb suctioning is unsuccessful, use mechanical suction for clearing the airway. Institute emergency procedures if the airway does not clear.

- The bulb syringe should be kept with the newborn, and the newborn's family should be instructed on its use. Family members should be asked to perform a demonstration to show that they understand bulb syringe techniques.
  - Compress bulb before insertion into one side of the mouth.
  - Avoid center of the mouth to prevent stimulating gag reflex.
  - Aspirate mouth first, one nostril, then second nostril.

Identification

Identification is applied to the newborn by the nurse immediately after birth. The nurse should ensure the information on the newborn's and parent's bracelets matches exactly. It is an important safety measure to prevent the newborn from being given to the wrong parents, switched, or abducted. Qs

- The newborn, client, and client's partner are identified by plastic identification wristbands with permanent locks that must be cut to be removed. Identification bands should include the newborn's name, sex, date, and time of birth, and client's health record number. The newborn should have one band placed on the ankle and one on the wrist. In addition, the newborn's footprints and client's thumb prints are taken. The above information is also included with the footprint sheet.
- Each time the newborn is given to the parents, the identification band should be verified against the client's identification band.
- All facility staff who assist in caring for the newborn are required to wear photo identification badges.
- The newborn is not given to anyone who does not have a photo identification that distinguishes that person as a staff member of the maternal-newborn unit.
- Many facilities have locked maternal-newborn units that require staff to permit entrance or exit. Some have a sensor device on the ID band or umbilical cord clamp that sounds an alarm if the newborn is removed from the facility.

Thermoregulation

Thermoregulation provides a neutral thermal environment that helps a newborn maintain a normal core temperature with minimal oxygen consumption and caloric expenditure. A newborn has a relatively large surface-to-weight ratio, reduced metabolism per unit area, blood vessels close to the surface, and small amounts of insulation.

- The newborn keeps warm by metabolizing brown fat, which is unique to newborns, but only within a very narrow temperature range. Becoming chilled (cold stress) can increase the newborn's oxygen demands and rapidly use up brown fat reserves. Therefore, monitoring temperature regulation is important.
- Monitor for hypothermia in the newborn.
  - Axillary temperature of less than 36.5° C (97.7° F)
  - Cyanosis
  - Increased respiratory rate
- Core temperature varies within newborns, but it should be kept at approximately 36.5° to 37.5° C (97.7° to 99.5° F).

INTERVENTIONS TO MAINTAIN THERMOREGULATION
- Heat loss occurs by four mechanisms.
  - **Conduction:** Loss of body heat resulting from direct contact with a cooler surface. Preheat a radiant warmer, warm a stethoscope and other instruments, and pad a scale before weighing the newborn. The newborn should be placed directly on the parent's chest and covered with a warm blanket, and a cap should be placed on the newborn's head.
  - **Convection:** Flow of heat from the body surface to cooler environmental air. Place the bassinet out of the direct line of a fan or air conditioning vent, swaddle the newborn in a blanket, and keep the head covered. Any procedure done with the newborn uncovered should be performed under a radiant heat source. Keep ambient temperature of the nursery or client's room at 22° to 26° C (72° to 78° F).
  - **Evaporation:** Loss of heat as surface liquid is converted to vapor. Gently rub the newborn dry with a warm, sterile blanket (adhering to standard precautions) immediately afterbirth. If thermoregulation is unstable, postpone the initial bath until the newborn's skin temperature is stable. When bathing, expose only one body part at a time, washing and drying thoroughly.
  - **Radiation:** Loss of heat from the body surface to a cooler solid surface that is close to but not in direct contact. Keep the newborn and examining tables away from windows and air conditioners.
- Temperature stabilizes at 37° C (98.6° F) within 12 hr after birth if chilling is prevented.
- The best method for promoting and maintaining the newborn's temperature is early skin-to-skin contact with the parent.

Bathing

- Bathing can begin once the newborn's temperature has stabilized to at least 36.5° C (97.7° F). A complete sponge bath should be postponed until thermoregulation stabilizes.
- Gloves should be worn until the newborn's first bath to avoid exposure to body secretions.

Feeding

Feedings can be started immediately following birth.
- Breastfeeding is initiated as soon as possible after birth as part of baby-friendly initiatives.
- Formula feeding usually is started at about 2 to 4 hr of age.
  - The newborn is fed on demand, which is normally every 3 to 4 hr for bottle-fed newborns and more frequently for breastfed newborns.
  - Monitor and document feedings per facility protocol.

Sleep

- Sleep-wake states are variations of consciousness in the newborn consisting of six states along a continuum comprised of deep sleep, light sleep, drowsy, quiet alert, active alert, and crying.
- Newborns sleep approximately 16 to 19 hr/day with periods of wakefulness gradually increasing. Newborns are positioned supine, "safe sleep," to decrease the incidence of sudden unexpected infant death (SUID). Qs
  - No bumper pads, loose linens, or toys should be placed in the bassinet.
  - Parents should sleep in close proximity but not in a shared space. Higher incidence rates are noted for SUID and suffocation with bed sharing/co-sleeping.
  - Educate parents about the need for immunizations as a measure to prevent SUID.

Elimination

- Monitor elimination habits.
  - Newborns should void once within 24 hr of birth. They should void 6 to 8 times per 24 hr after day 4.
  - Meconium should be passed within the first 24 hr to 48 hr after birth. The newborn will then continue to pass stool 3 to 4 times a day depending on whether they are being breastfed or bottlefed.
  - The stools of newborns who are breastfed can appear yellow and seedy. They should have at least 3 stools per day for the first few weeks. These stools are lighter in color and looser than the stools of newborns who are formula-fed.
- Monitor and document output.
- Keep the perineal area clean and dry. The ammonia in urine is irritating to the skin and can cause diaper rash.
  - After each diaper change, cleanse the perineal area with clear water or water with a mild soap. Diaper wipes with alcohol should be avoided. Pat dry, and apply triple antibiotic ointment, petroleum jelly, or zinc oxide, depending on facility protocol.

Infection control

Infection control is essential in preventing cross-contamination from newborn to newborn and between newborns and staff. Newborns are at risk for infection during the first few months of life because of immature immune systems.

- Provide individual bassinets equipped with diapers, T-shirts, and bathing supplies.
- All personnel who care for a newborn should scrub with antimicrobial soap from elbows to fingertips before entering the nursery. In between care of the newborn, the nurse should follow facility hygiene protocols. Cover gowns or special uniforms are used to avoid direct contact with clothes.

Family education

Reinforce family education and promote family-newborn attachment. QEBP

- Reinforce family education while performing all nursing care. Encourage family involvement, allowing the parent and family to perform newborn care with direct supervision and support by the nurse.
- Encourage parents and family to hold the newborn so that they can experience eye-to-eye contact and interaction.
- Foster sibling interaction in newborn care.

Umbilical cord care

Goal of cord care is to prevent or decrease risk for infection and hemorrhage.

NURSING ACTIONS

- Cord clamp stays in place for 24 to 48 hr.
- Recommendations for cord care include cleaning the cord with water (using cleanser sparingly if needed to remove debris) during the initial bath of the newborn.
- Check stump and base of cord for erythema, edema, and drainage with each diaper change.
- The newborn's diaper should be folded down and away from the umbilical stump.
- Bathing newborn by submerging in water should not occur until the cord has fallen off.
- Most cords fall off within the first 10 to 14 days, although it can take up to 3 weeks.

MEDICATIONS

Erythromycin

- Current recommendations regarding prophylactic eye care include the instillation of antibiotic ointment into the eyes to prevent ophthalmia neonatorum.
- Infections can be transmitted during descent through the birth canal. Ophthalmia neonatorum is caused by *Neisseria gonorrhoeae* or *Chlamydia trachomatis* and can cause blindness.

NURSING ACTIONS

- Use a single-dose unit to avoid cross-contamination.
- Apply a 1- to 2-cm ribbon of ointment to the lower conjunctival sac of each eye, starting from the inner canthus and moving outward.
- A possible side effect is chemical conjunctivitis, causing redness, swelling, drainage, and temporarily blurred vision for 24 to 48 hr. Reassure the parents that this will resolve on its own.
- Application can be delayed for 1 to 2 hr after birth to facilitate baby-friendly activities during the first period of newborn reactivity.

Vitamin K (phytonadione)

Administered to prevent hemorrhagic disorders. Vitamin K is not produced in the gastrointestinal tract of the newborn until around day 7. Vitamin K is produced in the colon by bacteria once formula or breast milk is introduced.

NURSING ACTIONS: Administer 0.5 to 1 mg intramuscularly into the vastus lateralis (where muscle development is adequate) within 1 hr after birth.

Hepatitis B immunization

Provides protection against hepatitis B

NURSING ACTIONS
- Recommended to be administered to all newborns.
- Informed consent must be obtained.
- For newborns born to healthy clients, recommended dosage schedule is at birth, 1 month, and 6 months.
- For parents infected with hepatitis B, hepatitis B immunoglobulin and the hepatitis B vaccine are given within 12 hr of birth. The hepatitis B vaccine is given alone at 1 month, 2 months, and 12 months.

   ! It is important NOT to give the phytonadione and the hepatitis B injections in the same thigh.

COMPLICATIONS

Cold stress

Ineffective thermoregulation can lead to hypoxia, acidosis, and hypoglycemia. Newborns who have respiratory distress are at a higher risk for hypothermia.

NURSING ACTIONS
- Monitor for manifestations of cold stress (skin pallor with mottling and cyanotic trunk; tachypnea).
- The newborn should be warmed slowly over a period of 2 to 4 hr. Correct hypoxia by administering oxygen. Correct acidosis and hypoglycemia. Q EBP

Hypoglycemia

- An initial drop in blood glucose after birth is a common occurrence due to the cessation of the maternal supply of glucose.
- Blood glucose levels are not usually checked in healthy term newborns as they have adequate glycogen stores to compensate for this physiological change.
  - A healthy term newborn can tolerate an initial decrease in their blood glucose level to as low as 30 mg/dL.
- Newborns who have risk factors for hypoglycemia should have a blood glucose level checked within the first hour after birth. This includes newborns who are preterm, small or large for gestational age, and newborns of diabetic mothers.
  - Interventions are indicated for at-risk newborns when their blood glucose levels are less than 40 to 45 mg/dL.

NURSING ACTIONS
- Monitor for manifestations of hypoglycemia (jitteriness, tremors, weak or high-pitched cry, decreased tone, poor feeding, apnea, respiratory distress, low temperature, seizures, and blood glucose level less than 40 to 45 mg/dL).
- Initiate feedings with breastmilk or formula in clinically stable newborns to maintain or increase blood glucose levels.
- Continue to monitor blood glucose levels and feed every 2 to 3 hr for at least the first 24 hr of life in at-risk newborns and those who have demonstrated hypoglycemia, as per facility protocol.
- Skin-to-skin contact will promote breastfeeding and thermoregulation to stabilize blood sugar levels.

Hemorrhage

Due to improper cord care or placement of clamp

NURSING ACTIONS
- Ensure that the clamp is tight. If seepage of blood is noted, a second clamp should be applied.
- Notify the provider if bleeding continues.

Newborn nutrition

Understanding the nutritional needs of newborns (breastfeeding, human pasteurized milk, human donor milk, formula feeding, bottle feeding) is essential. This includes nutrition considerations, complications, and interventions.

NUTRITIONAL NEEDS FOR THE NEWBORN

Desirable growth and development of the newborn is enhanced by good nutrition. Feeding the newborn provides an opportunity for parents to meet the newborn's nutritional needs as well as an opportunity for them to bond with the newborn. Whether the client breastfeeds, uses donor milk, or formula (bottle) feeds, nurses should provide education and support.
- Normal newborn weight loss immediately after birth and subsequent weight gain should be as follows.
  - **Loss of 5% to 10% after birth (regain 10 to 14 days after birth)**
  - **Gain of 110 to 200 g/week for first 3 months**
- During the first 2 days of life, healthy newborns need a fluid intake of 60 to 80 mL/kg/24 hr. From 3 to 7 days, the fluid requirement is 100 to 150 mL/kg/24 hr.
- Adequate caloric intake is essential to provide energy for growth, digestion, metabolic needs, and activity. For the first 3 months, the newborn requires 110 kcal/kg/day. Both breast milk and formula provide 20 kcal/oz.
- Carbohydrates should make up 40% to 50% of the newborn's total caloric intake. The most abundant carbohydrate in breast milk or formula is lactose.
- The fat in breast milk is easier to digest than the fat in cow's milk.

- For adequate growth and development, a newborn should receive 9.1 g per day of protein from birth to 6 months of age.
- Breast milk contains the vitamins necessary to provide adequate newborn nutrition. According to the American Academy of Pediatrics, all newborns who are breastfed or partially breastfed or formula fed should receive 400 IU of vitamin D daily beginning in the first few days of life if consuming less than 28 ounces of milk. Parents who are breastfeeding and do not consume meat, fish, and dairy products should provide vitamin B_{12} supplementation to their newborns. Ⓠ EBP
- The mineral content of commercial newborn formula and breast milk is adequate with the exception of iron and fluoride.
  - Iron is low in all forms of milk, but it is absorbed better from breast milk.
  - Newborns who only breastfeed may be prescribed iron supplements at 4 months of age and until they can consume iron-containing foods. Newborns who are formula-fed should receive iron-fortified newborn formula until 12 months of age.
  - Fluoride levels in breast milk and formulas are low. A fluoride supplement should be considered after 6 months of age, depending on the water supply.
- Solids can be introduced at 6 months of age. Solid food choices may be introduced in any order. Introduce one single-ingredient new food from any food group every 3 to 5 days and monitor for allergy or intolerance, which can include fussiness, rash, upper respiratory distress, vomiting, diarrhea, or constipation.

BREASTFEEDING

Breastfeeding is the optimal source of nutrition for newborns. The Centers for Disease Control and Prevention (CDC), World Health Organization (WHO), and the American Academy of Pediatrics (AAP) recommend that infants receive breast milk solely until 6 months of age and breastfeeding should be continued while introducing complementary foods up to 2 years of age or longer. Newborns should be breastfed every 2 to 3 hr. Parents should awaken the newborn to feed at least every 3 hr during the day and at least every 4 hr during the night until the newborn is feeding well and gaining weight adequately. Breastfeeding should occur eight to 12 times within 24 hr. Then, a feed-on-demand schedule can be followed.

- For the first few days after birth, the baby receives colostrum (early milk). Colostrum is secreted from the postpartum client's breasts during postpartum days 1 to 3. It contains immunoglobulin A (IgA), which provides passive immunity to the newborn.
- Nursing interventions can help a new parent be successful in breastfeeding. This includes the provision of adequate calories and fluids to support breastfeeding. The practice of rooming-in (allowing clients and newborns to remain together) should be encouraged as part of baby-friendly initiatives. Lactation consultants can improve success in breastfeeding. Encourage breastfeeding through the first 24 months of life or longer if desired. Ⓠ TC

ADVANTAGES OF BREASTFEEDING

Parents should receive with factual information about the nutritional and immunological needs of their newborn. Present information about both breastfeeding and bottle feeding in a nonjudgmental manner. The optimal time to provide newborn nutritional information is during pregnancy, so that the parents can make a decision prior to hospital admission.

BENEFITS OF BREASTFEEDING
- Reduces the risk of infection by providing IgA antibodies, lysozymes, leukocytes, macrophages, and lactoferrin that prevents infections
- Promotes rapid brain growth due to large amounts of lactose
- Provides protein and nitrogen for neurologic cell building and improves the newborn's ability to regulate calcium and phosphorus levels
- Contains electrolytes and minerals
- Easy for the newborn to digest
- Reduces incidence of sudden unexpected infant death (SUID), allergies, and childhood obesity
- Promotes maternal-infant bonding and attachment

Benefits specific to the newborn: Decreased risk for gastrointestinal infections, celiac disease, asthma, lower respiratory tract infections, otitis media, sudden unexpected infant death (SUID), obesity in adolescence and adulthood, diabetes mellitus types 1 and 2, acute lymphocytic and myeloid leukemia, childhood inflammatory bowel disease, and necrotizing enterocolitis in preterm infants

Benefits specific to the nursing parent: Decreased postpartum bleeding and more rapid uterine involution; decreased risk for ovarian and breast cancer, diabetes mellitus type 2, hypertension, hypercholesterolemia, cardiovascular disease, and rheumatoid arthritis

Benefits specific to families and society: Less expensive than formula, reduces annual health care costs, and reduces environmental effects related to disposal of formula packaging and equipment

NURSING INTERVENTIONS

- Place the newborn skin-to-skin on the parent's chest immediately after birth. Initiate breastfeeding as soon as possible or within the first 30 min following birth.
- Reinforce breastfeeding techniques to the parent. Have the parent wash their hands, get comfortable, and have caffeine-free, nonalcoholic fluids to drink during breastfeeding.
- Reinforce the let-down reflex (stimulation of maternal nipple releases oxytocin that causes the let-down of milk).
- Express a few drops of colostrum or milk and spread it over the nipple to lubricate the nipple and entice the newborn.

- Show the parent the proper latch-on position. Have them support the breast in one hand with the thumb on top and four fingers underneath. With the newborn's mouth in front of the nipple, the newborn can be stimulated to open their mouth by tickling the lower lip with the tip of the nipple. The parent pulls the newborn to the nipple with the newborn's mouth covering all or as much of the areola as possible, as well as the nipple.
- Demonstrate the four basic breastfeeding positions: football hold (under the arm), cradle (most common) or modified cradle (across the lap), and side-lying.
- Tell the parents to observe the newborn for cues of fullness rather than being concerned about the time the feeding takes.
- To prevent nipple trauma, show the parent how to insert a finger in the side of the newborn's mouth to break the suction from the nipple prior to removing the newborn from the breast.
- Promote rooming-in efforts.
- Offer referral to breastfeeding support groups.
- Contact a lactation consultant to offer additional recommendations and support, especially to parents who have concerns about adequate breast milk or parents who have been unsuccessful with breastfeeding in the past.

CLIENT EDUCATION

- Uterine cramps are normal during breastfeeding, resulting from oxytocin, and promote uterine involution.
- When the newborn is latched on correctly, the nose, cheeks, and chin will be touching the breast.
- Hunger cues include hand to mouth or hand to hand movements, sucking motions, and rooting reflex. Newborns will nurse on demand after a pattern is established.
- Breastfeed at least 15 to 20 min per breast to ensure that the newborn receives adequate fat and protein, which is richest in the breast milk as it empties the breast.
- Newborns need to be breastfed on demand, at least 8 to 12 times in 24 hr. Parents should awaken the newborn to feed at least every 3 hr during the day and at least every 4 hr at night.
- Observe for indications that the newborn has completed the feeding (slowing of newborn suckling, softened breast, sleeping). Offer both breasts to ensure that each breast receives equal stimulation and emptying.
- Burp the newborn when alternating breasts. The newborn should be burped either over the shoulder or in an upright position with the chin supported. Gently pat the newborn on the back to elicit a burp.
- Begin the newborn's next feeding with the breast you stopped feeding with in the previous feeding.

- The newborn is receiving adequate feeding if they are gaining weight, voiding 6 to 8 diapers per day, and are content between feedings.
- Loose, pale, and/or yellow stools are normal during breastfeeding.
- Avoid nipple confusion in the newborn by not offering supplemental formula, pacifier, or soothers until breastfeeding has been established (typically 3 to 4 weeks). Supplementation can be provided using a supplemental device or syringe feeding, if needed. If supplementation is necessary, expressed breast milk is best.
- Always place the newborn on the back after feedings.
- Herbal products (fenugreek, blessed thistle) and prescription medications (metoclopramide) have been reported to increase breast milk production. There is insufficient data to confirm or deny their effect on lactation. Check with a provider before taking over-the-counter or prescription medications. Q EBP
- Breast milk can be expressed using hand expression or a pump so the newborn can be fed using bottle or supplemental device.
  ○ Breast pumps can be manual, electric, or battery-operated and pumped directly into a bottle or freezer bag.
  ○ One or both breasts can be pumped, and suction is adjustable for comfort.
- Breast milk must be stored according to guidelines for proper containers, labeling, refrigerating, and freezing.
  ○ Breast milk can be stored at room temperature for up to 4 hr. It can be refrigerated in clean bottles and bags for use within 4 days, or it can be frozen in clean containers in the freezer compartment of a refrigerator for up to 6 months. Breast milk can be stored in a deep freezer for 12 months.
  ○ Thawing the milk in the refrigerator for 24 hr is the best way to preserve the immunoglobulins present in it. It also can be thawed by holding the container under running lukewarm water or placing it in a container of lukewarm water. The bottle should be rotated often but not shaken when thawing in this manner.
  ○ Thawing by microwave is contraindicated because it destroys some of the immune factors and lysozymes contained in the milk. Microwave thawing also leads to the development of hot spots in the milk because of uneven heating, which can burn the newborn.
- Do not refreeze thawed milk.
  ○ Unused portions of breast milk must be discarded after thawing or warming.

16.2 Breastfeeding positions

Football hold

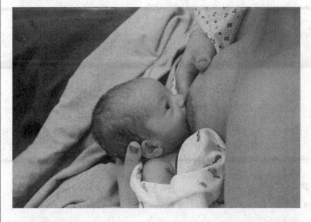

Cradle

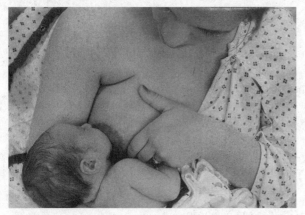

Modified cradle

The parent positions the baby as in the cradle position shown above, but reverses the function of each arm.

Side-lying

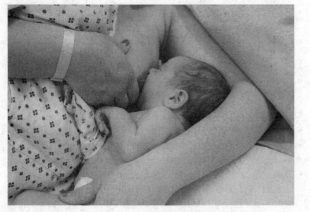

BOTTLE FEEDING

Formula

Formula feeding can be an adequate source of nutrition if the client does not breastfeed. The newborn should be fed every 3 to 4 hr. Parents should awaken the newborn to feed at least every 3 hr during the day and at least every 4 hr during the night until the newborn is feeding well and gaining weight adequately. Then, a feed-on-demand schedule can be followed.

NURSING ACTIONS
- Reinforce teaching with the parents about how to prepare formula (mix according to instructions), bottles, and nipples. Review the importance of hand hygiene prior to formula preparation.
- Reinforce teaching with the parents about the different forms of formula (ready-to-feed, concentrated, and powder) and how to prepare each correctly.

CLIENT EDUCATION
- Bottles and accessories can be put in the dishwasher, boiled, or washed by hand in hot, soapy water using a good bottle and nipple brush.
- Wash the lid of a can of formula with hot, soapy water, and shake before opening it.
- Use tap water to mix concentrated or powder formula. If the water source is questionable, tap water should be boiled first.
- Prepared formula can be refrigerated for up to 48 hr.
- Check the flow of formula from the bottle to ensure it is not coming out too slow or too fast.
- Do not use formula past the expiration date on the container.
- Cradle the newborn in the arms in a semi-upright position. The newborn should not be placed in the supine position during bottle feeding because of the danger of aspiration. Newborns who bottle feed do best when held close and at a 45° angle.
- Place the nipple on top of the newborn's tongue.
- Keep the nipple filled with formula to prevent the newborn from swallowing air.
- Always hold the bottle and never prop the bottle for feeding.
- Give the newborn opportunities to burp several times during a feeding.
- Place the newborn on the back after feedings.
- Discard any unused formula remaining in the bottle when the newborn is finished feeding due to the possibility of bacterial contamination. Qs
- The newborn is being adequately fed if they are gaining weight; bowel movements are yellow, soft, and formed; and they are satisfied between feedings.
  ○ Newborns usually have 6 or more wet diapers a day.
  ○ Newborns who consume breast milk usually have three or more bowel movements a day. Infants who receive formula have less frequent bowel movements.

RISK FACTORS FOR IMPAIRED NEWBORN NUTRITION

Risk factors for failure to thrive (newborn) can be related to the newborn or parent.

NEWBORN FACTORS
- Inadequate breastfeeding
- Illness/infection
- Malabsorption
- Other conditions that increase energy needs

MATERNAL FACTORS
- Inadequate or slow milk production
- Inadequate emptying of the breast
- Inappropriate timing of feeding
- Inadequate breast tissue
- Pain with feeding
- Hemorrhage
- Illness/infection

MONITORING NEWBORN FOR ADEQUATE GROWTH

- Monitor the newborn for adequate growth and weight gain.
  - Weights are done daily in the newborn nursery. Every newborn should be seen and examined at the provider's office within 3 to 5 days after discharge from the hospital and again at 2 weeks. Growth is evaluated by placing the newborn's weight on a growth chart. Adequate growth should be within the 10th to 90th percentile. Poor weight gain is below 10th percentile, and too much weight gain is above 90th percentile.
  - The newborn's length and head circumference are also routinely monitored.
- Check the parent's ability to feed their newborn, whether by breast or bottle.
- Calculate the newborn's 24-hr I&O, if indicated, to ensure adequate nutrition.

DATA COLLECTION OF NEWBORN NUTRITION

Data collection of newborn nutrition begins during pregnancy and continues after birth by reviewing parent and newborn factors that affect feeding.

NEWBORN
- Maturity level
- History of labor and delivery
- Birth trauma
- Congenital defects
- Physical stability
- State of alertness
- Presence of bowel sounds

PARENT
- Previous experience with breastfeeding
- Knowledge about breastfeeding
- Cultural factors
- Feelings about breastfeeding
- Physical features of breasts
- Physical/psychological readiness
- Support of family and significant others

INTERVENING FOR NEWBORN NUTRITION

Provide the parent with education about feeding-readiness cues exhibited by newborns, and encourage the parent to begin feeding the newborn upon cues rather than waiting until the newborn is crying. Cues include the following.
- Hand-to-mouth or hand-to-hand movements
- Sucking motions
- Rooting
- Mouthing

COMPLICATIONS FOR NEWBORN NUTRITION

There can be special considerations when a newborn has difficulty receiving adequate nutrition. Nursing interventions can often help these newborns receive adequate nutrition.

NEWBORNS WHO ARE SLEEPY
- Unwrap the newborn.
- Change the newborn's diaper.
- Hold the newborn upright, and turn them from side to side.
- Talk to the newborn.
- Massage the newborn's back, and rub the hands and feet.
- Apply a cool cloth to the newborn's face.

NEWBORNS WHO ARE FUSSY
- Swaddle the newborn.
- Hold the newborn close, move, and rock them gently.
- Reduce the newborn's environmental stimuli.
- Place the newborn skin-to-skin.

FAILURE TO THRIVE: Failure to thrive is slow weight gain. A newborn usually falls below the 5th percentile on the growth chart.

NEWBORNS WHO ARE BREASTFEEDING
- Evaluate positioning and latch-on during breastfeeding.
- Massage the breast during feeding. ⓠEBP
- Determine feeding patterns and length of feedings.
- If the newborn is spitting up, the newborn can have an allergy to dairy products. Determine the maternal intake of dairy products. The parent might need to eliminate dairy from their diet. Instruct them to consume other food sources high in calcium or calcium supplements.

NEWBORNS WHO ARE FORMULA FEEDING
- Evaluate how much and how often the newborn is feeding.
- If the newborn is spitting up or vomiting, they can have an allergy or intolerance to cow's milk-based formula and can require a soy-based formula.

Nursing care and reinforcing discharge teaching

Reinforcing discharge teaching and newborn care includes providing education about bathing, umbilical cord care, circumcision, car seat safety, environmental safety, newborn behaviors, feeding, elimination, and clinical findings of illness to report to the provider.

Prior to discharge, a nurse should provide anticipatory guidance to prepare new parents to care for their newborn at home. Clients and newborns are normally discharged 48 hr following a vaginal birth or 72 hr following a cesarean birth. Serious complications can result if improper discharge instructions are given to the parents prior to taking the newborn home.

A nurse should inquire about the family's experience and knowledge regarding newborn care, anticipate the learning needs of the parents, and evaluate their readiness for learning to provide education about newborn care.

Parents should be made aware of general guidelines about newborn behavior and care. These guidelines include causes of crying in the newborn; quieting techniques; sleeping patterns; hunger cues; and feeding, bathing, and clothing the newborn.

Parents need to be aware of the importance of well-newborn checkups, immunization schedules, and when to call the provider for manifestations of illness.

Providing a safe, protective environment at home should be stressed to new parents and should include instruction about proper car seat usage, which is a very important part of the discharge instruction process. Qs

DETERMINATION OF FAMILY READINESS FOR HOME CARE OF THE NEWBORN

- Previous newborn experience and knowledge
- Parent-newborn attachment
- Adjustment to the parental role
- Social support
- Educational needs
- Sibling rivalry issues
- Readiness of the parents to have their home and lifestyle altered to accommodate their newborn
- Parents' ability to verbalize and demonstrate newborn care following teaching

INTERVENTIONS FOR HOME CARE OF THE NEWBORN

Through discussion, pamphlets, and demonstration, provide education to the client and family regarding newborn behavior, quieting techniques, newborn care, findings of newborn well-being and illness, and issues of newborn safety. Qpcc

CRYING

CLIENT EDUCATION
- Newborns cry when they are hungry, overstimulated, wet, cold, hot, tired, bored, or need to be burped. In time, parents learn what the newborn's cry means.
- Do not feed the newborn every time they cry. Overfeeding can lead to stomach aches and diarrhea.
- Newborns often have a fussy time of day when they cry for no reason. In this case, it is not always possible to stop a newborn's crying, and the newborn might cry themselves to sleep.

Quieting Techniques
- Swaddling
- Close skin contact
- Nonnutritive sucking with pacifier
- Rhythmic noises to simulate utero sounds
- Movement (car ride, vibrating chair, infant swing, rocking newborn)
- Placing the newborn on the stomach across a holder's lap while gently bouncing legs
- En face position for eye contact (when parents' and newborns' faces are about 30 cm [12 in] apart and on the same plane)
- Stimulation

SLEEP-WAKE CYCLE

- Newborns sleep approximately 16 to 19 hr/day with periods of wakefulness gradually increasing.
- Many parents believe that adding solid food to the newborn's diet will help with sleep patterns. During the first 6 months of life, the American Academy of Pediatrics (AAP) recommends only breastfeeding. Most newborns will sleep through the night without a feeding by 4 to 5 months of age. The provider will instruct the parents when to add solid food to the newborn's diet.

CLIENT EDUCATION
- Placing the newborn in the supine position for sleeping greatly decreases the risk of sudden unexpected infant death (SUID).
- Keep the newborn's environment quiet and dark at night.
- Place the newborn in a crib or bassinet to sleep. The newborn should never sleep in the parents' bed due to the risk of suffocation.
- When awake, the newborn can be placed on the abdomen to promote muscle development for crawling. The newborn should be supervised.
- For nighttime feedings and diaper changes, keep a small night-light on to avoid having to turn on bright lights. Speak softly, and handle the newborn gently so that they go back to sleep easily.

ORAL AND NASAL SUCTIONING

Review correct technique with the parents. The bulb is compressed before inserting into the baby's mouth. The mouth should be suctioned first, then the nose to prevent aspiration.

POSITIONING AND HOLDING OF THE NEWBORN (HEAD SUPPORT)

CLIENT EDUCATION

- The newborn has minimal head control.
- The head should be supported when the newborn is lifted because the head is larger and heavier than the rest of the body.

Basic ways to hold a newborn

- **Cradle hold:** Cradle the newborn's head in the bend of the elbow. This permits eye-to-eye contact and is a good position for feeding.
- **Upright position:** Hold the newborn upright, and face them toward the holder while supporting the head, upper back, and buttocks.
- **Football hold:** Support half of the newborn's body in the holder's forearm with the newborn's head and neck resting in the palm of the hand. This is a good position for breastfeeding and when shampooing the newborn's hair.

SWADDLING

Parents should be shown how to swaddle their newborn. Swaddling the newborn snugly in a receiving blanket helps the newborn to feel more secure. Swaddling brings the newborn's extremities in closer to the trunk, which is similar to the intrauterine position. **QEBP**

BATHING

- Instruct the parents about proper newborn techniques by a demonstration. Have the parents return the demonstration.
- After the initial bath, the newborn's face, diaper area, and skin folds are cleansed daily. Complete bathing is performed two to three times per week using a mild soap.

CLIENT EDUCATION

- Bathing by immersion is not done until the newborn's umbilical cord has fallen off and the circumcision has healed, if applicable. Wash the area around the cord, taking care not to get the cord wet. Move from the cleanest to dirtiest part of the newborn's body, beginning with the eyes, face, and head; proceed to the chest, arms, and legs; and wash the groin area last.
- Bathing should take place at the convenience of the parents but not immediately after feeding to prevent spitting up and vomiting.
- Organize all equipment so that the newborn is not left unattended. Never leave the newborn alone in the tub or sink.

- Make sure the hot water heater is set at 49° C (120.2° F) or less. Test water for comfort with your elbow prior to bathing the newborn.
- Avoid drafts or chilling of the newborn. Expose only the body part being bathed, and dry the newborn thoroughly to prevent chilling and heat loss.
- Clean the newborn's eyes using a clean portion of the wash cloth. Use clear water to clean each eye, moving from the inner to the outer canthus.
- Each area of the newborn's body should be washed, rinsed, and dried, with no soap left on the skin.
- Wrap the newborn in a towel, and swaddle them in a football hold to shampoo the head. Rinse shampoo from the newborn's head, and dry to avoid chilling.
- To cleanse an uncircumcised penis, wash with soap and water and rinse the penis. The foreskin should not be forced back or constriction can result.
- To cleanse a circumcised penis, use warm water. Do not use soap until the circumcision is healed.
- Wash the vulva by wiping from front to back to prevent contamination of the vagina or urethra from rectal bacteria.
- Applying a fragrance-free, hypoallergenic, moisturizing emollient immediately after bathing can help prevent dry skin.

DIAPERING

To avoid diaper rash, the newborn's diaper area should be kept clean and dry. Diapers should be changed frequently and the perineal area cleaned with warm water or wipes and dried thoroughly to prevent skin breakdown.

CORD CARE

- Before discharge, the cord clamp is removed.
- Prevent cord infection by keeping the cord dry, and keep the top of the diaper folded underneath it.

CLIENT EDUCATION

- Sponge baths are given until the cord falls off, which occurs around 10 to 14 days after birth or can take up to 3 weeks. Tub bathing and submersion can follow.
- Cord infection (a complication of improper cord care) can result if the cord is not kept clean and dry.
  - Monitor for manifestations of a cord that is moist and red, has a foul odor, or has purulent drainage.
  - Notify the provider immediately if findings of cord infection are present.

CLOTHING

Instruct the parents about care for and choice of newborn clothing.

CLIENT EDUCATION

- Choose flame-retardant fabrics.
- Wash clothes separately with mild detergent and hot water.
- Dress newborns lightly for indoors and on hot days. Too many layers of clothing or blankets can make the newborn too hot.
- On cold days, cover the newborn's head when outdoors.
- A general rule is to dress the newborn as the parents would dress themselves. Parents should add no more than one additional layer.

HOME SAFETY

Provide community resources to clients who might need ongoing assessment and instruction on newborn care (adolescent parents).

CLIENT EDUCATION

- Never leave the newborn unattended with pets or other small children.
- Keep small objects (coins) out of the reach of newborns due to choking hazard.
- Never leave the newborn alone on a bed, couch, or table. Newborns move enough to reach the edge and fall off.
- Never place the newborn on the stomach to sleep during the first few months of life. The back-lying position is the position of choice. Reinforce education on the importance of tummy time, which is allowing the infant to lie in the prone position for 3 to 5 minutes, 2 to 3 times each day.
- Never provide a newborn with a soft surface to sleep on (pillows or water bed). The newborn's mattress should be firm. Never put pillows, toys, bumper pads, or loose blankets in a crib. Crib linens should be tight-fitting.
- Do not tie anything around the newborn's neck.
- Monitor the safety of the newborn's crib. The space between the mattress and sides of the crib should be less than 2 fingerbreadths. The slats on the crib should be no more than 5.7 cm (2.25 in) apart.
- The newborn's crib or playpen should be away from window blinds and drapery cords. Newborns can become strangled in them.
- The bassinet or crib should be placed on an inner wall, not next to a window, to prevent cold stress by radiation.
- Eliminate potential fire hazards. Keep a crib and playpen away from heaters, radiators, and heat vents. Linens could catch fire if they come into contact with heat sources.
- Control the temperature and humidity of the newborn's environment by providing adequate ventilation.
- Avoid exposing the newborn to cigarette smoke in a home or elsewhere. Secondhand exposure increases the newborn's risk of developing respiratory illnesses.
- All visitors should wash their hands before touching the newborn. Any individual who has an infection should be kept away from the newborn.
- Carefully handle the newborn. Do not toss the newborn up in the air or swing them by their extremities. Do not shake the newborn.

CAR SEAT SAFETY

CLIENT EDUCATION

- Use an approved rear-facing car seat in the back seat, preferably in the middle (away from air bags and side impact), to transport the newborn.
- Keep infants in rear-facing car seats until age 2 or until the child reaches the maximum height and weight for the seat. Qs

NEWBORN WELLNESS CHECKUPS

- Every newborn should be seen and examined at the provider's office within 72 hr (2 to 3 days) after discharge. The AAP recommends wellness checks at 2 to 5 days, 1 month, 2 months, 4 months, 6 months, 9 months, 12 months, 15 months, 18 months, 2 years, 2.5 years, 3 years, 4 years, and every year thereafter.

16.3 Case study

Scenario introduction

A nurse is reinforcing discharge teaching with a newly licensed nurse; they are discussing instructing parents about manifestations of illness to report to the provider.

Scene 1

Devon: "As you prepare to talk to the parents of the newborn you will be discharging home, there is certain information you need to include in the education."

Cotina: "I will review the information in our discharge paperwork and see if I have any questions I feel we need to discuss."

Devon: "Sounds like a good plan. Please let me know if you have something you do not understand."

Scene 2

Devon: "So, do you feel like you understand the content you should discuss with the parents regarding illness manifestations they should report to the provider?"

Cotina: "Yes, Devon. I will let you know if I have any trouble or if they have questions I cannot answer.:

Scene 3

Cotina: "Good morning to both of you. I know you are excited to be going home. I have a few things I need to discuss with you both about what to report to the provider if they should occur."

Parent : "Sounds good. We are so ready to go home and care for our baby."

Scenario conclusion

The nurse should discuss the following information with the parents and validate understanding for manifestations to report to the provider. These include:

- Temperature greater than 38° C (100.4° F) or less than 36.5° C (97.7° F)
- Poor feeding or little interest in food
- Forceful vomiting or frequent vomiting
- Decreased urination
- Diarrhea or decreased bowel movements
- Labored breathing with flared nostrils or an absence of breathing for greater than 15 seconds
- Jaundice
- Cyanosis
- Lethargy
- Inconsolable crying
- Difficulty waking
- Bleeding or purulent drainage around umbilical cord or circumcision
- Drainage developing in eyes

- Review the schedule for immunizations with the parents. Stress the importance of receiving these immunizations on a schedule for the newborn to be protected against diphtheria, tetanus, pertussis, hepatitis B, *Haemophilus influenzae*, polio, measles, mumps, rubella, influenza, rotavirus, pneumococcal, and varicella.

MANIFESTATIONS OF ILLNESS TO REPORT

Instruct parents regarding the manifestations of illness and to report them immediately.

- Temperature greater than 38° C (100.4° F) or less than 36.5° C (97.9° F)
- Poor feeding or little interest in food
- Forceful vomiting or frequent vomiting
- Decreased urination
- Diarrhea or decreased bowel movements
- Labored breathing with flared nostrils or an absence of breathing for greater than 15 seconds
- Jaundice
- Cyanosis
- Lethargy
- Inconsolable crying
- Difficulty waking
- Bleeding or purulent drainage around umbilical cord or circumcision

CARDIOPULMONARY RESUSCITATION

Encourage parents to seek CPR training.

COMPLICATIONS RELATED TO NEWBORN HOME CARE

Complications stemming from improper understanding of discharge instructions can include the following.

- Infected cord or circumcision from improper care or tub bathing too soon
- Falls, suffocation, strangulation, burns resulting in injuries, fractures, aspiration, or death due to improper safety precautions
- Respiratory infections due to passive smoke or inhaled powders
- Improper or no use of a car seat, resulting in injuries or death
- Serious infections due to lack of nonadherence with immunization schedule

Application Exercises

1. A nurse is reviewing contraindications for circumcision with a newly hired nurse. Which of the following conditions are contraindications? (Select all that apply.)
   A. Hypospadias
   B. Hydrocele
   C. Family history of hemophilia
   D. Hyperbilirubinemia
   E. Epispadias

2. A nurse is taking a newborn to a parent following a circumcision. Which of the following actions should the nurse take for security purposes?
   A. Ask the parent to state their full name.
   B. Look at the name on the newborn's bassinet.
   C. Match the parent's identification band with the newborn's band.
   D. Compare name on the bassinet and room number.

3. A nurse is assisting with the care of a newborn immediately following birth. Which of the following nursing interventions is the highest priority?
   A. Initiating breastfeeding
   B. Performing the initial bath
   C. Giving a vitamin K injection
   D. Covering the newborn's head with a cap

4. A newborn was not dried completely after birth. This places the newborn at risk for which of the following types of heat loss?
   A. Conduction
   B. Convection
   C. Evaporation
   D. Radiation

5. A nurse is preparing to administer prophylactic eye ointment to a newborn to prevent ophthalmia neonatorum. Which of the following medications should the nurse anticipate administering?
   A. Ofloxacin
   B. Nystatin
   C. Erythromycin
   D. Ceftriaxone

6. A nurse is reinforcing teaching with a group of new parents about proper techniques for bottle feeding. Which of the following instructions should the nurse provide?
   A. Burp the newborn at the end of the feeding.
   B. Hold the newborn close in a supine position.
   C. Keep the nipple full of formula throughout the feeding.
   D. Refrigerate any unused formula.

7. As a nurse, what should you instruct the parents of a newborn about home safety?

Application Exercises Key

1. **A, C, E. CORRECT:** The nurse should identify that the following conditions are contraindications for circumcisions: hypospadias, epispadias, and a family history of hemophilia. However, a hyperbilirubinemia and a hydrocele, which is a collection of fluid in the scrotal sac, are not contraindications for a circumcision.

   Ⓝ *NCLEX® Connection: Reduction of Risk Potential, Potential for Complications From Surgical Procedures and Health Alterations*

2. **C. CORRECT:** The nurse should verify the parent's identification band against the newborn's identification band each time the newborn is taken to the parent. Asking the parent to state their full name, looking at the name on the bassinet, and comparing the name on the bassinet with the room number are not appropriate means of verification because they do not include two identifiers involving the parent and the newborn.

   Ⓝ *NCLEX® Connection: Safety and Infection Control, Accident/Error/Injury Prevention*

3. **D. CORRECT:** The greatest risk to the newborn is cold stress. Therefore, the highest priority intervention is to prevent heat loss. Covering the newborn's head with a cap prevents cold stress due to excessive evaporative heat loss. Initiating breastfeeding is important following birth, but it is not the priority action. Initial baths are not given until the newborn's temperature is stable. Vitamin K can be given immediately after birth, but this is not the priority action.

   Ⓝ *NCLEX® Connection: Health Promotion and Maintenance, Ante-/Intra-/Postpartum and Newborn Care*

4. **C. CORRECT:** Evaporation is the loss of heat that occurs when a liquid is converted to a vapor. In a newborn, heat loss by evaporation occurs as a result of vaporization of the moisture from the skin. Therefore, the nurse should identify that the newborn is at risk for heat loss due to evaporation because they were not completely dried following birth. Conduction is the loss of heat from the body surface area to cooler surfaces that the newborn can be in contact with. Convection is the flow of heat from the body surface area to cooler air. Radiation is the loss of heat to a cooler surface that is not in direct contact with the newborn.

   Ⓝ *NCLEX® Connection: Health Promotion and Maintenance, Ante-/Intra-/Postpartum and Newborn Care*

5. **C. CORRECT:** One medication of choice for ophthalmia neonatorum is erythromycin ophthalmic ointment 0.5%. This antibiotic provides prophylaxis against *Neisseria gonorrhoeae* and *Chlamydia trachomatis*. The nurse should plan to administer this medication within 1 to 2 hr following birth. Ceftriaxone is an antibiotic, but it is not used for ophthalmia neonatorum. Nystatin is used to treat *Candida albicans*, an oral yeast infection. Ofloxacin is an antibiotic, but it is not used for ophthalmia neonatorum.

   Ⓝ *NCLEX® Connection: Pharmacological Therapies, Medication Administration*

6. **C. CORRECT:** The nurse should reinforce proper bottle-feeding techniques with the parent, which include always keeping the nipple full of formula to prevent the newborn from sucking in air during the feeding. The newborn should be burped after each ½ oz of formula, cradled in a semi-upright position, and any unused formula should be discarded due to the possibility of bacterial contamination.

   Ⓝ *NCLEX® Connection: Health Promotion and Maintenance, Ante-/Intra-/Postpartum and Newborn Care*

7. The nurse should inform the parents about the following home safety information prior to discharge. Never leave the newborn unattended with pets or other small children. Keep small objects (e.g., coins) out of the reach of newborns due to choking hazard. Never leave the newborn alone on a bed, couch, or table. Never place the newborn on the stomach to sleep during the first few months of life. The back-lying position is the position of choice. Reinforce education on the importance of tummy time, which is allowing the infant to lie in the prone position for 3 to 5 minutes per day, 2 to 3 times each day. Never provide a newborn with a soft surface to sleep on (pillows or water bed). The newborn's mattress should be firm. Never put pillows, toys, bumper pads, or loose blankets in a crib. Do not tie anything around the newborn's neck. Monitor the safety of the newborn's crib. The space between the mattress and sides of the crib should be less than 2 fingerbreadths. The slats on the crib should be no more than 5.7 cm (2.25 in) apart. The newborn's crib or playpen should be away from window blinds and drapery cords. The bassinet or crib should be placed on an inner wall, not next to a window, to prevent cold stress. Eliminate potential fire hazards. Keep a crib and playpen away from heaters, radiators, and heat vents.

   Ⓝ *NCLEX® Connection: Health Promotion and Maintenance, Ante-/Intra-/Postpartum and Newborn Care*

Active Learning Scenario

A nurse is reinforcing teaching about the use of a breast pump and storing breast milk with a group of new parents. What information should the nurse include in the teaching? Use the ATI Active Learning Template: Basic Concept to complete this item.

RELATED CONTENT

- List the types of breast pumps.
- Describe use of the pump.

NURSING INTERVENTIONS

- Describe storage and freezing of milk.
- Describe procedures for thawing milk.

Active Learning Scenario Key

Using the ATI Active Learning Template: Basic Concept

RELATED CONTENT

Types of breast pumps
- Manual
- Electric
- Battery-operated

Use of the pump: Pumping of one or both breasts using adjustable suction for comfort to obtain breast milk for storage in a bottle or freezer bag

NURSING INTERVENTIONS

Storage
- Store at room temperature under very clean conditions for up to 4 hr.
- Refrigerate in sterile bottles for use within 4 days.
- Freeze in sterile containers in the freezer of a refrigerator for up to 6 months.
- Store in a deep freezer for up to 12 months.

Thawing
- Thaw milk in the refrigerator for 24 hr to preserve immunoglobulins.
- Hold container under running lukewarm water or place in a pan of lukewarm water; bottle should be rotated but not shaken.
- Do not thaw in a microwave.

Ⓝ *NCLEX® Connection: Health Promotion and Maintenance, Ante-/Intra-/Postpartum and Newborn Care*

When reviewing the following chapters, keep in mind the relevant topics and tasks of the NCLEX outline.

Pharmacological Therapies

EXPECTED ACTIONS/OUTCOMES
Apply knowledge of pathophysiology when addressing client pharmacological agents.

Evaluate client response to medication.

Reduction of Risk Potential

POTENTIAL FOR COMPLICATIONS OF DIAGNOSTIC TESTS/TREATMENTS/PROCEDURES: Use precautions to prevent injury or complications associated with a procedure or diagnosis.

LABORATORY VALUES: Monitor diagnostic or laboratory test results.

Physiological Adaptation

ALTERATIONS IN BODY SYSTEMS
Identify signs and symptoms of an infection.

Provide care for a client experiencing complications of pregnancy/labor or delivery.

FLUID AND ELECTROLYTE IMBALANCES: Identify signs and symptoms of client fluid or electrolyte imbalances.

CHAPTER 17 ## Complications of the Newborn

Management of newborn complications includes data collection, identification of risk factors, and collaborative care. It is essential for a nurse to immediately identify complications and assist with performing appropriate interventions. Ongoing emotional support to a client and their significant other is also imperative to the plan of care.

Complications include neonatal substance withdrawal, hypoglycemia, respiratory distress syndrome (RDS)/asphyxia/meconium aspiration, preterm newborn, small-for-gestational-age (SGA) newborn, large-for-gestational-age (LGA)/macrosomic newborn, postmature newborn, newborn infection/sepsis (sepsis neonatorum), birth trauma or injury, hyperbilirubinemia, and congenital anomalies.

Neonatal substance withdrawal

Maternal substance use during pregnancy consists of any use of alcohol or drugs. Intrauterine drug exposure can cause anomalies, neurobehavioral changes, and evidence of withdrawal in the neonate. These changes depend on the specific drug or combination of drugs used, dosage, route of administration, metabolism and excretion by the parent and fetus, timing of drug exposure, and length of drug exposure.
- Substance withdrawal in the newborn occurs when the parent uses drugs that have addictive properties during pregnancy. This includes illegal drugs, alcohol, tobacco, and prescription medications.
- Fetal alcohol syndrome (FAS) results from the chronic or periodic intake of alcohol during pregnancy. Alcohol is considered teratogenic, so the daily intake of alcohol increases the risk of FAS. Newborns who have FAS are at risk for specific congenital physical defects and long-term complications.

LONG-TERM COMPLICATIONS
- Central nervous system dysfunction (cognitive impairment, cerebral palsy)
- Attention deficit disorder
- Language abnormalities
- Microcephaly
- Delayed growth and development
- Poor maternal-newborn bonding

DATA COLLECTION

RISK FACTORS
- Maternal use of substances prior to knowing they are pregnant
- Maternal substance use during pregnancy

EXPECTED FINDINGS

Monitor the newborn for abstinence syndrome (withdrawal), also referred to as neonatal opioid withdrawal syndrome (NOWS), and increased wakefulness using the neonatal abstinence scoring system that determines and scores the following.
- **CNS:** High-pitched, shrill cry; incessant crying; irritability; tremors; hyperactivity with an increased Moro reflex; increased deep-tendon reflexes; increased muscle tone; disturbed sleep pattern; hypertonicity; convulsions
- **Metabolic, vasomotor, and respiratory findings:** Nasal congestion with flaring, frequent yawning, skin mottling, retractions, apnea, tachypnea greater than 60/min, sweating, temperature greater than 37.2° C (99° F)
- **Gastrointestinal:** Poor feeding; regurgitation (projectile vomiting); diarrhea; excessive, uncoordinated, constant sucking

OPIATE WITHDRAWAL: Manifestations of neonatal abstinence syndrome

HEROIN WITHDRAWAL
- Low birth weight
- Small for gestational age (SGA)
- Manifestations of neonatal abstinence syndrome
- Increased risk of sudden unexpected infant death (SUID)

METHADONE WITHDRAWAL
Manifestations of neonatal opioid withdrawal syndrome (NOWS): Increased incidence of seizures, sleep pattern disturbances, stillbirth, SUID, higher birth weights (compared with heroin exposure)

MARIJUANA WITHDRAWAL
- Preterm birth, intrauterine growth restriction
- Long-term effects, such as deficits in attention, cognition, memory, and motor skills

METHAMPHETAMINE WITHDRAWAL: Preterm or SGA, drowsiness, jitteriness, sleep pattern disturbances, respiratory distress, frequent infections, poor weight gain, emotional disturbances, delayed growth and development

ALCOHOL WITHDRAWAL: Jitteriness, irritability, increased tone and reflex responses, seizures

FETAL ALCOHOL SYNDROME

- Facial anomalies: small eyes, flat midface, smooth philtrum, thin upper lip, eyes with a wide-spaced appearance, epicanthal folds, strabismus, ptosis, poor suck, small teeth, cleft lip or palate
- Many vital organ anomalies, such as heart defects, including atrial and ventricular septal defects, tetralogy of Fallot, patent ductus arteriosus
- Developmental delays and neurologic abnormalities
- Prenatal and postnatal growth delays
- Sleep disturbances

TOBACCO: Prematurity, low birth weight, increased risk for SUID, increased risk for bronchitis, pneumonia, and developmental delays

LABORATORY TESTS

Blood tests should be done to differentiate between neonatal drug withdrawal and central nervous system disorders.
- CBC
- Blood glucose
- Thyroid-stimulating hormone, thyroxine, triiodothyronine
- Drug screen of urine or meconium to reveal the substance used by the parent
- Hair analysis

DIAGNOSTIC PROCEDURES

Chest x-ray for FAS to rule out congenital heart defects

PATIENT-CENTERED CARE

NURSING CARE

Nursing care for maternal substance use and neonatal effects or withdrawal include the following in addition to normal newborn care.
- Elicit the newborn's reflexes.
- Monitor the newborn's ability to feed and digest intake. Offer small frequent feedings.
- Swaddle the newborn with legs flexed.
- Offer non-nutritive sucking.
- Monitor the newborn's fluids and electrolytes with skin turgor, mucous membranes, fontanels, daily weights, and I&O.
- Reduce environmental stimuli (decrease lights, lower noise level).

MEDICATIONS

Based on withdrawal manifestations

Morphine sulfate
CLASSIFICATION: Opioid

Methadone
CLASSIFICATION: Opioid analgesic

Phenobarbital
CLASSIFICATION: Anticonvulsant

INTENDED EFFECT: Decrease CNS irritability and control seizures for newborns who have alcohol or opioid withdrawal

NURSING ACTIONS
- Check for any medication incompatibilities.
- Decrease environmental stimuli.
- Cluster care to minimize stimulation.
- Swaddle the newborn to reduce self-stimulation and protect the skin from abrasions.
- Monitor and maintain fluids and electrolytes.
- Administer frequent, small feedings of high-calorie formula; can require gavage feedings.
- Elevate the newborn's head during and following feedings, and burp the newborn to reduce vomiting and aspiration. Qs
- Try various nipples to compensate for a poor suck reflex.
- Have suction equipment available to reduce the risk for aspiration.
- For newborns who are withdrawing from cocaine, avoid eye contact and use vertical rocking and a pacifier.
- Prevent infection.
- Assist with initiating a consult with child protective services.
- Consult lactation services to evaluate whether breastfeeding is desired or contraindicated to avoid passing narcotics in breast milk. Methadone or buprenorphine is not contraindicated during breastfeeding.
- Pharmacological treatment is prescribed based on the severity of the withdrawal symptoms and assessment scoring tools. In addition to methadone, morphine, and/or phenobarbital, clonidine may be prescribed.

CLIENT EDUCATION

- Utilize a drug and/or alcohol treatment center.
- Understand the importance of SUID prevention activities due to the increased rate in newborns of parents who used methadone.

Hypoglycemia

The newborn's source of glucose stops when the umbilical cord is clamped. If newborns have other physiological stress, they can experience hypoglycemia due to inadequate gluconeogenesis or increased use of glycogen stores.

- An initial drop in blood glucose after birth is a common occurrence due to the cessation of the maternal supply of glucose. Healthy term newborns can compensate for this change by utilizing their glycogen stores to mobilize free fatty acids and ketones to provide energy.
  - Healthy term newborns can tolerate a decrease in glucose levels to as low as 30 mg/dL within the first 2 hr after birth.
- Newborns who are at risk for inadequate glycogen stores to compensate for this physiological change should have their glucose levels closely monitored after birth.
  - This includes newborns who are preterm, small or large for gestational age, newborns of diabetic mothers, and any who display manifestations of hypoglycemia or experienced difficulty transitioning to extra-uterine life.
- Interventions to raise blood glucose levels are usually indicated when glucose levels fall below 40 to 45 mg/dL.
- Untreated hypoglycemia can result in seizures and neurological injury.

DATA COLLECTION

RISK FACTORS

- Maternal diabetes mellitus
- Preterm infant
- LGA or SGA
- Stress at birth (cold stress, asphyxia)

EXPECTED FINDINGS

- Poor feeding
- Jitteriness/tremors
- Hypothermia
- Abnormal cry
- Lethargy
- Flaccid muscle tone
- Seizures/coma
- Irregular respirations
- Cyanosis
- Apnea

LABORATORY TESTS

Obtain a laboratory specimen to verify a bedside blood glucose level of less than 40 to 45 mg/dL, dependent upon facility protocol.

PATIENT-CENTERED CARE

NURSING CARE

- Perform blood glucose monitoring by heel stick for all newborns who are identified as being at-risk or displaying manifestations of hypoglycemia.
- Initiate early feedings, within the first hour of life, if the newborn is clinically stable.
  - Newborns who are unstable or unable to feed can require intravenous glucose infusions to maintain blood glucose levels.
- Continue to monitor blood glucose levels and feed every 2 to 3 hr for at least the first 24 hr of life, dependent on facility protocol.
- Skin-to-skin contact will promote breastfeeding and thermoregulation to stabilize blood sugar levels.

Respiratory distress syndrome, asphyxia, and meconium aspiration

- RDS occurs as a result of surfactant deficiency in the lungs and is characterized by poor gas exchange and ventilatory failure.
- Surfactant is a phospholipid that assists in alveoli expansion. Surfactant keeps alveoli from collapsing and allows gas exchange to occur.
- Atelectasis (collapsing of a portion of lung) increases the work of breathing. As a result, respiratory acidosis and hypoxemia can develop.
- Birth weight alone is not an indicator of fetal lung maturity.
- Complications from RDS are related to oxygen therapy and mechanical ventilation.
  - Pneumothorax
  - Pneumomediastinum
  - Retinopathy of prematurity
  - Bronchopulmonary dysplasia
  - Infection
  - Intraventricular hemorrhage

DATA COLLECTION

RISK FACTORS

- Preterm gestation
- Perinatal asphyxia (meconium staining, cord prolapse, nuchal cord)
- Maternal diabetes mellitus
- Premature rupture of membranes
- Maternal use of barbiturates or narcotics close to birth
- Maternal hypotension
- Cesarean birth without labor
- Hydrops fetalis (massive edema of the fetus caused by hyperbilirubinemia)
- Maternal bleeding during the third trimester
- Hypovolemia
- Genetics: white males and second-born twin

EXPECTED FINDINGS

- Tachypnea (respiratory rate greater than 60/min)
- Nasal flaring
- Expiratory grunting
- Retractions
- Labored breathing with prolonged expiration
- Fine crackles on auscultation
- Cyanosis
- Unresponsiveness, flaccidity, and apnea with decreased breath sounds (manifestations of worsened RDS)

LABORATORY TESTS

- ABGs
- Complete blood count with differential
- Culture and sensitivity of the blood, urine, and cerebrospinal fluid
- Blood glucose

DIAGNOSTIC PROCEDURES

Chest x-ray

PATIENT-CENTERED CARE

NURSING CARE

- Maintain thermoregulation.
- Provide mouth and skin care.
- Correct respiratory acidosis with ventilatory support.
- Correct metabolic acidosis by administering sodium bicarbonate.
- Maintain adequate oxygenation, prevent lactic acidosis, and avoid the toxic effects of oxygen.
- Monitor pulse oximetry.
- Provide parenteral nutrition as prescribed.
- Monitor laboratory results, I&O, and weight to evaluate hydration status.
- Decrease stimuli.

MEDICATIONS

Beractant, calfactant, lucinactant

CLASSIFICATION: Lung surfactant

INTENDED EFFECT: Restores surfactant and improves respiratory compliance for newborns who are premature and have RDS

NURSING ACTIONS

- Monitor respiratory effort, including ABGs, respiratory rhythm, and rate and skin color before and after administration of agent.
- Provide suction to the newborn prior to administration of the medication.
- Monitor endotracheal tube placement.
- Avoid suctioning of the endotracheal tube for 1 hr after administration of the medication.

> Factors that can accelerate lung maturation in the fetus while in utero include increased gestational age, intrauterine stress, exogenous steroid use, and ruptured membranes.

Preterm newborn

- A preterm newborn's birth occurs after 20 weeks of gestation and before completion of 37 weeks of gestation.
- A late preterm newborn's birth occurs from 34 0/7 to 36 6/7 weeks of gestation.
- Preterm newborns are at risk for a variety of complications due to immature organ systems. The degree of complications depends on gestational age. There is a decreased risk for complications the closer the newborn is to 40 weeks of gestation.
  - Goals include meeting the newborn's growth and development needs and anticipating and managing associated complications (RDS, sepsis).
  - The main priority in treating newborns who are preterm is supporting the cardiac and respiratory systems as needed. Most newborns who are preterm are cared for in a neonatal intensive care unit (NICU). Meticulous care and observation in the NICU is necessary until the newborn can receive oral feedings, can maintain body temperature, and weighs approximately 2 kg (4.4 lb.).

COMPLICATIONS

Respiratory distress syndrome: Decreased surfactant in the alveoli occurs, regardless of a newborn's birth weight.

Bronchopulmonary dysplasia (BPD): Causes the lungs to become stiff and noncompliant, requiring a newborn to receive mechanical ventilation and oxygen. BPD is also commonly caused by mechanical ventilation. It is sometimes difficult to remove the newborn from ventilation and oxygen after initial placement.

Aspiration: A result of a newborn who is premature not having an intact gag reflex or the ability to effectively suck or swallow

Apnea of prematurity: A result of immature neurological and chemical mechanisms

Intraventricular hemorrhage: Bleeding in or around the ventricles of the brain

Retinopathy of prematurity: Disease caused by abnormal growth of retinal blood vessels and is a complication associated with oxygen administration to the newborn; can cause mild to severe eye and vision problems

Patent ductus arteriosus: Occurs when the ductus arteriosus fails to close after birth due to neonatal hypoxia, or when the ductus arteriosus does not close after birth

Necrotizing enterocolitis: An inflammatory disease of the gastrointestinal mucosa due to ischemia. It results in necrosis and perforation of the bowel. (Short-gut syndrome can be the result secondary to removal of most or part of the small intestine due to necrosis.)

Additional complications: Infection, hyperbilirubinemia, anemia, hypoglycemia, and delayed growth and development

DATA COLLECTION

RISK FACTORS

- Maternal gestational hypertension
- Multiple pregnancies that are closely spaced
- Adolescent pregnancy
- Lack of prenatal care
- Maternal substance use, smoking
- Previous history of preterm birth
- Abnormalities of the uterus
- Cervical incompetence
- Placenta previa
- Preterm labor
- Preterm premature rupture of membranes

EXPECTED FINDINGS

- Ballard assessment showing a physical and neurological data collection totaling less than 37 weeks of gestation
- Periodic breathing consisting of 5- to 10-second respiratory pauses, followed by 10- to 15-second compensatory rapid respirations
- Manifestations of increased respiratory effort and/ or respiratory distress, including nasal flaring or retractions of the chest wall during inspirations, expiratory grunting, and tachypnea
- Apnea: a pause in respirations 20 seconds or greater
- Low birth weight
- Minimal subcutaneous fat deposits
- Head that is large in comparison with the body, and small fontanels
- Wrinkled features with abundance of lanugo covering back, forearms, forehead, and sides of face, and few or no creases on soles of feet
- Skull and rib cage that feel soft
- Eyes closed if the newborn is born at 22 to 24 weeks of gestation
- Weak grasp reflex
- Inability to coordinate suck and swallow; weak or absent gag, suck, and cough reflex; weak swallow
- Hypotonic muscles, decreased level of activity, and a weak cry for more than 24 hr
- Lethargy, tachycardia, and poor weight gain

LABORATORY TESTS

- CBC showing decreased Hgb and Hct as a result of slow production of RBCs
- Urinalysis and specific gravity
- Increased PT and aPTT time with an increased tendency to bleed
- Serum glucose
- Calcium
- Bilirubin
- ABGs

DIAGNOSTIC PROCEDURES

- Chest x-ray
- Head ultrasounds
- Echocardiography
- Eye exams

PATIENT-CENTERED CARE

NURSING CARE

- Perform initial collection of data.
- Assist with resuscitative measures if needed.
- Monitor the newborn's vital signs.
- Determine the newborn's ability to consume and digest nutrients. Before feeding by breast or nipple, the newborn must have an intact gag reflex and be able to suck and swallow to prevent aspiration.
- Monitor I&O and daily weight.
- Monitor the newborn for bleeding from puncture sites and the gastrointestinal tract.
- Ensure and maintain thermoregulation in a newborn who is preterm by using a radiant heat warmer.
  - Manifestations of hypothermia: Apnea, cyanosis, hypoglycemia, feeding intolerance, lethargy, irritability, bradycardia
- Assist with the administration of respiratory support measures, such as surfactant and/or oxygen administration.
- Assist with the administration of parental or enteral nutrition and fluids as prescribed (most preterm newborns who are less than 34 weeks of gestation will receive fluids either by IV and/or gavage feedings). Provide for nonnutritive sucking, such as using a pacifier while gavage feeding.
- Minimize the newborn's stimulation. Cluster nursing care. Touch the newborn very smoothly and lightly. Keep lighting dim and noise levels reduced.
- Position the newborn in neutral flexion with the extremities close to the body to conserve body heat. Prone and side-lying positions are preferred to supine with body containment using blanket rolls and swaddling, but only in the nursery under monitored supervision.
- Examine skin daily to minimize risk of breakdown.
- Encourage skin-to-skin contact (Kangaroo care) whenever possible to reduce preterm infant stress.

- Protect the newborn against infection by enforcing hand hygiene and gowning procedures.
  ○ Equipment should not be shared with other newborns.
  ○ **Evidence of infection:** Temperature instability, lethargy, irritability, cyanosis, bradycardia or tachycardia, apnea or tachypnea, feeding intolerance, glucose instability
- Observe the newborn for findings of dehydration or overhydration (resulting from IV nutrition and fluid administration).
  ○ **Dehydration**
    ▪ Urine output less than 1 mL/kg/hr
    ▪ Urine-specific gravity greater than 1.015
    ▪ Weight loss
    ▪ Dry mucous membranes
    ▪ Absent skin turgor
    ▪ Depressed fontanel
  ○ **Overhydration**
    ▪ Urine output greater than 3 mL/kg/hr
    ▪ Urine-specific gravity less than 1.001
    ▪ Edema
    ▪ Increased weight gain
    ▪ Crackles in lungs
    ▪ Intake greater than output

CLIENT EDUCATION

Remain engaged in the care of the preterm newborn.

Small-for-gestational-age newborn

- SGA describes a newborn whose birth weight is at or below the 10th percentile and who has intrauterine growth restriction.
- Common complications of newborns who are SGA are perinatal asphyxia, meconium aspiration, hypoglycemia, polycythemia, and instability of body temperature.

DATA COLLECTION

RISK FACTORS

- Congenital or chromosomal anomalies
- Maternal infections, disease, or malnutrition
- Gestational hypertension and/or diabetes
- Maternal smoking, drug, or alcohol use
- Multiple gestations
- Placental factors (small placenta, placenta previa, decreased placental perfusion)
- Fetal congenital infections (rubella, toxoplasmosis)

EXPECTED FINDINGS

- Weight below 10th percentile
- Normal skull, but reduced body dimensions
- Hair is sparse on scalp.
- Wide skull sutures from inadequate bone growth
- Dry, loose skin
- Decreased subcutaneous fat
- Decreased muscle mass, particularly over the cheeks and buttocks
- Thin, dry, yellow, and dull umbilical cord rather than gray, glistening, and moist
- Drawn abdomen rather than well-rounded
- Respiratory distress and hypoxia
- Wide-eyed and alert appearance, which is attributed to prolonged fetal hypoxia
- Hypotonia
- Evidence of meconium aspiration
- Hypoglycemia

LABORATORY TESTS

- Blood glucose for hypoglycemia
- CBC will show polycythemia resulting from fetal hypoxia and intrauterine stress.
- ABGs can be prescribed due to chronic hypoxia in utero due to placental insufficiency.

DIAGNOSTIC PROCEDURES

Chest x-ray to rule out meconium aspiration syndrome

PATIENT-CENTERED CARE

NURSING CARE

- Support respiratory efforts, and suction the newborn as necessary to maintain an open airway. Qs
- Provide a neutral thermal environment for the newborn (isolette or radiant heat warmer) to prevent cold stress.
- Assist with early feedings. (A newborn who is SGA will require feedings that are more frequent.)
- Monitor parenteral nutrition if necessary.
- Maintain adequate hydration.
- Conserve the newborn's energy level.
- Prevent skin breakdown.
- Protect the newborn from infection.
- Provide support to the newborn's parents and extended family.

CLIENT EDUCATION

Participate in caring for the newborn. Anticipate home care needs.

Large-for-gestational-age (macrosomic) newborn

- LGA occurs in neonates who weigh above the 90th percentile or more than 4,000 g (8.8 lb).
- Neonates who are LGA can be preterm, postmature, or full-term.
- Newborns who are macrosomic are at risk for birth injuries (shoulder dystocia, clavicle fracture or a cesarean birth, asphyxia, hypoglycemia, polycythemia and Erb-Duchenne paralysis due to birth trauma).
- Uncontrolled hyperglycemia during pregnancy (leading risk factor for LGA) can lead to congenital defects with the most common being congenital heart defects and CNS anomalies.

DATA COLLECTION

RISK FACTORS

- Newborns who are postmature
- Maternal diabetes mellitus during pregnancy (High glucose levels stimulate continued insulin production by the fetus.)
- Genetic factors
- Maternal obesity

EXPECTED FINDINGS

- Weight above 90th percentile (4,000 g)
- Large head
- Plump and full-faced (cushingoid appearance) from increased subcutaneous fat
- Manifestations of hypoxia, including tachypnea, retractions, cyanosis, nasal flaring, and grunting
- Birth trauma (fractures, shoulder dystocia, intracranial hemorrhage, CNS injury)
- Sluggishness, hypotonic muscles, and hypoactivity
- Tremors from hypocalcemia
- Hypoglycemia
- Respiratory distress from immature lungs or meconium aspiration

Findings of increased intracranial pressure: dilated pupils, vomiting, bulging fontanels, high-pitched cry

LABORATORY TESTS

- Blood glucose levels to monitor closely for hypoglycemia
- ABGs can be prescribed due to chronic hypoxia in utero secondary to placental insufficiency.
- CBC shows polycythemia (Hct greater than 65%) from in utero hypoxia.
- Hyperbilirubinemia resulting from polycythemia as excessive RBCs break down after birth
- Hypocalcemia can result in response to a long and difficult birth.

DIAGNOSTIC PROCEDURES

Chest x-ray to rule out meconium aspiration syndrome

PATIENT-CENTERED CARE

NURSING CARE

Prior to birth

- Prepare the client for a possible vacuum-assisted or cesarean birth.
- Prepare to place the client in McRoberts position (lithotomy position with legs flexed to chest to maximize pelvic outlet).
- Prepare to apply suprapubic pressure to aid in the delivery of the anterior shoulder, which is located inferior to the maternal symphysis pubis.

For a newborn who is LGA following birth

- Obtain blood glucose level within the first hour of life.
- Initiate early feedings or IV therapy to maintain glucose levels within the expected reference range.
- Examine the newborn for birth trauma (broken clavicle, Erb-Duchenne paralysis).
- Identify and treat any birth injuries.

Postmature infant

- A newborn who is postmature is born after the completion of 42 weeks of gestation. Postmaturity of the infant can be associated with either of the following.
  - **Dysmaturity from placental degeneration and uteroplacental insufficiency** (placenta functions effectively for approximately 40 weeks) resulting in chronic fetal hypoxia and fetal distress in utero. The fetal response is polycythemia, meconium aspiration, and/or neonatal respiratory problems. Perinatal mortality is higher when a postmature placenta fails to meet increased oxygen demands of the fetus during labor.
  - **Continued growth of the fetus in utero** because the placenta continues to function effectively, and the newborn becomes LGA at birth. This leads to a difficult delivery, cephalopelvic disproportion, as well as high insulin reserves and insufficient glucose reserves at birth. The neonatal response can be birth trauma, perinatal asphyxia, a clavicle fracture, seizures, hypoglycemia, and/or temperature instability (cold stress).
- A newborn who is postmature can be either SGA or LGA depending on how well the placenta functions during the last weeks of pregnancy.
- Newborns who are postmature have an increased risk for aspirating the meconium passed by the fetus in utero.
- Persistent pulmonary hypertension (persistent fetal circulation) is a complication that can result from meconium aspiration. There is an interference in the transition from fetal to neonatal circulation, and the ductus arteriosus (connecting the main pulmonary artery and the aorta) and foramen ovale (shunt between the right and left atria) remain open, and fetal pathways of blood flow continue.

DATA COLLECTION

RISK FACTORS

In most cases, the cause of a pregnancy that extends beyond 40 weeks of gestation is unknown, but there is a higher incidence in first pregnancies and in clients who have had a previous postmature pregnancy.

EXPECTED FINDINGS

- Wasted appearance, thin with loose skin, having lost some of the subcutaneous fat
- Peeling, cracked, and dry skin; leathery from decreased protection of vernix and amniotic fluid
- Long, thin body
- Meconium staining of fingernails and umbilical cord
- Hair and nails can be long.
- Alertness similar to a 2-week-old newborn
- Difficulty establishing respirations secondary to meconium aspiration
- Hypoglycemia due to insufficient stores of glycogen
- Clinical findings of cold stress
- Neurological manifestations that become apparent with the development of fine motor skills
- Macrosomia

LABORATORY TESTS

- Blood glucose levels to monitor for hypoglycemia
- ABGs secondary to chronic hypoxia in utero due to placental insufficiency
- CBC to show polycythemia from decreased oxygenation in utero
- Hct elevated from polycythemia and dehydration

DIAGNOSTIC PROCEDURES

Chest x-ray to rule out meconium aspiration syndrome

PATIENT-CENTERED CARE

NURSING CARE

- Monitor vital signs.
- Monitor IV fluids.
- Moisturize the skin with a petrolatum-based ointment.
- Monitor mechanical ventilation if necessary.
- Administer oxygen as prescribed.
- Assist with exchange transfusion if hematocrit is high.
- Provide thermoregulation in an isolette to avoid cold stress.
- Provide early feedings to avoid hypoglycemia.
- Identify and treat any birth injuries.

Tracheoesophageal fistula (TEF)

TEF is a gastrointestinal anomaly that can occur independently or together with an EA. TEF alone can include a variety of abnormal connections between the esophagus and trachea. TEF and EA combined include a blind esophagus pouch and/or abnormal connection between the esophagus and trachea. The presence of a TEF places the newborn at risk for aspiration and respiratory complications.

HEALTH PROMOTION AND DISEASE PREVENTION

TEF can be detected and diagnosed during a prenatal ultrasound.

DATA COLLECTION

RISK FACTORS

- History of polyhydramnios
- Cardiac anomaly
- Cleft lip/palate
- Neural tube defects

EXPECTED FINDINGS

- Depends on specific defect present
- Excessive oral secretions
- Drooling
- Feeding intolerance (gagging, coughing during feeding, spitting up, gastric distention)
- Respiratory distress and cyanosis

DIAGNOSTIC PROCEDURES

Prenatal ultrasound

PATIENT-CENTERED CARE

Maintain thermoregulation, electrolyte balance, and acid-base balance.

NURSING CARE

- Position supine with head of bed elevated.
- Ensure orogastric tube is set to low-continuous suction.
- Monitor for findings of respiratory distress. Qs

  ! Do not feed any newborn who has excessive oral secretions with respiratory distress until a provider is consulted.

MEDICATIONS

- Antireflux medications
- Antacids

THERAPEUTIC PROCEDURES

Surgical intervention to correct specific defect

COMPLICATIONS

- Respiratory distress
- Depends upon other anomalies present

Newborn infection, sepsis (sepsis neonatorum)

- Infection can be contracted by the newborn before, during, or after birth. Newborns are more susceptible to micro-organisms due to their limited immunity and inability to localize infection. The infection can spread rapidly into the bloodstream.
- Newborn sepsis is the presence of micro-organisms or their toxins in the blood or tissues of the newborn during the first month after birth. Manifestations of sepsis are subtle and can resemble other diseases; the nurse often notices them during routine care of the newborn.
- Organisms frequently responsible for newborn infections include *Staphylococcus aureus*, *Staphylococcus epidermidis*, *Escherichia coli*, *Haemophilus influenzae*, and group B streptococcus beta-hemolytic.
- Prevention of infection and newborn sepsis starts perinatally with maternal screening for infections, prophylactic interventions, and the use of sterile and aseptic techniques during delivery. Prophylactic antibiotic treatment of the eyes of all newborns and appropriate umbilical cord care also help to prevent newborn infection and sepsis.

DATA COLLECTION

RISK FACTORS

- Premature rupture of membranes
- Prolonged labor
- Toxoplasmosis, rubella, cytomegalovirus, and herpes (TORCH)
- Chorioamnionitis
- Preterm birth
- Low birth weight
- Maternal substance use
- Maternal urinary tract infection
- Meconium aspiration
- HIV transmitted from the parent to the newborn perinatally through the placenta and postnatally through the breast milk

EXPECTED FINDINGS

- Temperature instability
- Suspicious drainage (eyes, umbilical stump)
- Poor feeding pattern (weak suck, decreased intake)
- Vomiting and diarrhea
- Hypoglycemia, hyperglycemia
- Abdominal distention
- Apnea, retractions, grunting, nasal flaring
- Decreased oxygen saturation
- Color changes (pallor, jaundice, petechiae)
- Tachycardia or bradycardia
- Tachypnea
- Low blood pressure
- Irritability and seizure activity
- Poor muscle tone and lethargy

LABORATORY TESTS

- CBC with differential, C-reactive protein
- Blood, urine, and cerebrospinal fluid cultures and sensitivities
- Chemical profile to show a fluid and electrolyte imbalance

PATIENT-CENTERED CARE

NURSING CARE

- Determine infection risk. (Review maternal health record.)
- Monitor for findings of opportunistic infection.
- Monitor vital signs continuously.
- Monitor I&O and daily weight.
- Monitor fluid and electrolyte status.
- Monitor the newborn's visitors for infection.
- Obtain specimens (blood, urine, stool) to assist in identifying the causative organism.
- Maintain IV therapy as prescribed to administer electrolyte replacements, fluids, and medications.
- Isolation precautions as indicated
- Administer medications as prescribed (antibiotics, antivirals, or antifungals).
- Maintain respiratory support as needed.
- Monitor IV site for evidence of infection.
- Provide newborn care to maintain temperature.
- Clean and sterilize all equipment to be used.
- Provide emotional support to the family.

CLIENT EDUCATION

DISCHARGE INSTRUCTIONS
- Breastfeeding is encouraged due to the protective properties of the breast milk.
- Understand and adhere to infection control.
  - Use clean bottles and nipples for each feeding.
  - Discard any unused formula.
  - Perform proper hand hygiene.
- Promote adequate rest for newborn, and decrease physical stimulation.

Birth trauma or injury

Birth injury occurs during childbirth, resulting in physical injury to a newborn. Most injuries are minor and resolve rapidly. Other injuries can require some intervention. A few are serious enough to be fatal.

TYPES OF BIRTH INJURIES
- **Skull:** Linear fracture, depressed fracture
- **Scalp:** Caput succedaneum, hemorrhage
- **Intracranial:** Epidural or subdural hematoma, contusions
- **Spinal cord:** Spinal cord transaction or injury, vertebral artery injury
- **Plexus:** Brachial plexus injury, Klumpke's palsy
- **Cranial and peripheral nerve:** Radial nerve palsy, diaphragmatic paralysis

DATA COLLECTION

RISK FACTORS
- Maternal age: younger than 16 or older than 35
- Fetal macrosomia
- Abnormal or difficult presentations
- Prolonged labor
- Precipitous labor
- Oligohydramnios
- Cephalopelvic disproportion
- Multifetal gestation
- Congenital abnormalities
- Internal FHR monitoring
- Forceps or vacuum extraction
- External version
- Cesarean birth

EXPECTED FINDINGS
- Irritability, seizures within the first 72 hr, and decreased level of consciousness are manifestations of a subarachnoid hemorrhage.
- Facial flattening and unresponsiveness to grimace that accompanies crying or stimulation, as well as eyes remaining open, are findings to monitor for facial paralysis.
- A weak or hoarse cry is characteristic of laryngeal nerve palsy from excessive traction on the neck.
- Flaccid muscle tone can signal joint dislocations and separation during birth.
- Flaccid muscle tone of the extremities suggests nerve-plexus injuries or long bone fractures.
- Limited motion of an arm, crepitus over a clavicle, and absence of the Moro reflex on the affected side are manifestations of clavicular fractures.
- A flaccid arm with the elbow extended and the hand rotated inward, absence of the Moro reflex on the affected side, sensory loss over the lateral aspect of the arm, and intact grasp reflex are manifestations of Erb-Duchenne paralysis (brachial paralysis).
- Localized discoloration, ecchymosis, petechiae, and edema over the presenting part are seen with soft-tissue injuries.

DIAGNOSTIC PROCEDURES

Birth injuries are normally diagnosed by a CT scan, x-ray of suspected area of fracture, or neurological exam to determine paralysis of nerves.

PATIENT-CENTERED CARE

NURSING CARE
- Review maternal history for factors that can predispose the newborn to injuries.
- Review Apgar scoring that might indicate a possibility of birth injury.
- Perform frequent head-to-toe examinations.
- Obtain vital signs and temperature.
- Promote parent-newborn interaction as much as possible.
- Administer treatment to the newborn based on the injury and according to the provider's prescriptions.

CLIENT EDUCATION

DISCHARGE INSTRUCTIONS
- Understand the injury and management of the injury.
- Perform parent-newborn bonding.

Hyperbilirubinemia

Hyperbilirubinemia is an elevation of serum bilirubin levels resulting in jaundice. Jaundice normally appears on the head (especially the sclera and mucous membranes), and then progresses down the thorax, abdomen, and extremities.

Jaundice can be physiologic or pathologic.
- **Physiologic jaundice** is considered benign (resulting from normal newborn physiology of increased bilirubin production due to the shortened lifespan and breakdown of fetal RBCs and liver immaturity). The newborn who has physiological jaundice exhibits an increase in unconjugated bilirubin levels 72 to 120 hr after birth, with a rapid decline to 3 mg/dL 5 to 10 days after birth.
- **Pathologic jaundice** is a result of an underlying disease. Pathologic jaundice appears before 24 hr of age or is persistent after day 14. In the term newborn, bilirubin levels increase more than 0.5 mg/dL/hr, peaks at greater than 12.0 mg/dL, or is associated with anemia and hepatosplenomegaly. Pathologic jaundice is usually caused by a blood group incompatibility or an infection, but can be the result of RBC disorders.

Acute bilirubin encephalopathy is when the bilirubin is deposited in the brain. This occurs once all of the binding sites for the bilirubin are used within the body, resulting in necrosis of neurons. Bilirubin levels higher than 25 mg/dL place the newborn at risk. This can result in permanent damage, including dystonia and athetosis, upward gaze, hearing loss, and cognitive impairments.

Kernicterus is an irreversible, chronic result of bilirubin toxicity. The newborn demonstrates many of the same manifestations of bilirubin encephalopathy with hypotonia, severe cognitive impairments, and spastic quadriplegia.

DATA COLLECTION

RISK FACTORS

- Increased RBC production or breakdown
- Rh or ABO incompatibility
- Decreased liver function
- Maternal ingestion of diazepam, salicylates, or sulfonamides close to birth
- Maternal diabetes
- Oxytocin during labor
- Neonatal hyperthyroidism
- Ecchymosis or hemangioma
- Cephalohematomas
- Prematurity

EXPECTED FINDINGS

- Yellowish tint to skin, sclera, and mucous membranes.
- To verify jaundice, press the newborn's skin on the cheek or abdomen lightly with one finger. Then, release pressure, and observe the newborn's skin color for yellowish tint as the skin is blanched.
- Note the time of jaundice onset.
- Monitor the underlying cause by reviewing the maternal prenatal, family, and newborn history.
- Hypoxia, hypothermia, hypoglycemia, and metabolic acidosis can occur as a result of hyperbilirubinemia and can increase the risk of brain damage.

LABORATORY TESTS

- An elevated serum bilirubin level can occur (direct and indirect bilirubin). Monitor the newborn's bilirubin levels every 4 hr until the level returns to normal. Qs
- Monitor maternal and newborn blood type to determine whether there is ABO incompatibility. This occurs if the newborn has blood type A or B and the parent is type O.
- Review Hgb and Hct.
- A direct Coombs' test reveals the presence of antibody-coated (sensitized) Rh-positive RBCs in the newborn.
- Check electrolyte levels for dehydration from phototherapy.

DIAGNOSTIC PROCEDURES

Transcutaneous bilirubin level is a noninvasive method to measure a newborn's bilirubin level.

PATIENT-CENTERED CARE

NURSING CARE

- Observe the skin and mucous membranes for jaundice.
- Monitor vital signs.
- Set up phototherapy if prescribed.
  - Maintain an eye mask over the newborn's eyes for protection of corneas and retinas.
  - Keep the newborn undressed. For a male newborn, a surgical mask should be placed (like a bikini) over the genitalia to prevent possible testicular damage from heat and light waves. Be sure to remove the metal strip from the mask to prevent burning.
  - Avoid applying lotions or ointments to the skin because they absorb heat and can cause burns.
  - Remove the newborn from phototherapy every 4 hr, and unmask the newborn's eyes, checking for inflammation or injury.
  - Reposition the newborn every 2 hr to expose all of the body surfaces to the phototherapy lights and prevent pressure sores.
  - Check the lamp energy with a photometer per facility protocol.
  - Turn off the phototherapy lights before drawing blood for testing.
- Observe the newborn for effects of phototherapy.
  - Bronze discoloration: not a serious complication
  - Maculopapular skin rash: not a serious complication
  - Development of pressure areas
  - Dehydration: poor skin turgor, dry mucous membranes, decreased urinary output
  - Elevated temperature
- Encourage the parents to hold and interact with the newborn when phototherapy lights are off.
- Monitor elimination and daily weights, watching for evidence of dehydration.
- Check the newborn's axillary temperature every 4 hr during phototherapy because temperature can become elevated.
- Feed the newborn early and frequently, every 3 to 4 hr. This will promote bilirubin excretion in the stools.
- Encourage continued breastfeeding of the newborn. Supplementation with donor milk or formula can be prescribed.
- Maintain adequate fluid intake to prevent dehydration.
- Reassure the parents that most newborns experience some degree of jaundice.
- Explain hyperbilirubinemia, its causes, diagnostic tests, and treatment to parents.
- Explain that the newborn's stool contains some bile that will be loose and green.
- Assist with the administration of an exchange transfusion for newborns who are at risk for kernicterus.

THERAPEUTIC PROCEDURES

Phototherapy: The newborn's bilirubin should start to decrease within 4 to 6 hr after starting treatment.

CLIENT EDUCATION

DISCHARGE INSTRUCTIONS
- Remember and adhere to the newborn's plan of care.
- Newborns who have low to moderate risk of hyperbilirubinemia should receive follow-up care within two days. Newborns at higher risk should be seen within 24 hr.

Congenital anomalies

Newborns can be born with congenital anomalies involving all systems. Anomalies are often diagnosed prenatally. A nurse should provide emotional support to the parents whose newborn is facing procedures or surgeries to correct the defects.

When congenital anomalies are present at birth, they can involve any of the body systems. Major anomalies causing serious problems include the following.

- **Congenital heart disease (CHD):** Atrial septal defects, ventricular septal defects, coarctation of the aorta, tetralogy of Fallot, transposition of the great vessels, stenosis, atresia of valves
- **Neurological defects:** Neural tube defects, hydrocephalus, anencephaly, encephalocele, meningocele, myelomeningocele
- **Gastrointestinal problems:** Cleft lip/palate, diaphragmatic hernia, imperforate anus, tracheoesophageal fistula/esophageal atresia (EA), duodenal atresia, omphalocele, gastroschisis, umbilical hernia, intestinal obstruction
- **Musculoskeletal deformities:** Clubfoot, polydactyly, developmental dysplasia of the hip
- **Genitourinary deformities:** Hypospadias, epispadias, exstrophy of the bladder, ambiguous genitalia
- **Metabolic disorders:** Phenylketonuria, galactosemia, hypothyroidism
- **Chromosomal abnormalities**

Congenital anomalies are generally identified soon after birth by Apgar scoring and a brief data collection indicating the need for further investigation. Once identified, congenital anomalies are treated in a pediatric setting.

- **Cleft lip/palate:** Failure of the lip or hard or soft palate to fuse
- **Tracheoesophageal atresia:** Failure of the esophagus to connect to the stomach
- **Phenylketonuria (PKU):** Inability to metabolize the amino acid phenylalanine
- **Galactosemia:** Inability to metabolize galactose into glucose
- **Hypothyroidism:** Slow metabolism caused by maternal iodine deficiency or maternal antithyroid medications during pregnancy
- **Neurologic anomalies (spina bifida):** A neural tube defect in which the vertebral arch fails to close

- **Hydrocephalus:** Excessive spinal fluid accumulation in the ventricles of the brain
- **Patent ductus arteriosus:** A noncyanotic heart defect in which the ductus arteriosus connecting the pulmonary artery and the aorta fails to close after birth
- **Tetralogy of Fallot:** Cyanotic heart defect characterized by a ventricular septal defect, the aorta positioned over the ventricular septal defect, stenosis of the pulmonary valve, and hypertrophy of the right ventricle
- **Down syndrome:** Trisomy 21, which is the most common trisomic abnormality with 47 chromosomes in each cell

DATA COLLECTION

RISK FACTORS

GENETIC AND/OR ENVIRONMENTAL FACTORS
- Maternal age greater than 40 years
- Chromosome abnormalities, such as Down syndrome
- Viral infections, such as rubella
- Excessive body heat exposure during the first trimester (neural tube defects)
- Medications and substance use during pregnancy
- Maternal obesity
- Radiation exposure
- Maternal metabolic disorders (phenylketonuria, diabetes mellitus)
- Poor maternal nutrition such as folic acid deficiency (neural tube defects)
- Newborns who are preterm
- Newborns who are SGA
- Oligohydramnios or polyhydramnios

EXPECTED FINDINGS

Monitor the newborn for evidence of congenital anomalies.

Cleft lip/palate: Opening in the lip or palate

Tracheoesophageal atresia: Excessive mucous secretions and drooling, periodic cyanotic episodes and choking, abdominal distention after birth, immediate regurgitation after birth

Duodenal atresia: Abdominal distention, bilious vomiting, failure to pass meconium in the first 24 hr

PKU: Can result in cognitive impairment if untreated; not evident at birth but will be identified with neonatal screening

Galactosemia: Can result in failure to thrive, cataracts, jaundice, cirrhosis of the liver, sepsis, and cognitive impairment if untreated; this will not be evident at birth, but will be identified with neonatal screening

Hypothyroidism: Can result in hypothermia, poor feeding, lethargy, jaundice, and cretinism if untreated; not evident at birth but can be identified at 6 weeks by manifestations of bradycardia, abdominal distention, coarse dry hair, and thick dry skin, which can progress to delayed CNS development

Neurologic anomalies (spina bifida): Protrusion of the meninges and/or spinal cord

Hydrocephalus: Enlarged head and bulging fontanels; sun-setting sign is common in which the whites of the eyes are visible above the iris

Patent ductus arteriosus: Murmurs, abnormal heart rate or rhythm, breathlessness, and fatigue while feeding

Tetralogy of Fallot: Respiratory difficulties, cyanosis, tachycardia, tachypnea, and diaphoresis

Down syndrome: Oblique palpebral fissures or upward slant of eyes; epicanthal folds; flat facial profile with a depressed nasal bridge and a small nose; protruding tongue; small, low-set ears; short broad hands with a fifth finger that has one flexion crease instead of two; a deep crease across the center of the palm (frequently referred to as a simian crease); hyperflexibility; hypotonic muscles

DATA COLLECTION

- Newborn's ability to take in adequate nourishment
- Newborn's ability to eliminate waste products
- Vital signs and axillary temperature
- Newborn-parental bonding, observing the parent's response to the diagnosis of a congenital defect, and encouraging the parents to verbalize concerns Qpcc

DIAGNOSTIC AND THERAPEUTIC PROCEDURES

- Prenatal screening for congenital anomalies can be done by ultrasound and multiple-marker screening (triple and quad screen).
- Confirmation of a diagnosis depends on the anomaly.
- Prenatal diagnosis or confirmation of congenital anomalies is often made by amniocentesis, chorionic villi sampling, or ultrasound.
- Pulse oximetry readings for CHD.
- Routine testing of newborns for metabolic disorders (inborn errors of metabolism):
  ○ A Guthrie test for PKU is done to show elevations of phenylalanine in the blood and urine. It is not reliable until the newborn has ingested sufficient amounts of protein.
  ○ Monitor blood and urine levels of galactose (galactosemia).
  ○ Measure thyroxine (hypothyroidism).
  ○ Cytologic studies (karyotyping of chromosomes), such as a buccal smear, use cells scraped from the mucosa from inside the newborn's mouth.

PATIENT-CENTERED CARE

NURSING CARE

Nursing interventions for congenital anomalies are dependent upon the type and extent of the anomaly.
- Maintain adequate respiratory status.
- Maintain extrauterine circulation.
- Maintain adequate thermoregulation.

- Administer medications as prescribed, such as thyroid replacement for hypothyroidism.
- Reinforce education with the parents regarding preoperative and postoperative treatment procedures.
- Encourage the parents to hold, touch, and talk to the newborn.
- Ensure that parents provide consistent care to the newborn.
- Provide parents with information about parent groups or support systems.

Neurologic anomalies (spina bifida)

- Protect the membrane with a sterile, moist, non-adherent dressing to prevent drying.
- Observe for leakage of cerebrospinal fluid.
- Handle the newborn gently by placing them in a prone-kneeling position to prevent trauma.
- Prevent infection by keeping the area free from contamination by urine and feces.
- Measure the circumference of the newborn's head to identify hydrocephalus.
- Observe the newborn for indications of increased intracranial pressure.

Hydrocephalus

- Frequently reposition the newborn's head to prevent sores.
- Measure the newborn's head circumference daily.
- Observe for manifestations of increased intracranial pressure (vomiting, shrill cry).

Patent ductus arteriosus

Reinforce education with the parents about surgical treatment.

Tetralogy of Fallot

- Conserve the newborn's energy to reduce the workload on the heart.
- Administer gavage feedings, or give oral feedings with a specialized nipple.
- Elevate the newborn's head and shoulders to improve respirations and reduce the cardiac workload.
- Prevent infection.
- Place the newborn in a knee-chest position during respiratory distress.

Cleft lip/palate

- Encourage expression of parental concerns, grief, and fears.
- Monitor the newborn's weight daily while hospitalized.
- Monitor for manifestations of dehydration.
- Encourage parental attachment.
- Suction nose and mouth gently with bulb syringe as needed to clear airway.
- Position infant to facilitate drainage of sections.
- Reinforce education with the parents on feeding requirements of infants.

NUTRITION

Provide adequate nutrition.

Cleft lip/palate: Determine the most effective nipple for feeding. Can use specialized bottles, cups, or syringes to feed the newborn. Newborns who have cleft lip can achieve breastfeeding with changes in positioning. Feed the newborn in the upright position to decrease aspiration risk. Feed the newborn slowly, and burp them frequently so that they do not swallow air. Cleanse the mouth after feedings.

Tracheoesophageal atresia: Withhold feedings until esophageal patency is determined. Elevate the head of the newborn's crib to prevent gastric juice reflux. Supervise the first feeding to observe for this anomaly.

Duodenal atresia: Withhold feedings until surgical repair is done and the newborn has begun to pass stools. Administer IV fluids as prescribed. Monitor for jaundice.

PKU: Specialized synthetic formula in which phenylalanine is removed or reduced. The parent should restrict meat, dairy products, diet drinks (artificial sweeteners), and protein during pregnancy. Aspartame must be avoided.

Galactosemia: Give the newborn a soy-based formula because galactose is present in milk. Eliminate lactose and galactose in the newborn's diet. Breastfeeding is also contraindicated.

Active Learning Scenario

A nurse is reviewing hyperbilirubinemia with a newly hired nurse. What should the nurse include in this review? Use the ATI Active Learning Template: System Disorder to complete this item.

ALTERATION IN HEALTH (DIAGNOSIS): Describe the difference between physiologic and pathologic jaundice, acute bilirubin encephalopathy, and kernicterus.

DIAGNOSTIC PROCEDURES: Describe the procedure that can be used to verify the presence of jaundice.

NURSING CARE: Describe care of the newborn receiving phototherapy.

Application Exercises

1. A nurse is assisting with an in-service for newly licensed nurses about neonatal opioid withdrawal syndrome (NOWS) in newborns. Which of the following statements by a newly licensed nurse indicates an understanding of the teaching?

   A. "The newborn will have decreased muscle tone."

   B. "The newborn will have a continuous, high-pitched cry."

   C. "The newborn will sleep for 2 to 3 hours after a feeding."

   D. "The newborn will have mild tremors when disturbed."

2. A nurse is assisting with the care of a newborn who is preterm and has respiratory distress syndrome. Which of the following should the nurse monitor to evaluate the newborn's condition following administration of synthetic surfactant?

   A. Oxygen saturation

   B. Body temperature

   C. Serum bilirubin

   D. Heart rate

3. A nurse is assisting with the care of a newborn who was born at 32 weeks of gestation. The newborn's birth weight is 1,100 g. Which of the following are expected findings in this newborn? (Select all that apply.)

   A. Lanugo

   B. Long nails

   C. Weak grasp reflex

   D. Translucent skin

   E. Plump face

4. A nurse is assisting with the care of a client who is at 42 weeks gestation and in labor. The client asks the nurse what to expect because the baby is postmature. Which of the following statements should the nurse make?

   A. "Your baby will have excess body fat."

   B. "Your baby will have flat areola without breast buds."

   C. "Your baby's heels will easily move to their ears."

   D. "Your baby's skin will have a leathery appearance."

5. A nurse is assisting with the care of an newborn who has a high bilirubin level and is receiving phototherapy. Which of the following findings is the priority for the nurse to report to the charge nurse?

   A. Conjunctivitis

   B. Bronze skin discoloration

   C. Sunken fontanels

   D. Maculopapular skin rash

Application Exercises Key

1. B. **CORRECT:** The nurse should identify that the newly licensed nurse understands the findings associated with neonatal opioid withdrawal syndrome (NOWS) when they state the newborn will have a high-pitched, continuous cry. These newborns also exhibit an increased muscle tone. Sleep pattern disturbances and difficulty sleeping for 2 to 3 hours after a feeding is common. Also, they often have moderate to severe tremors when undisturbed.

Ⓝ *NCLEX® Connection: Physiological Adaptation, Alterations in Body Systems*

2. A. **CORRECT:** Surfactant administration has no direct effect on heart rate.

Ⓝ *NCLEX® connection: Pharmacological Therapies, Expected Actions/Outcomes*

3. A, C, D. **CORRECT:** The nurse should identify that characteristics of preterm newborns include: the presence of abundant lanugo, a weak grasp reflex, and skin that is thin, smooth, shiny, and translucent. Long nails are a finding in a newborn who is postmature. A plump face is observed in a newborn who is macrosomic.

Ⓝ *NCLEX® Connection: Health Promotion and Maintenance, Data Collection Techniques*

4. D. **CORRECT:** The nurse should tell the parents to expect their baby to have leathery, cracked, and wrinkled skin, which is seen in the postmature newborn because of placental insufficiency. Postmature newborns have excess body fat. Flat areolas without breast buds are seen in a newborn who is preterm. Heels that are movable fully to the ears are seen in a newborn who is preterm.

Ⓝ *NCLEX® Connection: Reduction of Risk Potential, Potential for Alterations in Body Systems*

5. C. **CORRECT:** Using the safety and risk reduction framework, the nurse should identify that sunken fontanels is the priority finding. Newborns receiving phototherapy are at risk for dehydration from loose stools due to increased bilirubin excretion. Conjunctivitis, bronze skin discoloration, and maculopapular skin rash are important findings but not the priority.

Ⓝ *NCLEX® Connection: Physiological Adaptation, Alterations in Body Systems*

Active Learning Scenario Key

Using the ATI Active Learning Template: System Disorder

ALTERATION IN HEALTH (DIAGNOSIS)

- Physiologic jaundice is considered benign (resulting from normal newborn physiology of increased bilirubin production due to the shortened lifespan and breakdown of fetal RBCs and liver immaturity). The newborn who has physiological jaundice exhibits an increase in unconjugated bilirubin levels 72 to 120 hr after birth, with a rapid decline to 3 mg/dL 5 to 10 days after birth.
- Pathologic jaundice is a result of an underlying disease. Pathologic jaundice appears before 24 hr of age or is persistent after day 14. In the term newborn, bilirubin levels increase more than 0.5 mg/dL/hr, peak at greater than 12.9 mg/dL, or are associated with anemia and hepatosplenomegaly. Pathologic jaundice is usually caused by a blood group incompatibility or an infection but can be the result of RBC disorders.
- Acute bilirubin encephalopathy is when the bilirubin is deposited in the brain. This occurs once all of the binding sites for the bilirubin are used within the body, resulting in necrosis of neurons. Bilirubin levels greater than 25 mg/dL place the newborn at risk for permanent damage, including dystonia, athetosis, upward gaze, hearing loss, and cognitive impairments.
- Kernicterus is an irreversible, chronic result of bilirubin toxicity. The newborn demonstrates many of the same manifestations of bilirubin encephalopathy with hypotonia, severe cognitive impairments, and spastic quadriplegia.

DIAGNOSTIC PROCEDURES: Press the newborn's skin on the cheek or abdomen lightly with one finger. Then release pressure, and observe for a yellowish tint to the skin as the skin is blanched.

NURSING CARE

- Maintain an eye mask over the newborn's eyes.
- Keep the newborn undressed. Place a mask (like a bikini) over the genitalia of a male newborn.
- Remove the newborn from phototherapy every 4 hr, and unmask the eyes.
- Reposition the newborn every 2 hr to expose all body surfaces to the phototherapy lights and prevent pressure sores.
- Check the lamp energy with a photometer following facility protocol.
- Turn off the phototherapy lights before drawing blood for testing.

Ⓝ *NCLEX® Connection: Physiological Adaptation, Alterations in Body Systems*

Academy of Nutrition and Dietetics. (2021). *Do's and don'ts for baby's first foods.* https://www.eatright.org/food/nutrition/eating-as-a-family/dos-and-donts-for-babys-first-foods

American Academy of Pediatrics (2022). *Breastfeeding recommendations.* https://www.cdc.gov/breastfeeding/recommendations/index.htm

American Academy of Pediatrics. (2022). *Back to sleep, tummy to play.* https://www.healthychildren.org/English/ages-stages/baby/sleep/Pages/Back-to-Sleep-Tummy-to-Play.aspx

American Academy of Pediatrics. (2022). *Policy statement: Breastfeeding and the use of human milk.* https://doi.org/10.1542/peds.2022-057988

American Academy of Pediatrics. (2022). *Starting solid foods.* https://www.healthychildren.org/English/ages-stages/baby/feeding-nutrition/Pages/Starting-Solid-Foods.aspx

American College of Obstetricians and Gynecologists. (2020). Prelabor rupture of membranes. *Practice Bulletin Number 217.* https://www.acog.org/clinical/clinical-guidance/practice-bulletin/articles/2020/03/prelabor-rupture-of-membranes#

American College of Obstetrics and Gynecology. (2022). *COVID-19, pregnancy, childbirth, and breastfeeding: Answers from Ob-Gyns.* https://www.acog.org/womens-health/faqs/coronavirus-covid-19-pregnancy-and-breastfeeding

Analgesia and anesthesia in the intrapartum period: evidence-based clinical practice guideline, 2020. (2020). *AWHONN, 24*(S1). https://doi.org/10.1016/j.nwh.2019.12.002

Burchum, J.R. & Rosenthal, L.D. (2022). *Lehne's pharmacology for nursing care* (11th ed.). Elsevier.

Centers for Disease Control and Prevention. (2021). *STD treatment guidelines.* https://www.cdc.gov/std/treatment-guidelines/default.htm

Centers for Disease Control and Prevention. (2021). *When, what, and how to introduce solid foods.* https://www.cdc.gov/nutrition/infantandtoddlernutrition/foods-and-drinks/when-to-introduce-solid-foods.html

Centers for Disease Control and Prevention. (2021, July 23). *Sexually transmitted infections treatment guidelines, 2021.* https://www.cdc.gov/std/treatment-guidelines/STI-Guidelines-2021.pdf

Centers for Disease Control and Prevention.(2022). *Coronavirus 2019.* https://www.cdc.gov/coronavirus/2019-ncov/your-health/about-covid-19.html

Centers for Disease Control and Prevention. (2022). *Frequently asked questions: What are the benefits of breastfeeding?* https://www.cdc.gov/breastfeeding/faq/index.htm#howlong

Cleveland Clinic. (2022). *Benefits of tummy time and how to do it safely: A few minutes a day can go a long way for your newborn.* https://health.clevelandclinic.org/3-benefits-of-tummy-time-for-newborns-how-to-do-it-safely/

Dudek, S. G. (2022). *Nutrition essentials for nursing practice* (9th ed.). Lippincott, Williams & Wolter.

Duryea, T. K., & Fleischer, D. M. (2022, March 17). *Patient education: Starting solid foods during infancy (Beyond the Basics).* https://www.uptodate.com/contents/starting-solid-foods-during-infancy-beyond-the-basics

Grodner, M., Escott-Stump, S., & Dorner, S. (2020). *Nutritional foundations and clinical applications: A nursing approach.* (7th Ed.). Elsevier.

Gulbransen, K., Thiessen, K., Pidutti, J., Watson, H., & Winkler, J. (2022). Scoping review of best practice guidelines for care in the labor and birth setting of pregnant women who use methamphetamines. *JOGNN, 51*(2). https://doi.org/10.1016/j.jogn.2021.10.008

Healthy People 2030. (n.d.). *Reduce the rate of mother-to-child HIV transmission-HIV-06.*https://health.gov/healthypeople/objectives-and-data/browse-objectives/sexually-transmitted-infections/reduce-rate-mother-child-hiv-transmission-hiv-06

HIV.gov. (2023). *Preventing perinatal transmission of HIV.* https://www.hiv.gov/hiv-basics/hiv-prevention/reducing-mother-to-child-risk/preventing-mother-to-child-transmission-of-hiv

Hurt, K., Kodym, P., Stejskal, D., Zikan, M., Mojhova, M., & Rakovic, J. (2022). Toxoplasmosis impact on prematurity and low birth weight. *PLOS ONE, 17*(1), e0262593. https://doi.org/10.1371/journal.pone.0262593

Lowdermilk, D., Perry, S. E., Cashion, K., Rhodes Alden, K. & Olshansky, E. (2020). *Maternity and women's health care* (21th ed.). Elsevier.

Makker, K., Alissa, R., Dudek, C., Travers, L., Smotherman, C., & Hudak, M. (2018). Glucose gel in infants at risk for transitional neonatal hypoglycemia. *American Journal of Perinatal, 35*(11). https://doi.org/10.1055/s-0038-1639338

Marcellus, L. (2018). Social Ecological Examination of Factors that Influence the Treatment of Newborns with Neonatal Abstinence Syndrome. *JOGNN, 47*(4). https://doi.org/10.1016/j.jogn.2018.04.135

National Institutes of Health. (2022). *Babies need tummy time.* https://safetosleep.nichd.nih.gov/safesleepbasics/tummytime#ways

Pagana, K. D., Pagana, T. J., & Pagana, T. N. (2022). *Mosby's manual of diagnostic and laboratory tests* (7th ed.). Elsevier.

Palylyk-Colwell, E., & Campbell, K. (2018). Oral glucose gel for neonatal hypoglycemia: A review of clinical effectiveness, cost-effectiveness and guidelines. *Canadian Agency for Drugs and Technologies in Health.*

Sharma, A., Davis, A., & Shekhawat, P. (2017). Hypoglycemia in the preterm neonate: Etiopathogenesis, diagnosis, management and long-term outcomes. *Translational Pediatrics, 6*(4). https://doi.org/10.21037%2Ftp.2017.10.06

Silbert-Flagg, J. & Pillitteri, A., (2023). *Maternal and child health nursing: Care of the childbearing and childrearing family* (9th ed.). Lippincott Williams & Wilkins.

Smithers-Sheedy, H., Swinburn, K., Waight, E., King, R., Hui, L., Jones, C.A., Daly, K., Rawlinson, W., Mcintyre, S., Webb, A., Badawi, N., Bowen, A., Britton, P.N., Palasanthiran, P., Lainchbury, A. & Shand, A. (2022), eLearning significantly improves maternity professionals' knowledge of the congenital cytomegalovirus prevention guidelines. *The Australian and New Zealand Journal of Obstetrics and Gynaecology.* https://doi.org/10.1111/ajo.13500

Stanzo, K., Desai, S., & Chiruvolu A. (2019). Effects of dextrose gel in newborns at risk for neonatal hypoglycemia in a baby-friendly hospital. *JOGNN, 49*(1). https://doi.org/10.1016/j.jogn.2019.11.006

Vallerand, A. H. & Sanoski, C. A. (2021). *Davis's drug guide for nurses* (17th ed). F.A. Davis.

Velez, M., Jordan, C., & Jansson, L. (2021). *Reconceptualizing non-pharmacologic approaches to neonatal abstinence syndrome (NAS) and neonatal opioid withdrawal syndrome (NOWS): A theoretical and evidence-based approach.* Elsevier. https://www.sciencedirect.com/science/article/abs/pii/S089203622100074X?via%3Dihub

Wallin, L., & Ghidini, A. (2020). Use of sequential compression devices for prevention of maternal hypotension after epidural analgesia in birth. *JOGNN, 49*(5). https://doi.org/10.1016/j.jogn.2020.09.033

World Health Organization. (2022). *Breastfeeding.* https://www.who.int/health-topics/breastfeeding#tab=tab_2

Wyckoff, A. S. (Ed.). (2022, June). *Updated AAP guidance recommends longer breastfeeding due to benefits.* American Academy of Pediatrics. https://publications.aap.org/aapnews/news/20528/Updated-AAP-guidance-recommends-longer

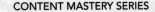

STUDENT NAME _____

CONCEPT_____ REVIEW MODULE CHAPTER_____

Related Content

(E.G., DELEGATION, LEVELS OF PREVENTION, ADVANCE DIRECTIVES)

Underlying Principles

Nursing Interventions

WHO? WHEN? WHY? HOW?

STUDENT NAME _____

PROCEDURE NAME _____   REVIEW MODULE CHAPTER_____

Description of Procedure

Indications

CONSIDERATIONS

Nursing Interventions (pre, intra, post)

Interpretation of Findings

Client Education

Potential Complications

Nursing Interventions

Growth and Development

STUDENT NAME _____

DEVELOPMENTAL STAGE _____ REVIEW MODULE CHAPTER_____

EXPECTED GROWTH AND DEVELOPMENT

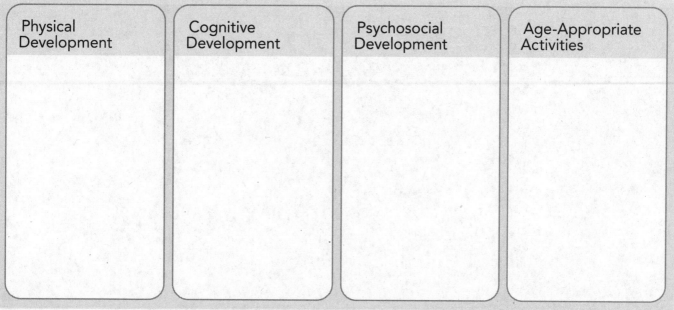

Physical Development	Cognitive Development	Psychosocial Development	Age-Appropriate Activities

Health Promotion

Immunizations	Health Screening	Nutrition	Injury Prevention

STUDENT NAME _____

MEDICATION _____   REVIEW MODULE CHAPTER_____

CATEGORY CLASS_____

PURPOSE OF MEDICATION

Expected Pharmacological Action

Therapeutic Use

Complications

Medication Administration

Contraindications/Precautions

Nursing Interventions

Interactions

Client Education

Evaluation of Medication Effectiveness

STUDENT NAME _____

SKILL NAME_____   REVIEW MODULE CHAPTER_____

Description of Skill

Indications

CONSIDERATIONS

Nursing Interventions (pre, intra, post)

Outcomes/Evaluation

Client Education

Potential Complications

Nursing Interventions

STUDENT NAME _____

DISORDER/DISEASE PROCESS _____ REVIEW MODULE CHAPTER_____

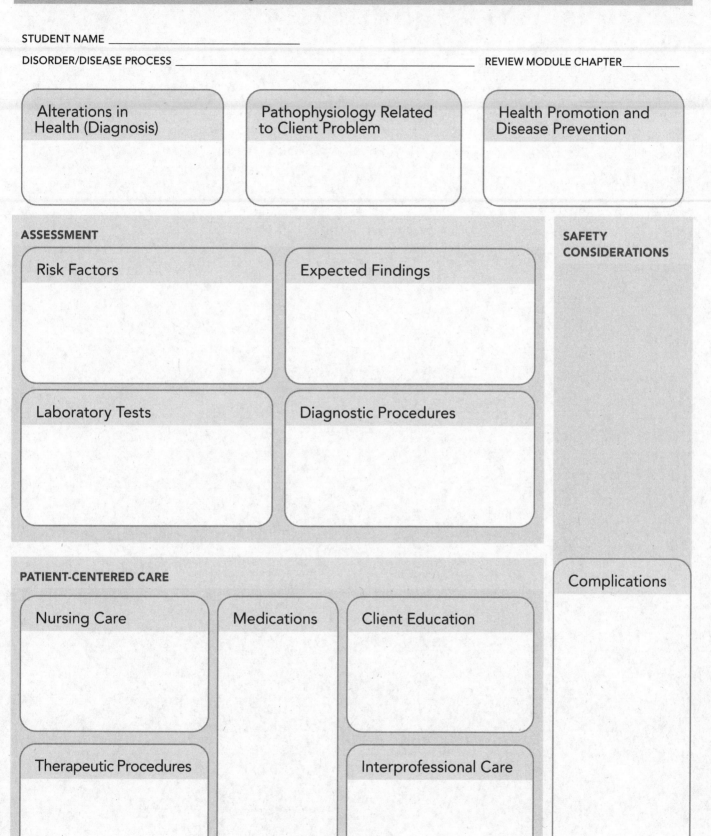

Alterations in
Health (Diagnosis)

Pathophysiology Related
to Client Problem

Health Promotion and
Disease Prevention

ASSESSMENT

Risk Factors

Expected Findings

Laboratory Tests

Diagnostic Procedures

SAFETY CONSIDERATIONS

PATIENT-CENTERED CARE

Nursing Care

Medications

Client Education

Therapeutic Procedures

Interprofessional Care

Complications

STUDENT NAME _____

PROCEDURE NAME _____ REVIEW MODULE CHAPTER_____

Description of Procedure

Indications

CONSIDERATIONS

Nursing Interventions (pre, intra, post)

Outcomes/Evaluation

Client Education

Potential Complications

Nursing Interventions

Concept Analysis

STUDENT NAME _____

CONCEPT ANALYSIS_____

Defining Characteristics

Antecedents

(WHAT MUST OCCUR/BE IN PLACE FOR
CONCEPT TO EXIST/FUNCTION PROPERLY)

Negative Consequences

(RESULTS FROM IMPAIRED ANTECEDENT —
COMPLETE WITH FACULTY ASSISTANCE)

Related Concepts

(REVIEW LIST OF CONCEPTS AND IDENTIFY, WHICH
CAN BE AFFECTED BY THE STATUS OF THIS CONCEPT
— COMPLETE WITH FACULTY ASSISTANCE)

Exemplars